CANCER: AN ENIGMA IN BIOLOGY AND SOCIETY

CANCER

AN ENIGMA IN BIOLOGY AND SOCIETY

R. Nery, DSc, FRSC,

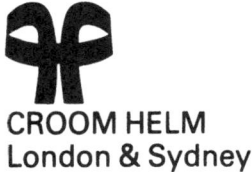

CROOM HELM
London & Sydney

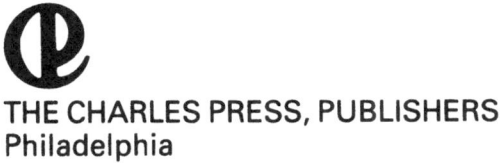

THE CHARLES PRESS, PUBLISHERS
Philadelphia

© 1986 R. Nery
Softcover reprint of the hardcover 1st edition 1986

Croom Helm Ltd, Provident House, Burrell Row,
Beckenham, Kent BR3 1AT
Croom Helm Australia Pty Ltd, Suite 4, 6th Floor,
64–76 Kippax Street,
Surry Hills, NSW 2010, Australia

British Library Cataloguing in Publication Data

Nery, R.
  Cancer : an enigma in biology and society.
  1. Cancer
  I. Title
  616.99′4   RC261

ISBN-13: 978-1-4684-8093-1   e-ISBN-13: 978-1-4684-8091-7
DOI: 10.1007/978-1-4684-8091-7

and
The Charles Press, Publishers, Suit 14K,
1420 Locust Street, Philadelphia,
Pennsylvania 19102

Library of Congress Catalog Card Number: 85-0728-52

ISBN-13: 978-1-4684-8093-1

CONTENTS

List of Tables

Preface

1 Outline of the Cancer Enigma   1

2 Historical Perspectives: Concepts   32

3 Historical Perspectives: Practices   83

4 Hormones and Cancer   138

5 Heredity and Cancer: Comparative Aspects   177

6 Heredity and Cancer: Human Aspects   206

7 Chromosomes and Cancer: General Principles   235

8 Chromosomes and Cancer: Human Aspects   279

9 Interpretations: Facts, Fancies and the Future in Oncology   319

Bibliography   371

Index   431

TABLES

1.1 Proportional Occurrence among all New Cases of 23
Cancer and Cancer Deaths, by Sex and Site, in the
United States in 1978

4.1 Some Landmarks in the History of Hormones and 142
Cancer

4.2 Some Hormone Preparations in Common Use 156

5.1 Differential Susceptibility of Common Laboratory 198
Strains of Inbred Mice and of Their Breast Tissues
to Spontaneous Mammary Neoplasia

6.1 Some of the Polyposis and Related Syndromes 215
Associated with Heritable Colon Cancer

6.2 Some Cancer-associated Conditions Showing 216
Autosomal Dominant Inheritance

6.3 Some Cancer-associated Conditions Showing 218
Autosomal Recessive Inheritace

6.4 Some Cancer-associated Conditions Showing 219
Sex-linked Recessive Inheritance

6.5 Some Miscellaneous Cancer-associated Disorders 220
with Mixed or Unknown Modes of Inheritance, or
with Unknown Heritability

7.1 The Gene Map of Human Chromosomes 1 and 17 240

7.2 Chromosomal Distribution in the Four 267
Near-haploid Human Leukemic Cell Lines Which
Are Currently Known

7.3 Some Recent Examples of Chromosomal 270
Anomalies Occurring in Families

7.4 The Principal Chromosome-breakage Neoplasia- 272
predisposing Syndromes, All Autosomal Recessive,
and Their Major Associated Neoplasms, Anomalies,
and Sensitivities (with Related Features)

8.1 Various Non-Hodgkin Lymphomas Showing 286
Significant Morphological Similarities

8.2	Some Karyotypes Found in Banding Studies of Preleukemias and Acute Lymphocytic Leukemia	292
8.3	A Partial List of the Known Translocations Involving Chromosome 1 in Some Lympho- and Myeloproliferative Disorders	295
8.4	Chromosomes and Their Anomalies Showing Preferential Involvements in Various Human Neoplasms	298
9.1	Proportions of Human Cancer Incidence or Mortality Attributed to Various Different Factors According to Three Independent Estimates	332
9.2	A Complete List of Chemicals or Industrial Processes for Which There is Sufficient Evidence for Their Association with Risk of Human Cancers at Specific Body Sites	334
9.3	Some Epidemiologically Derived Risk Factors for Various Human Cancers	336

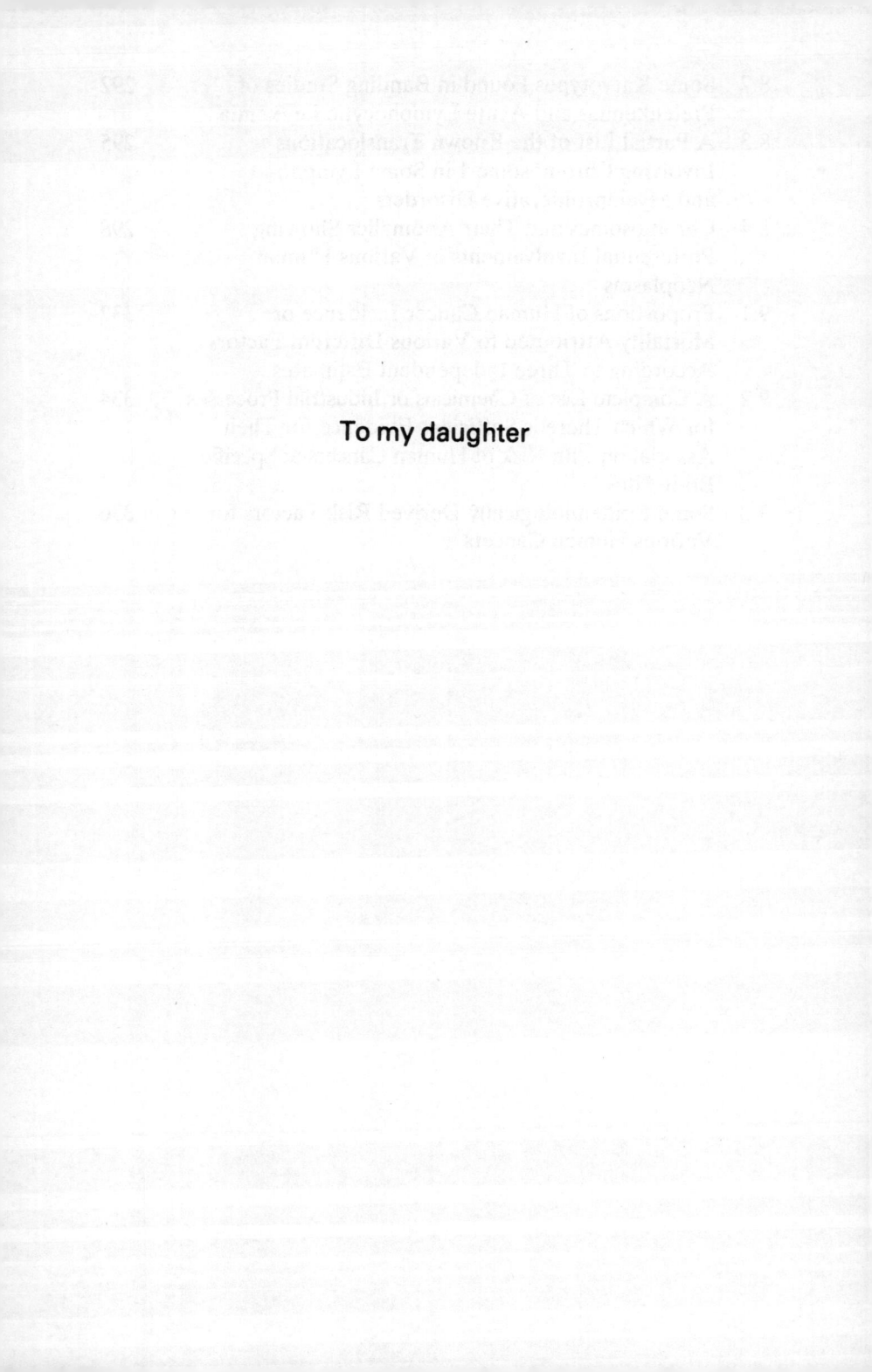

To my daughter

PREFACE

For obvious practical reasons the subject of oncology has increasingly been becoming artificially subdivided, e.g. into epidemiology, experimental carcinogenesis, pathology, immunology, genetics, and even microbiology. Most extant treatments of the subject are multi-authored, even when they deal with just one of these various subdivisions. Moreover, the corresponding specialists have seen the cancer problem as one within the purview of their own calling. In nature, however, the problem is a unity: its immunology, biochemistry, genetics, and cell biology, for example, are closely interdependent. Consequently, its proper appraisal requires detailed examination of all of the major parts, but with the primary aim of a single-minded and hence unified survey of the whole.

The present work is an offering in this direction. It is addressed specifically to all practising oncologists, whether clinical or experimental, and generally to all serious students of the growth of oncology and medicine from ancient to modern times.

The author is indebted to his many colleagues at the Institute of Cancer Research and elsewhere for valuable discussions, to the Institute's library and other offices for their unstinting help, and to the Institute for financial support during the many long and arduous years of preparation of this work.

1 OUTLINE OF THE CANCER ENIGMA

1.1 Introduction : The General Scope of the Enigma

In Greek mythology, Proteus, an ancient demi-god of the seas, was guardian of the seals (the animal variety) of Poseidon, that lord of the waters and earthquakes whom the Romans later called Neptune. Among his divinatory and other attributes, Proteus could readily assume any one of countless forms, all of which were different but all intended for one specific purpose: to confound detection and questioning. So elusive was he said to have been that all who would learn his secrets had first to find and identify him and then to devise means for holding him fast. Only then could any meaningful dialogue with Proteus even begin. Not surprisingly, they usually failed, even in these preliminary efforts.

In the light of these attributes, Proteus could well be regarded as the mythical father of cancer, but with due allowances made for the fact that the chip has far surpassed the block in variety, quality and extent of such protean arts and crafts. Thus, the disease occurs in many distinct or overlapping forms, actually or potentially involving all known species of multicellular organisms and all of the latters' tissues, most likely from the very dawn of metazoan evolution. Not even plants, nor the insects with which they developed the most ancient, universal, and impressive of symbiotic relationships known to evolutionary biology, are free of the disease. Neither are adult nervous and muscular tissues of higher organisms, despite the fact that cancer cannot become evident in the absence of cell division which, normally, does not occur in such tissues. Moreover, in its various basic manifestations, cancer so closely emulates the similarities and differences which characterize normal tissues and normal developmental processes that it is, at least on current information, impossible to distinguish it unequivocally from normalcy on the basis of any known single feature.

For present purposes, usage of the terms 'neoplasia', 'tumour' and 'cancer' is simply conventional. Accordingly, *neoplasia* (literally 'new growth') refers to all neoplasms or tumours. In-

1

itially, *tumours* denoted swellings caused mainly by inflammation but they now only indicate those which are neoplastic, whether benign *or* malignant. *Cancer* refers to all *malignant* tumours, although it is rarely still distinguished from leukemia (literally 'white blood'). Perhaps the best of the available definitions of a neoplasm is that of Willis (1952), as 'an abnormal mass of tissue, the growth of which exceeds and is uncoordinated with that of the normal tissues and persists in the same excessive manner after cessation of the stimuli which evoked the change'. In a recent discussion of this definition, Robbins *et al.* (1984) added that the abnormal mass 'is purposeless, preys on the host, and is virtually autonomous'. However, even such definitions are, at best, approximations (Section 1.2.1). For instance, *in vivo*, tumour autonomy develops slowly and perhaps never completely; and a feature of the 'conditional' neoplasms such as those caused in the ears of rabbits by the dye Scarlet Red (cf. Chapter Three, Section 3.6.3.5) is their tendency to regress with disappearance of the inciting stimuli.

It is for such reasons as outlined above that the fundamental problems posed by cancer have remained those centred around questions of specificity, e.g. in definition, diagnosis, and treatment. In the entirety of their scope, nature, and implications to health and society, though not in any of their specifics, the problems set cancer apart from any other known disease, whether the latter is a frankly environmentally caused disease such as smallpox, or a disease such as xeroderma pigmentosum whose cause is thought to be a specific, heritable genetic defect.

From ancient times, there have been multifarious intranational and international attempts, recently becoming increasingly interdisciplinary, concerted, and accelerated, at delineation of the etiology and the developmental course of cancer in man, other animals, and plants. In their outcome, these attempts have implicated the same heritable, adaptive, and other factors by which, naturally, species evolve, individuals develop, and both diversify. These factors include a large compendium of inherited genes or genetic traits which may be defined with some accuracy or be simply surmised, be single or multiple, or be common ('normal') or rare ('abnormal'). Sharing similar features is an even larger compendium of implicated, non-heritable factors. Within this second category are environmental factors, which may, additionally, be specific or non-specific, public or private, or static or changing;

as well as a variety of personal practices related, particularly, to sex and reproduction. In fact, this second category, in its totality, bestrides practically every aspect of society, e.g. its aspects of leisure, pleasure, industry, medicine, nutrition, and reproduction. Most importantly, the factors are those involved in multiple genetic–environmental interactions. The latter may themselves vary during the multiple stages that almost certainly mark both the neoplastic transformation (or *initiation*) of the normal target tissue or cell(s) and the subsequent processes (*promotion* and *progression*) that lead to the establishment of frank neoplasms and, eventually, fatal malignancy. As if to exacerbate this already bewildering complexity, the pattern of operation involving any set of these factors even in the same histological type of the disease may itself vary both within and between species of organisms. Then also, a particular neoplasm may rarely display a distinguishing feature such as an unusual (or *marker*) chromosome, but it is even rarer for that feature to be faithfully reproduced in other neoplasms even in those sharing the histogenesis and host species of the former.

In view of such a complexity, it need hardly be stressed, nor can it be too surprising, that the keyword description of the factors is 'implicated'. That is, at best, the factors may show significant statistical associations with the excess incidence of specific types of cancer, but they are rarely, if ever, proven causes of the disease itself. For instance, the cancers forming part of even the most well-documented of the associations such as colon cancer associated with the inherited polyposis trait or lung cancer with the habit of cigarette smoking, neither develops in all correspondingly affected individuals nor only in such individuals. This may be considered together with features such as the well-known difficulties in proper identification and correction of such a trait and in control of such a habit. When this is done, it becomes only too obvious that the scope of the enigma posed by cancer extends far beyond the realms mentioned above, i.e. those of definition, diagnosis, and treatment. It also bestrides prevention which, potentially, is the most utilitarian of all current approaches to the disease, at least until the latter's biochemical and related features have become sufficiently well understood to be exploited beneficially.

Both cancer and Proteus represent historic enigmas, but cancer, unlike Proteus, is no myth. Despite its stark reality, however, the disease occurs non-uniformly, afflicting some but not others belonging to the same species, or even to the same ethnic, familial, exposure or other category. Yet, there is no known means whereby any individual, except perhaps one already nearing death from some non-cancerous cause, can be sure of not already harbouring an incipient neoplasm which will eventually develop clinically and prove fatal.

This uncertainty is a major source of the great fear and mystique that surround cancer. Together, these may then contribute to the type of psychosomatic stress to which man is peculiarly susceptible, he being the species with the most highly developed awareness and capacity for projective (rational and irrational) thinking that may even see spectres where none exist. There are indications that this stress, in turn, may itself sometimes contribute to the development of some forms of cancer (Riley, 1978; Kets de Vries, 1980; Sklar *et al.*, 1980). This depicts a vicious cycle in which cancer, with its attendant mystique, uncertainty, and fear, can generate a stress that then exacerbates both the disease and its associated clinical and societal problems. It is a cycle in which the hope that 'springs eternal' is regularly knocked about by despair. This is well exemplified by the enthusiasm with which some new 'promising' discovery in cancer research is periodically hailed in the popular media but only, more often than not, never to be heard of again. Had this frustrating discipline of chronically unfulfilled promises not been so vital, it would certainly have been abandoned long ago.

As it relates to cancer, stress is biochemically extremely complex. It is almost certainly centrally controlled, but little is known about the biochemical mechanism(s) involved. Three major theories (psychoanalytic, behavioural, metabolic) have been variously proposed, and there is some indication that a major central control point is the locus ceruleus, the small dark blue streak located at the base of the fourth ventricle with abundant norepinephrine-containing neurones (Redmond and Huang, 1979; Brown *et al.*, 1984). Stress stimulates brain production of opiate peptides which, in turn, stimulate the synthesis of growth effectors such as prolactin (PRL) (Rossier *et al.*, 1980). This hypothalamus-controlled pituitary hormone has been associated with the development of breast cancer (Chapter Four). In turn, PRL production is influenced by various agents, e.g. estradiol, which seems to stimulate it, and the estradiol metabolite 2-hydroxyestrone, which inhibits it (Fishman and Tulchinsky, 1980). PRL production is also sometimes inhibited by dopamine, and dopamine agonists such as the ergot alkaloids ergocryptine and bromoergocryptine (Maurer, 1980; Dannies and Rudnick, 1980). The situation is further complicated by factors such as the capacity of dopamine in high or low levels to respectively inhibit or stimulate PRL production (Denef *et al.*, 1980). Also, control of PRL synthesis occurs at many stages including gene transcription; processing of the primary transcript of the PRL gene, which has four introns (Chien and Thompson, 1980); translation; and post-translational proteolytic modifications of pre-PRL, different peptide portions of which may carry different activities (Mittra, 1980). Thus, in the case of PRL alone, stress-induced opiates may influence PRL production through direct or indirect effects upon the various enzymes that catalyze the synthesis and metabolism of a variety of hormones (cf. Malcolm, 1981). The major sites of synthesis of both the steroidal and catechol hormones, respectively the cortex and medulla of the adrenal gland, may themselves be affected by stress, e.g. stress causes extensive cortical lipid depletion (Neville and O'Hare, 1982).

To cap this bewildering complexity, the neoplasm itself may produce, either ectopically or eutopically, unbalanced amounts of the body's own mediators of stress (Imura, 1980; see also Chapter Nine, Section 9.2.5). Adrenocorticotropic hormone (ACTH) produced ectopically by cancers of the lung and several other tissues can, for instance, produce all of the symptoms constituting Cushing's syndrome. This hormone shares its molecular biosynthetic precursor with lipotrophin, which has considerable sequence homology with the centrally active opioid neuropeptides β-endorphin and methionine enkephalin. These and other psychoactive products usually of the anterior pituitary can all be produced in deranged fashion by carcinoid and/or other neoplasms to cause what has been called *biochemical* or *psychiatric* malignancy (cf. Pullan *et al.*, 1980).

Overall, the problems posed by cancer centre around the extent and proximity of its mimicry of the fundamentals of normal biological and societal evolution and development. Indeed, this is sufficiently great to justify recognition of cancer, in its multifarious ramifications, as the prime caricature of life on this planet; and, by analogy with Proteus, as the prime but unwelcome guardian of the seals (the stamping variety) used by Nature to authorize the various stages in life evolution from events in the ancient seas. Proteus might have rivalled cancer in properties such as the polymorphism and general slipperiness that preclude proper detection and questioning. In matters of general cunning, however, Proteus was no match for the disease, presumably not even in the wildest dreams of those admirable Greeks who invented him. The salient features of some of the more prominent of the problems posed by cancer are outlined below, to set the stage for their more detailed discussions in the later chapters of this work.

1.2   The Salient Features of the Enigma

1.2.1   Problems of Definition and Diagnosis

1.2.1.1   Mimicries of Normal Features. As indicated above, it has already become an established principle of oncology that the basic manifestations of naturally occurring neoplasia are close mimicries of the normal analogues. It is largely for this reason that neither neoplasia (inclusive of its so-called preneoplastic states) nor the processes by which the disease develops from normal tissues can, for the present at least, be defined or diagnosed specifically. Accordingly, the associated problems of definition and diagnosis are essentially identical.

A commonly encountered version of this principle is that the basic differences so far observed between normal and neoplastic states are quantitative rather than qualitative. It should be stressed, however, that the validity of this statement is unquestionable only when the appropriate intercomparisons involve these states in a single individual but not necessarily in different individuals either intraspecifically or interspecifically. Thus, the important point of the principle is not whether the differences are qualitative or quantitative. Rather, it is whether or not they type-specifically match their evolved and/or developmentally expressed normal counterparts, whether in comparisons within or between individuals, or within or between species of organism.

This point is well illustrated by available data on some of the embryo-fetal re-expressions in cancer (cf. Coggin and Anderson, 1974; see also Chapter Nine, Sections 9.2.5 and 9.10.4), e.g. as represented by alpha-fetoprotein (AFP) and the so-called carcino-embryonic antigen (CEA). AFP occurs in many species of higher animals, inclusive of man, and all of the common laboratory animals. Among these it shows some structural differences, and it seems to be the fetal equivalent of adult albumin. Thus, the two substances share extensive structural homology; in their relative blood concentrations they show a reciprocal relationship with AFP levels reaching peak heights prenatally and albumin levels post-natally; and at least in the pig, they are synthesized by the same clone of cells. Embryologically, AFP is associated with the yolk sac and developing liver, occurring in low to undetectable concentrations in the adult liver and gonads. AFP levels in blood and/ or urine are significantly elevated in some neoplastic diseases, especially of the liver and gonads, but also in actively regenerating liver and in certain non-neoplastic disorders such as hepatitis and, in particular, neural tube defects for which it is a valuable aid in prenatal diagnosis (Summitt, 1980; Milunsky, 1980). Further, such structural differences that exist among the various AFPs from these various sources appear to be naturally evolved (e.g. inter-specifically) rather than to be due to any neoplastic or another diseased state itself (for reviews, see Abelev, 1974; Ruoslahti and Seppälä, 1979).

Analogously, immunoreactive CEA, first described by Gold and Freedman in 1965 as a specific antigen of human colorectal carcinomas, has subsequently been shown by numerous workers to represent a large family of cell surface-bound glycoproteins that may be shed into the circulation or urine (Nery *et al.*, 1974a,b) and sometimes filtered by the kidney in an even larger number of normal and pathologic (including neoplastic) states (Fuks *et al.*, 1974; Gold and Freedman, 1975). Like AFP, alkaline and acid phosphatases, and perhaps any other cellular product associated with human cancers, CEA can occur in elevated amounts even in the absence of any known signs of disease, e.g. in adolescents (Tabor *et al.*, 1981) and in certain groups of individuals in relation to factors such as sex, ethnicity, and smoking habits. For instance, serum CEA levels are higher in males than in females of both black and white races; among non-smokers, they are higher in black than white males but not females; they are higher in white but not black smokers than non-smokers; and smoking increases the levels in whites but not blacks (reviewed by Haines *et al.*, 1979).

Related natural complexities are even carried over to the clinical states requiring medical intervention. For instance, surgical or therapeutic reduction of the mass of a CEA-producing cancer of the large bowel, breast, or some other body site usually results in decreased serum CEA levels. However, in analogous situations, it is not always clear whether the manipulation itself rather than the mass reduction may sometimes influence the serum level of some tumour-associated biomarker. For instance, it was an almost traditional tenet of medical textbooks that serum acid phosphatase levels rise temporarily following prostatic manipulation in cases of metastatic carcinoma of the prostate. Within recent years, however, this tenet has been thoroughly disproved (Johnson *et al.*, 1979; Daar *et al.*, 1981).

To add to such complexities, a single neoplasm, or some but not all of a group of neoplasms of the same type, may produce more than one of the conventional tumour-associated biomarkers. Human bronchogenic carcinomas, for instance, can produce not only ACTH, usually of the 'big' variety (Yalow, 1979; Imura, 1980), but also a variety of placental proteins including chorionic gonadotrophin, placental lactogen, and alkaline phosphatase. Analogously, human colon cancers, which are usually associated with CEA, sometimes also produce a CEA-independent β_2-microglobulin-associated biomarker (Thompson *et al.*, 1980). This biomarker, insofar as it occurs on the cell surface intimately bound to the microglobulin, is but one of the new disproofs of yet another almost traditional tenet, i.e. that β_2-microglobulin occurs on cell surfaces exclusively as the light chain of HLA antigens (for review, see Peterson *et al.*, 1977). As a further complication, even the ectopic synthesis is not confined to neoplasia. ACTH, for instance, which is not known to be normally produced by the lung, is found in the lung of some heavy smokers lacking signs of lung cancer (Yalow, 1979).

For such reasons, and many others (e.g. the rarity of gene mutations in comparison with the commonness of recombinations), it seems that Nature relies upon what it has already evolved and/or developed rather than upon new structures for generation of its astounding diversity. This appears to apply equally whether the diversity is one of species, individual organisms, phenotypes, genotypes or cells, or of the cellular products or their combinations that occur in normal or neoplastic states. Thus it is not uncommon for such products to be capable of crossing species barriers, indicated by the well-defined classes of nucleic acids, proteins, lipids, carbohydrates and their various conjugates (e.g. glycolipids and lipoproteins) which are so widespread in nature. In some instances, even a substance as vital as insulin can be transferred interspecifically (e.g. from pig to man) without necessarily setting up reactions any more adverse than those of which the recipient's own analogues are capable (cf. Owens *et al.*, 1981). This, however, represents only one extreme of a broad spectrum, with the other represented by the strict operation of some of the interspecific, intraspecific and even intra-individual natural barriers. Thus, other than the familiar limitations of interspecific crosses and homografts, even human leucocyte interferon, such as that prepared by genetic engineering in bacteria, can be highly toxic in human recipients, causing headache, malaise, fever, influenza-like symptoms, and bone marrow depressive effects (Priestman, 1980; Scott *et al.*, 1981). Analogously, in cases of diabetes, even administered insulin, whether from animal or human sources, can be toxic, usually to the liver, kidney and/or cardiovascular system (Owens *et al.*, 1981). Features such as fine structural differences and as vagaries in dose, its timing, and its individual metabolic handling may contribute to such indications of the strict operation of the natural barriers. For instance, despite its apparent ubiquity in the animal kingdom, insulin from the dogfish, casiragua, porcupine, and guinea pig lack the zinc-binding capacity of insulin from most other sources including man, pig, and ox (Blundell *et al.*, 1972; Horuk *et al.*, 1980).

Neoplastic expressions can sometimes mimic even pre-embryonic features, e.g. the glycolytic and other metabolic features of the germ cells from which the neoplastic cells and their normal counterparts ultimately develop (Floridi *et al.*, 1981).

It is for such reasons of natural mimicries that neoplasia is yet to be defined in a way which sets it apart, unequivocally, from the non-neoplastic phenomena which characterize the host organism in which it occurs. Indeed, this is yet to be achieved even on the basis of extra-organismic comparative studies, such as those of normal and neoplastic cells or tissues in artificial cultures. From such studies, many 'transformed' phenotypes have been described, e.g. loss of contact inhibition, reduced serum requirement, lectin agglutination, growth in soft agar, anchorage independence, immortality *in vitro*, and cytogenetic and biochemical changes. However, none of these *in vitro*-determined phenotypes is restricted to or universal in the neoplastic state, nor is any of them (Jonasson *et al.*, 1977; Straus *et al.*, 1977), except perhaps extremely rarely

(Marshall and Dave, 1978), correlatable with ability to form neoplasms *in vivo*. This is despite the fact that, in nature, neoplastic transformation is most likely a part of a protracted host-controlled process that includes a long latency marked by many, though poorly understood, 'preneoplastic' stages.

1.2.1.2 Latency and Preneoplasia. The Creator, say the Jewish and Moslem Scriptures, charged Adam with the responsibility of giving names to what Adam saw, presumably to exercise his brain, and improve his knowledge. Since then, or whenever in evolutionary terms, man has been naming and defining, within his developing and expanding disciplines, in strict accordance with the state of his knowledge at any given time. In any given discipline, this state has reflected the accuracy of the definitions, and *vice versa*. Defining, in human terms, is a dynamic, developing, and changing art.

In oncology, the accuracy of definitions has depended almost entirely upon the known properties of observed, i.e. frank, neoplasms. Such neoplasms, however, represent end-stages of well-nigh completely mysterious multistage and multiphase but certainly protracted processes (cf. Foulds, 1969). For instance, tumour latency, as reflected in the period spanning inception and first overt appearance of the primary neoplasm, can span up to half the normal lifespan of the species of organism involved. In man, for instance, it is about 40 years for industrial bladder cancer (Hoover and Cole, 1973), and the cigarette smoking–lung cancer association became prominent between 30 and 40 years after the smoking habit became so popular (Hammond, 1975; Wynder and Hoffman, 1976). Consequently, the end-stages give little or no clue regarding important earlier phenomena such as those pertaining to the nature of cause, specificity, selectivity and 'preneoplastic' stages and phases. The imponderables of this situation are stressed by many well-known features ascertained epidemiologically, clinically, and/or experimentally. Among these are the appearance of neoplasm(s) long after disappearance from the body of any associated exogenously derived chemical or physical 'carcinogenic' stimulus; the latter's capacity to affect multiple tissues and multiple cell populations similarly, despite the tendency of the neoplasms to appear monoclonal in origin and/or to be restricted to one or very few of the body's tissues; and the closer structural and functional resemblance of the neoplasms to their parent normal tissues the 'earlier' the former happen to be at their stage of detection. Moreover, by the time the neoplasms, whether experimental or clinical, have caused recognizable disease or have reached recognizable size, they may or may not display cellular atypia but they most likely have already expressed their more-or-less characteristic capacity for localized infiltrative (*invasive*) growth, occurring with or without distant (*metastatic*) spread; and their less characteristic and even highly controversial capacity for 'rapid' and/or 'uncontrolled' (*autonomous*) growth. Worst of all, they have quite likely reached the brink of producing their most characteristic outcome, i.e. host death preceded by a suffering crescendo, usually by their *paraneoplastic* effects. Among these effects, that generalized wasting away of body and mind known as *cachexia* is not only the most prominent and serious but also the most problematical, particularly since, unlike anorexia nervosa, it can proceed inexorably to finality even in the presence of adequate food intake by the patient.

1.2.1.3 Some Definitions and the Question of Benign and Malignant Neoplasms. Such features related to atypia, spread, and fatality are the usual reliances in all serious attempts at definition of neoplasia and its associated terminologies such as benign and malignant. For instance, according to a recent issue of the American Cancer Society's *Cancer Facts and Figures* (1978), 'cancer is . . . uncontrolled growth and spread of abnormal cells', resulting in death 'if the spread is not controlled or checked'.

This definition restricts itself to the more serious of the clinical forms of the disease, i.e. to *cancer*, as defined earlier. This definition compares favourably with any other yet devised. None the less, it remains significantly equivocal in all of its features, despite the fact that it evades the issue of what is or is not neoplastic. The complexity of this issue is exemplified by the many known lesions, such as hyperplastic nodules and adenomatoses, that occupy the borderline between the patently normal and the more-or-less clearly neoplastic (cf. Foulds, 1969).

Such lesions are generally believed to represent intermediate stages in the process leading from normalcy to malignancy, as are at least some benign neoplasms. However, analogously with the distinction between normal and neoplastic, that between benign and malignant is far from clear-cut. Conventionally, benign neoplasms are discrete, encapsulated, and localized growths which neither invade their peritumoral tissues nor metastasize, and whose constitutent cells closely display the differentiated features of their normal counterparts. Some notable consequences of these features are that the neoplasms lack underlying anchorage and are hence movable within limits, e.g. under applied hand pressure; and that they may, like certain warts, lipomas, and sebaceous cysts, remain innocuous for years within their own limited domains. Conventionally also, malignant neoplasms (cancers) show contrasting features, e.g. they invade and usually metastasize, and their capacity to kill their hosts roughly parallels their degree of disorganization and cellular anaplasia.

Yet, these distinctions bridge an expansive no-man's-land. For instance, some patently benign neoplasms not only can subsequently develop all the features of malignancy but, even without this sequela, they can kill, e.g. meningiomas, killing their hosts through sheer physical pressure exerted in the brain. Like meningiomas, a variety of other neoplasms, including most of those occurring in rodents, remain encapsulated, and they neither invade nor metastasize. None the less, these 'benign' hallmarks are no guarantee that the neoplasms will not display the conventional features of malignancy. The rodent neoplasms, for instance, often match the worst of the malignant and metastasizing of human neoplasms in features such as complexity of morphology, heterogeneity of growth, cellular anaplasia, and ability to kill the host by cachexia or some other paraneoplastic effect. In contrast, albeit by far too rarely, some cancers which are usually highly malignant and highly fatal may differentiate spontaneously, mercifully to give their hosts the chance of a normal or near-normal life thereafter. A well-known example of this is neuroblastoma appearing in children of no more than around 30 months of age. In these cases, but almost never in the older analogues, the cancer all too rarely differentiates spontaneously to form the relatively harmless and benign ganglioneuroma (Pochedly, 1976; Coldman *et al.*, 1980; Adam and Hochholser, 1981).

1.2.1.4 Heterogeneity of Neoplasms. Attempts at accuracy in definition of neoplasia, and hence cancer, are further complicated by other features, some quite controversial, of this supra-protean disease. These include features such as structural, compositional, and expressional heterogeneity, as well as variability in properties related to growth and growth control.

For instance, it is not an uncommon notion that a neoplasm is a mass of homogeneous neoplastic cells and precious little else. However, the major source of this notion is artificiality, e.g. culturings of cells or tissues from neoplasms either *in vitro*, or *in vivo* in some 'privileged' site such as hamster cheek pouch, or in mouse peritoneal cavity, as ascites. All such culturings involve processes of extensive cellular selection and adaptation. As first demonstrated by the Kleins and others during the 1950s (cf. Klein and Klein, 1956), for instance, the mouse peritoneal cavity has anoxic and other properties which make it unusual among body sites, an equivalent of suspension culture medium *in vitro*, and an inhospitable place for growth and survival of all but the most competent and adaptable (or adapted) of the malignant cell populations. In humans, this situation has its counterpart in the highly malignant nature of the free-living neoplastic cells that through their sheer numbers can cause distension of the peritoneal cavity in some cases of severely invasive colon cancer. In all such rather unusual natural situations, as in their artificial counterparts, the neoplastic end products bear little or no resemblance to their primary, parent neoplasms.

In its natural state, even a highly malignant neoplasm is heterogeneous (Pitot *et al.*, 1974). It is usually composed of normal as well as neoplastic elements, both of which are, in turn, heterogeneous. Among the normal elements are infiltrating migratory cells such as macrophages (Levy and Wheelock, 1974; Svennevig *et al.*, 1979), cells of the involved tissue, and connective tissue stromal elements. The macrophages are themselves highly heterogeneous, and are also metabolically active in ways among which are some associated with carcinogenesis, for instance in production of hydrogen peroxide and superoxide (Johnston *et al.*, 1978) and of proximate and ultimate carcinogens from benzo(a)pyrene (Harris *et al.*, 1978). Among the stromal elements, some provide the vasculature and other supporting structures without which the neoplasm cannot outgrow a critical size. This is presumably because of the attendant inadequacy in supply of blood and oxygen, forcing the different cell populations of the neoplasm to adapt as best they can to these adverse conditions. One of the more well-known of the adaptive measures is the classical 'Warburg effect'. This effect, i.e. anaerobic glycolysis for energy requirements, utilizes large amounts of glycogen and/or glucose, usually accumulates lactate, and is less efficient at energy production than the more usual ATP-dependent oxidative mechanisms. Although almost traditionally regarded as a characteristic energy-yielding resort of neoplasms, glycolysis is now known to be common among developing or regenerating tissues, whether normal or neoplastic, and the tricarboxylic cycle to be basically intact in neoplastic tissues. In some organisms also, glycolysis is an adaptive measure. The goldfish, for instance, often resorts to glycolysis, producing ethanol·from glycogen through glucose and lactate. The resulting low accumulation of lactate prevents acidosis and thus allows the fish to live in essentially anoxic conditions for several days at a time (Shoubridge and Hochachka, 1980).

Among the neoplastic elements themselves, heterogeneity is the rule rather than the exception. This involves variable features such as state of differentiation; composition and variety of *stem* cells, i.e. poorly differentiated cells capable of both self-regeneration and of alternative modes of differentiation; and capacities for growth, invasion, metastatic spread, and biosynthesis of both parent-cell type-specific (*eutopic*) and non-specific (*ectopic*) products. (For detailed discussions, see Fidler *et al.*, 1978; Pierce *et al.*, 1978; Lord *et al.*, 1978; Imura, 1980; also Chapter Nine, Section 9.6.4). The demonstrations of significant heterogeneity in metastatic properties of cells of a single tumour that have been cloned and grown *in vitro* (Fidler *et al.*, 1978; Poste and Fidler, 1980) and *in vivo* (Chambers *et al.*, 1981) would suggest that this type of heterogeneity is not necessarily an artifact of the *in vitro* culturing.

In general, it is these cellular, subcellular, intercellular, functional, and other types of heterogeneity of naturally occurring neoplasms that make it so difficult for pathologists to define exactly which cell in an established neoplasm is or is not neoplastic or malignant.

1.2.1.5 Growth and its Control: the Question of Autonomy. There is currently no known way of ascertaining that a given neoplastic process is earmarked for malignant sequelae from its very beginning. Overt malignancy, whenever it appears, develops slowly and at different rates either among different neoplasms or different cell populations of single neoplasms. Moreover, malignant development does not necessarily involve all of the neoplastic cells of even a single neoplasm. It appears that the different cell populations in a given tissue undergoing neoplastic change are differently susceptible to this change, which may itself involve differential unmasking of embryonic and/or other genes that aid the neoplastic process. In the large bowel, for instance, cells with the polyposis gene unmasked may more readily progress through adenoma to carcinoma than cells without (Danes, 1979).

Many of the difficulties associated with accurate definition of neoplasia are well illustrated by the hepatomas (cf. Pierce *et al.*, 1978). Strictly, the suffix *oma* appended to the name of a tissue, e.g. in *hepatoma*, signifies a benign neoplasm; as distinct from *carcinoma*, which denotes a malignant neoplasm of epithelial tissue derivation, e.g. *hepatocarcinoma*. Strictly also, the related term *sarcoma*, popularly meaning a malignant neoplasm of mesenchymal tissue derivation, is as much a misnomer as the already mentioned *cancer* that additionally reflects the historical resemblance of all infiltrative growths to crab-like structures. None the less, all hepatomas show one or more of the usual stigmata of malignancy, despite the fact that they range in complexity from the poorly differentiated and non-functional to the well differentiated and functional. Moreover, these extremes are themselves morphologically and functionally heterogeneous; but the latter extreme more closely resembles normal liver tissue than the former, and more readily synthesizes bile. Despite these wide-ranging differences, it is likely that all hepatomas are derived primarily from the same tissue type, i.e. the hepatic parenchyma, and ultimately from the same embryologic source, i.e. the primitive ducts that differentiate from endodermal cells.

The hepatomas have been particularly well investigated in rodents. The results show that hepatoma development is multistaged, apparently passing through a common stage, that of hyperplastic nodules. This stage, however, represents no more than a clinical empiricism, being itself heterogeneous and difficult to define with any precision (Foulds, 1969). Furthermore, as in man, the rodent hepatomas show a wide range of differentiation in their final states, e.g. from the highly anaplastic *Novikoff* hepatoma (Novikoff, 1957) to the highly differentiated *minimal deviation* or *Morris* hepatomas (Morris, 1965). The latter, in many of their properties inclusive of biosynthetic functions, morphological appearance, and growth rate, are almost indistinguishable from normal liver tissues. In fact, their growth rates lag far behind those of regenerating normal liver, such as a partially hepatectomized liver which can regenerate itself completely within 48 hours. In comparison with the Novikoff hepatoma, these Morris hepatomas are, by far, more slow-growing. Yet, they too are malignant and they may even sometimes display that rare property of rodent neoplasms, the capacity to metastasize (Morris and Meranze, 1974).

Thus, neither a qualitative abnormality in appearance or in function nor rapid growth is a necessary component of the definition of neoplasia.

As mentioned above, the development of malignancy is a slow, step-wise, variable, and, almost certainly, highly selective and adaptive process (Foulds, 1969). Thus, at one extreme, there is the primary source of any neoplasm. This is a normal tissue or, more precisely, one or more of its component cell types, but all showing normal response to the homeostatic mechanisms of the host organism. At the other extreme, there are the manifest neoplasm(s) derived from this primary source and composed of, as discussed above, various cell types, both normal and neoplastic. Since the growth of such neoplasm(s) in their natural hosts is never an unlimited process, it seems reasonable that all of these cell types are also subject to the homeostatic mechanisms, albeit to different and variable extents. Between these two extremes, there is the already-mentioned long latency period. In addition, the manifest neoplasm(s) may then develop further, or *progress* in the terminology of Foulds (1969, 1975), through stages marked by adaptive loss or gain of characteristics, and by selection of those adapted cells which are most proficient at proliferation and survival under the prevailing conditions. It is felt in some quarters that the final state is characterized by an overgrowth of cells that no longer respond to the homeostatic mechanisms, i.e. that have become *autonomous*. However, within their natural host organisms, not even the most active of primary, invasive, or metastatic growths are quite unpatterned or unrestricted. Thus, malignant growth is restricted by factors such as availability of nutrients and space, lymphatic and blood circuitry, suitability of metastatic sites, and effects of various physiologic agents. For instance, even some highly malignant cancers, e.g. of breast and prostate, have been known since the 1890s to respond variably to certain manipulations of the body's hormones (cf. Chapter Four). In oncology, it would thus seem, *autonomy* is a misnomer that would be more meaningfully replaced by *relative autonomy*. This would reflect the general principle that neoplastic–non-neoplastic differences in independence of host controls are more questions of degree than of kind. For its immediate substantiation, one needs only to contemplate the well-known growths of supernumerary or ectopic organs or tissues in non-neoplastic states.

1.2.1.6 Section Summary. In summary, uncontrolled growth, except in relative terms, like rapid growth or any known qualitative abnormality in structure or function, is not a necessary component of the definition of neoplasia. Such an abnormality, were it to exist, remains to be discovered. Until this has been done, the exclusive and inclusive definition of neoplasia will remain as elusive as the mythical Proteus is thought to have been.

1.2.2 Incidence, Mortality, and Civilization

The not uncommon notion that cancer is a disease of modern civilization is clearly inconsistent with relevant evidence from available historical records (Chapter Two). This evidence shows that even the most ancient of known human civilizations, such as those of the Sumerians, Egyptians, Chinese, Hindus, Mayans, and Greeks, were familiar with, for obvious reasons, mainly the more easily recognized growths, many of which would now be called true neoplasms. In those ancient civilizations, a convergence of factors, such as loss of records and inadequacies of recording and diagnosis, has made the true incidence of the disease, particularly its internal forms, as uncertain as its true mortality. The oldest of the reliable and available epidemiological records date back to the 1840s, when Tanchou in France and Rigoni-Stern in Italy analyzed the collected incidence and mortality statistics in malignancies of body sites such as the breast, uterus, skin, and lung (Chapter Three).

In retrospect, these efforts of Tanchou and Rigoni-Stern could not have been more timely. In particular, they provided a fairly reliable baseline for comparative studies of causal statistics since the Industrial and Medical (especially infective disease-related) Revolutions of the latter part of the nineteenth century. This period marks the known beginning of significant improvements in general health, living standards, and life expectancy, but also of significant increases in industrial and other types of environmental pollution. Thus, in addition to the growth of industrial exhausts, factors such as food additives, pesticides, medications, and radiation, many now known to be cancer-associated through experimental or human epidemiological studies, have been increasingly added to the human environment during and since that period. It has been estimated that the synthetic chemicals alone numbered around 2 million by 1974, that about 250,000 new ones are now added annually, but that less than one per cent of the grand total have been subjected to carcinogenesis testing (Carter, 1974). Thus, a major problem in oncology centres around the relevance of these opposing factors (the improvements and the increases) to the marked rises in the true rates of overall cancer incidence which have been noted particularly in Europe and North America since around the turn of the present century.

By such rises, cancer has enforced not only its recognition as a growing menace to health and society but also, in consequence, acceleration and expansion, as never before, of the regional, national, and international anticancer effort. Among other factors, this effort has produced steady improvements in diagnosis of the disease and, hence, in recognition of the true incidence of both its internal and superficial forms. It is on this basis that the disease is now known to be capable of involving any of the normal tissues of the body at any stage in life, although with increasing incidence at older ages.

In overall terms, cancer incidence rates have, for decades, been rising almost in parallel with the growth of industrialization and urbanization. In details, however, the rates have been showing significant non-uniformities, e.g. in relation to age, sex, ethnicity, geography, time, and cancer-type (cf. Waterhouse *et al.*, 1976; Wynder and Gori, 1977; *Cancer Facts and Figures*, 1978; Devesa and Silverman, 1978; see also Chapter Nine, Sections 9.3 and 9.4). In the United States, for instance, cancer is the prime cause of death between ages 3 and 14 years, is three times as common in women as in men between ages 20 and 40 years, and is significantly more prevalent in men than in women between ages 60 and 80 years. The ethnic non-uniformity (cf. Chapter Six) is exemplified by the unusually high prevalance of stomach cancer among the Japanese, breast cancer among the Bombay Parsis and most Caucasian ethnic groups, esophageal cancer among the Iranians, Kaposi sarcoma among Africans, both this sarcoma and the cancer-predisposing Bloom's syndrome among the Ashkenazi Jews, nasopharyngeal cancer among the Cantonese Chinese, and cancer of the gall bladder among Amerindians. In temporal terms, the overall increases in cancer incidence that have been observed from around the turn of the century have been non-uniform, as exemplified by the continuing increases in most developing countries (cf. Mingxin *et al.*, 1980) but the slight declines, over the past two-to-three decades, in most developed countries.

These statistics represent a highly complex situation. In Japan, the United States, and most European countries, for instance, the past two-to-three decades have witnessed slow declines in the average age-adjusted incidence rates of few types of malignancy, mainly cancers of the stomach, uterus, rectum, and esophagus. However, during this same period, there have been significant increases in the rates of few others, mainly lung cancer in both sexes; but, with the recent rise in the liberation movements and smoking habits of women particularly in Western countries, the rate of lung cancer increases in women has, over the past decade or so, been surpassing that in men. For most of the remaining types of cancer, including the historical prototype of all human cancers, women's breast cancer, the mean age-adjusted rates of incidence in specific populations have remained essentially static for as long as reliable records have been kept and have remained available. To complicate the issue even further, the basic features of the incidence patterns in specific populations may remain unchanged or slowly, over generations, approach those of the host populations when migrants from the former settle in the latter. British migrants to South Africa and Cantonese migrants to Malaysia (Armstrong *et al.*, 1979), for instance, retain their characteristically high incidences of, respectively, lung cancer and nasopharyngeal carcinoma. In South Africa also, Negroes maintain their characteristically low incidence of colon cancer. This is despite not only their increasing urbanization but also their increasing use of Western-type diets (i.e., diets high in animal-derived protein and fat and low in fibre) with its resulting increase in fecal transit time, constipation, and accumulation of toxins and carcinogens, as well as its resulting decreases in dietary dilution and fecal volume. This represents the by now familiar listing of environmental risk factors in colon cancer. In contrast, Japanese migrants to the United States show some tendency towards the latter's characteristically low incidence of stomach cancer and high incidences of cancers of the breast and colon, the exact reverse of the situation in Japan.

There are clearly complex genetic and environmental involvements in such variations of cancer incidence among humans, as there are, indeed, among animals (Chapter Five). Among animals, for instance, the natural incidence of mammary neoplasia varies from practically none in pigs and sheep to 100 per cent in selected strains of mice; and there are also natural variations in the pattern of development and progression of the disease (cf. Nagasawa, 1979). Among humans at present, only the environmental involvements are capable of sensible manipulations; but, even then, they are usually too complex (e.g. multiple in character, combination, and activity at different stages and phases of neoplastic development) to be properly indentified and manipulated. Thus, the known variations in incidence of lung cancer are not correlatable with smoking habits alone, being dependent upon other factors including occupational exposure in the shipbuilding, chemical, petroleum, furniture; and papermaking industries (Fraumeni, 1979).

It thus seems as if humans are particularly primed to neoplastic development which can explode in the presence of triggers that are ubiquitous in the human environment.

1.2.3 Comparative Studies: A Special Predilection of the Human Species for Cancer

Man's unparalleled fear of cancer is correlatable with certain aspects of his highly developed mentality (Section 1.1). In one respect at least, this fear is not without some justification. This is that although no species of metazoan organisms is known to be incapable of developing cancer of one type or another, the human species has the dubious distinction of evincing the highest of all known species-specific predilections for the disease. This is evident in a variety of the disease-associated features, including not only the overall incidence and mortality discussed above but also features such as the extensiveness of histologic and embryologic type-specific neoplasms, and the degrees of malignancy. The human species might thus be forgiven for suspecting, as part of its fear, that cancer calculates and exacts its macabre toll in accordance with species-specific status within the evolutionary hierarchy of terrestrial life.

The principle can be illustrated by some comparisons between man and other animals. In man, the existence of over 100 distinct or overlapping types of cancer has long become a cliché in oncology. However, even this number is periodically having to be revised upwards with the continuing demonstrations, on structural, functional, embryologic, and/or other criteria, of additional types or subtypes of the disease. Moreover, over 90 per cent of the malignant neoplasms in man are carcinomas originating in the epithelial tissues such as those of the skin, and the respiratory, digestive, and urogenital systems. In contrast, carcinomas are relatively rare in non-human animals, inclusive of non-human primates, and of reptiles, birds, amphibians, and fishes. Although it is not clear to what extent this marked difference is due to lack of observation of sufficient numbers of animals to old ages, their predominant malignant neoplasms are sarcomas (inclusive of lymphomas and leukemias). Further, many of these neoplasms, and even some of the rare epithelial neoplasms such as the Lucke renal adenocarcinoma in the North American leopard frog and breast carcinomas in mice are, unlike the situation in man, causally associated with endogenous and/or exogenous viruses (Chapters Three and Five). Finally, in man, despite the predominance of carcinomas, sarcomas can hardly be regarded as rare. For instance, the latter, mainly in the forms of acute lymphoblastic leukemia in most countries and/or Burkitt's lymphoma in certain African and other countries, are the major cause of cancer mortality among children between the ages of three and fourteen years.

In plants, neoplasia does not appear to represent the problem, i.e. in incidence and mortality, it does in man and other animals (cf. Braun, 1977). This is despite the sustained embryonic (or poorly differentiated and multipotential) nature of most actively growing components of both normal plants and animal neoplasms. In both cases, such components have great potential longevity, as exemplified by the thousands-of-years-old trees such as some brimblecone pines and by the various neoplastic cell lines which have been successfully maintained through artificial subculturings already for many decades. Perhaps plants have evolved special protective devices related to the fact that they can, without suffering noticeably in consequence, shed and replace parts such as leaves, flowers, shoots, and even whole branches that may have become diseased.

However, as in all of its known features, neoplasia offers no simple answers short of death. Certain animals, or their body parts, such as starfish, the limbs of urodeles, and the heads of hydra, have remarkable self-regenerative capacities. However, such instances are conceptually not very different from the general regulative mechanisms by which early embryos develop (Wolpert, 1978).

In higher animals, neoplasms primarily involve epithelial tissues or mesenchymal tissues. Among the former tissues are those of the skin and small intestines which regularly desquamate and regenerate their cells as the latter become damaged or effete. Among the latter are similarly-behaving tissues such as those of the blood-forming organs. Yet, in the adult animals, the liver, the organ with the highest known potential for self-regeneration following serious damage such as that induced by partial hepatectomy, is rarely involved in neoplasia in man but quite commonly in animals. Finally, neoplastic involvement is no respecter of tissue-regenerative capacity: as indicated above (Section 1.1), it does not spare even adult nervous and muscular tissues, which normally display features such as regular turning over of subcellular elements and ageing-related cell-loss but not cell division.

In microorganisms, neoplasia cannot occur, i.e. in the sense of it being a disease of the type of intimate intercellular society that characterizes multicellular organisms only. In principle, however, certain other features of neoplasia, such as changes in growth rates and in dependence upon specific nutrients and other physiological factors, can be exhibited by different strains and substrains of the same species of microorganism. An important example of this is provided by the different *Salmonella* varieties developed by Ames and his colleagues for the study of the bacterial mutagenicity of chemical carcinogens (Ames *et al.*, 1973).

Such interspecific comparisons based upon aspects of biological evolution and development are not the only known indications of the preference of neoplasia for the human species. Other indications are intraspecific, e.g. those related to the cultural advances of mankind. Thus, as already indicated (Section 1.2.2), the disease was well known in ancient human populations, but it was almost certainly rarer than it is in their modern counterparts among which, in turn, it represents a greater menace in the developed than developing countries. In the developed countries, for instance, over one per cent of all the individuals now living have a history of the disease. Moreover, about one in four of these individuals will eventually develop the disease in one form or another, as it will in some one in three of all their families. In the United States, for instance, such a situation was already reached some years ago (cf. *Cancer Facts and Figures*, 1978).

1.2.4 Problems of Prevention and Treatment

To continue the analogy with Proteus, by the time a cancer has grown sufficiently or has caused sufficient disease symptoms to attract detection and questioning, the time is usually already too late to block the impending doom, let alone to restore the normal health previously enjoyed by the patient. This gloomy situation is exemplified in Table 1.1, which shows the close parallelisms in the incidence and mortality statistics for the major types of malignancy occurring in the United States in 1978.

Table 1.1: Proportional Occurrence among all New Cases of Cancer and Cancer Deaths, by Sex and Site, in the United States in 1978

Body Site	Incidence[a]		Mortality[a]	
	Men	Women	Men	Women
Prostate	16	—	10	—
Breast	—	26	—	19
Ovary	—	5	—	6
Uterus[b]	—	14	—	6
Lung	22	7	33	12
Colon and rectum	14	15	12	15
Urinary system	9	4	5	3
Blood and lymph systems	9	7	9	9
Mouth	5	2	3	1
Pancreas	3	3	5	5
Skin[c]	1	1	2	1
Others	21	16	21	23

Notes: a. Figures shown are estimated percentages of total (incidence or mortality), based upon data from the Third National Cancer Survey (1968–71). b. Excluding *in situ* carcinoma of the uterine cervix. c. Excluding non-melanoma skin cancer.

Despite the enforced preoccupation with therapy of the disease from ancient times, patient survival for five years after presentation of the clinical disease and/or after initiation of treatment by even the most advanced of available methods has now reached no more than around one-third of all cases (cf. *Cancer Facts and Figures*, 1978). Even in these 'cured' cases, their quality of life remains so highly compromised that they usually succumb to an overt recurrence of their initial malignancy, to an overt appearance of a different malignancy, to an intercurrent infection such as pneumonia, and/or to one or more of the various side effects of their therapy. Within the context of the individual patient, as discussed above (Section 1.2.1), the neoplastic cells do not differ qualitatively in any basic manner from their normal counterparts. It is mainly for this reason that there is no known basis for selectivity in the cytotoxicity upon which the treatment usually depends. Consequently, a commonly encountered statement such as 'the host cells and the cancer cells' is meaningless, for both types are host cells; i.e. the latter are not heterografts. More importantly in this context, that which is cytotoxic will kill some of both types of cells. In current cancer therapy, therapeutic efficacy is always complicated by unwanted side effects.

As a broad principle therefore, most clinical cancers are still fundamentally incurable. How feasible, then, is the preferred alternative, that of prevention? The basic requirement for the initiation of effective preventive measures is identification of causes which are as controllable as they are in the infectious and other diseases that might be termed 'outside jobs' rather than, as in the genetic or predominantly genetic diseases, 'inside jobs'. However, as already indicated (Section 1.1.), the outside causes of most types of human cancer remain problematical. Deliberate reductions in the incidence of certain types have depended upon 'early' detection, e.g. of cancer-predisposing conditions such as polyposis coli and xeroderma pigmentosum, or, by the Papanicolaou smear test, of cellular atypia in the uterine cervix in the case of cervical cancer.

There can be little doubt that commonsense health precautions, e.g. in hygiene, dietetics, and exercise, will maintain or improve health generally and even reduce the incidence of certain cancers perhaps non-specifically. In specific terms, however, the situation becomes more doubtful and highly problematical. For instance, the major cause of the near epidemic rises this century in the incidence of lung cancer has been traced by numerous epidemiological studies conducted in many countries to the smoking habit, i.e. generally to the growth, activities, and governmental and public support of the tobacco industry. To ensure its continuing prosperity, this industry, in blatant disregard of the rising cost in human lives and suffering, has been peddling its deadly wares, particularly since the recent smoking–lung cancer scare publicized mainly in the developed countries, increasingly in the developing countries of Africa, Asia, and South America (cf. Wickström, 1979; Taha and Ball, 1980).

Despite all this, however, the prime fact remains that smoking, sniffing, and/or chewing of tobacco, and other products, including the smoking of cow-dung in some instances, are such widespread, ancient, ingrained, and uniquely human habits (Chapter Three) that they may well have played a role in the cultural evolution of mankind. Indeed, these habits have been fabricated in the same mould used for many of the other human habits with which cancer has been variously associated, e.g. drinking of alcoholic beverages, eating of cooked or pyrolyzed foodstuffs especially those of animal origin, exposure to strong sunlight, and certain sexual and reproductive practices. The entire situation has been well epitomized in Mark Twain's immortal: 'The only way to keep your health is to eat what you don't want, drink what you don't like, and do what you'd rather not'. Prerequisites for rendering obsolete both the smoking habit and the tobacco industry may well include proper understanding and sensible exploitation of the process of human habituation and effectuation of the necessary cultural (and genetic?) changes in man himself. It is a tall order which, most likely, will never be filled. Were prima facie consideration given to the totality of 'causes' of human neoplasia as they have been implicated by epidemiology and experimentation (Chapters Three and Nine), effective cancer prevention would require drastic changes in practically every aspect of present-day human society, not to mention the even more difficult requisite changes in poorly-defined human genetic features (Chapter Eight).

Even were effectuation of the changes feasible, this would sometimes present difficulties of choice. For instance, early sexual intercourse, particularly with multiple partners, is thought to increase the risk of cervical cancer, but early first parity and multiparity to reduce that of breast cancer. Controversially, reduced risk of fibrocystic breast disease is also associated with the use of oral contraceptives which, however, may increase the risk of cancer of the liver and certain other organs (Chapter Four). Also the same socioeconomic factor (e.g. income or education) may show strong but opposite associations with different cancers, e.g.

cancers of the cervix and breast (Devesa and Diamond, 1980); and it may show no association with others, e.g. pancreatic cancer (Levin *et al.*, 1981). Analogously, low levels of serum cholesterol have been associated, though not without some controversy, with increased risk of several cancers including those of the colon, lung, liver, and stomach (Rose and Shipley, 1980; Williams *et al.*, 1981), but high levels with increased risk of heart disease, one of the major killers in Western societies. Even that most notorious of the risk factors, tobacco smoking, which is probably the worst of the preventable causes of ill-health known to medicine, shows a negative association with colon cancer (Williams *et al.*, 1981). To exacerbate the difficulties even further, many of the environmental factors which are known or suspected to increase the cancer risk in man are themselves useful in agricultural and other industries, and also in medicine inclusive of cancer therapy itself (Chapters Three and Four).

The list of such difficulties is practically endless. Thus, comparative studies aimed at identification of the risk factors are often of little extrapolative significance (Chapter Five). For instance, in contrast with the above-mentioned associations involving early first parity or multiparity, breeders compared with virgin rodents may show, depending upon species or strain, either increased or decreased risk of breast cancer. Analogously, many of the most important of the epidemiologically ascertained environmental risks of human cancer, such as tobacco smoke, betel quid, and alcohol, have consistently failed to produce experimental cancers, or such cancers of the types with which they are associated in man, i.e. respectively bronchogenic, oral, and upper gastrointestinal cancers. It is as much an impossibility to eliminate from the environment all of the cancer-risk factors (cf. ultraviolet radiation, the prime associate of skin cancer) which have been pinpointed or implicated by epidemiology and/or experimentation, as it is to abolish the environment itself. Even were the former possible and effectuated, it seems unlikely that cancer would also be abolished in consequence. None the less, there can be little doubt of the outcome that, thereby, the mean incidence of many types of cancer would be significantly reduced. Such an outcome is greatly to be desired, even more so than the eventual rendering of the worst risk factors, such as the smoking, chewing, and drinking habits, totally unacceptable socially. Ideally, both the outcome and the rendering would be less feasible in relation to populations at large than to individuals at unusually high risk of specific cancers. For instance, individuals with xeroderma pigmentosum, upon learning of their associated high risk of ultraviolet light-induced skin cancer, would be more inclined than others to avoid sunlight as much as possible. In the annals of oncology, however, this instance is unique insofar as it involves a readily identifiable condition or individual, a specific environmental factor, and a particular type of cancer. In other instances, such as a female member of a breast-cancer-prone family, the corresponding knowledge may well become a source of great fear and emotional distress, which may turn out to have been unfounded.

Herein lies another of the great difficulties in preventive oncology, that of uncertainty about which member of an at-risk group will and which will not develop cancer and, if so, when. For instance, heavy smokers cannot but know of their increased risk of developing lung cancer in a lifetime. However, they probably also know that their individual risk is only about 10 per cent, and that the disease occurs mainly in old age by when non-cancerous death might already have intervened. So, as a calculated gamble, many opt to keep on smoking. By the time it has become clear that the gamble has been lost, it is already too late for the option of kicking the habit to be effective.

1.2.5 Problems of Etiology

Since the major known manifestations of cancer are close mimicries of many of the essentials of general biology and medicine (Section 1.2.1), it is hardly surprising that the historical growth of carcinogenic theories has paralleled that of basic understanding or of theories in these general disciplines, or even in religion, economics, and sociology. Thus, as discussed by Thorwald (1962), the ancient Egyptians saw a close parallelism between the people's diseases and the behaviour of the Nile Valley with its seasonal floodings regulated by the complex system of irrigation channels. They thus equated disease with disturbances in the normal flow of juices in the body's channels. To the Hebrews, the cause of their afflictions was a visitation either of the Jobian type (for the testing of faith), or of the sins of forefathers. To the Hindus, the cause was the errors of a previous existence or, as reminiscent of the Egyptian channels, disturbances in the flow of the various yogistic winds or juices (humours) along passages emanating from the navel. To the Chinese, it was disturbances in the paired, counterbalancing forces of Yin and Yang, the concept behind their acupuncture. From some of these older notions, the Greeks developed their familiar medical philosophy based upon the four body humours, among them atrabilis or black bile, their reputed cause of all tumours. This Greek version of pathogenesis was destined to dominate medical thinking around the Mediterranean for well over a thousand years after the Greeks. Indeed, in various modifications, its basic principle, that of pathologic formations from formless elements, persisted well into the nineteenth century before it finally gave way to the cellular theories of Johannes Müller and his most illustrious student, Rudolph Virchow. Then, during the latter part of this century, the heyday of microbiology, the indisputable cause of cancer was parasites in polluted air, water, and other public amenities especially of conurbations, or in sources such as bogs and marshes. In the meantime, at least from the days of Paracelsus in the sixteenth century, various other environmental factors, mainly chemicals, became implicated in the etiology of cancer.

The majority of the implicated environmental factors have been elucidated by human cancer epidemiology, a discipline initiated in the 1840s by Tanchou in France and Rigoni-Stern in Italy (Chapter Three). However, one of the major results of the modern discipline is the age-relatedness of cancer. In overall terms, age correlates better with the incidence of the disease than any other known factor. Not only do many types of the disease gain in prominence with increasing age, except in childhood, but it is or was also more prevalent in older than younger populations such as those of the present than of the past, or of the developed than developing countries (Section 1.2.2). For the first time in known human history, human populations have been becoming progressively older, e.g. in the West since around the time of the Industrial and Medical Revolutions of the nineteenth century. In China not many decades ago, the mean at-birth life expectancy was under 30 years; but it has since been rising, and so has the incidence of neoplasia (Mingxin *et al.*, 1980).

This worldwide phenomenon of increasingly older populations would have been presenting a novel experience to evolutionary adaptation. The latter is an extremely slow process in comparison with the great rapidity, especially in recent times, of cultural change. This has led to the not uncommon notion that cancer etiology is related to age and, in particular, to the ageing process itself. Against this notion, however, is the fact that cancer usually involves one or few of an individual's tissues, whatever his age. In contrast, the ageing process is a generalized phenomenon, one occurring from or before birth and affecting practically all of the body's tissues and functions, and with marked differences in specific rate, order, quality, and quantity. Briefly, from its earliest stages, the ageing process leads to recognizable positions on the chronological growth scale. For instance, visual and auditory acuities reach peak at around the age of 10 years, intellectual power around 21 years, and muscular power and co-ordination around 25 years. The degenerations within the nervous and muscular systems that lead to conditions such as presbyopia, presbycusis, slowed reaction time, and reduced muscular strength and co-ordination become prominent at around 75 years, at which time brain mass decreases by about 150 grams. From around age 40–50 years, skeletal bone mass declines. This occurs faster in women than men, and at different rates in different parts, e.g. faster in metacarpals and femoral neck than in the femoral midshaft, the tibia, or skull. Ageing-related changes in collagen and elastin cause widespread deterioration, e.g. in skin, muscle, bone, joint, and blood vessels. Changes occur in respiratory functions such as oxygen uptake, ventilation volume, and vital capacity; and gonads deteriorate, earlier in women than men. Cells of non-dividing tissues (muscles and nerves) accumulate cytoplasmic lipofuchsin or lipochrome, and undergo decreases in cellular and nuclear volumes and in oxidative phosphorylative capacity. Fibroblasts develop reduced capacity to divide, e.g. at infancy, they divide about 50 times; at age 20 years, about 30 times; and about 20 times at age 80 years.

Just by itself, the fact of such a patterned, generalized uniformity would suggest strongly that ageing is a genetically programmed process of finite duration. Among such widespread and complex degenerative ageing-associated changes are increases in chromosome aberrations and instability (cf. Chapter Seven) and interference with hematopoiesis (Lipschitz *et al.*, 1984). Yet, some gerontologists and oncologists have singled out just these increases as the prime causes of both ageing and cancer. There are also the traditional medical notions that, despite this apparently inexorable running down of practically all of the body's cells, tissues, and vital functions, natural death is never due to ageing but to some disease, and that ageing itself is the cumulative effect of disease. It seems inconceivable that elimination of all diseases could ever make the individual immortal, or even extend the average human lifespan to, say, 100 years. Also, it is obvious that many old people, like many old trees, show no signs of cancer and eventually die, peacefully, as the nature-prescribed end of their allotted life cycle.

The simplest answer to the question of age and cancer is thus that the older populations afford longer intervals for the disease to become overt in those individuals harbouring it incipiently. This, however, is oversimplification of an obviously very complex problem. For instance, studies of the latency of the naturally-occurring neoplastic disease (lymphoid leukosis) of chickens have suggested that the latency is an intrinsic property of the target B cells and is unrelated to maturational events of the host physiology (Fadly *et al.*, 1981). As discussed above, much evidence also suggests that ageing is a genetically programmed process non-uniformly affecting different cell populations at different stages and phases of the life cycle. This may well mean that the stage-and-phase-specific on-off gene switchings which are known to occur during prenatal development is a continuous process, but one involving different sets of genes at different developmental stages and phases, e.g. embryofetal sets and various later-acting sets. This is the essence of differentiation, which is also widely believed to be at the core of both normal and neoplastic development (Markert, 1968; Graham and Wareing, 1976; Pierce *et el.*, 1978; Lord *et al.*, 1978). Although this does not mean that the three processes are identical, ageing may none the less exert a highly variable and complex array of influences, differing in quality and timing, upon whatever intrinsic interphenotypic susceptibilities to cancer may exist in the individual.

1.3 Summary and Outlook

The problems posed by cancer are many, varied, and difficult, but they are certainly not new. As a general disease, cancer in one form or another is probably as old as multicellular evolution. As a human disease, it has been known throughout the recorded history of mankind. During this period, the fortunes of thought and practice upon which modern oncology has been built have been largely dependent upon those of many of the major aspects of mysticism, philosophy, science, technology, and medicine. This has led to the growth of oncology into its present complex state, now bestriding disciplines as diverse as pathology, medicine, embryology, chemistry, biochemistry, genetics, immunology, epidemiology, microbiology, and even the behavioural sciences. In all of these, various practitioners have already laid claims upon neoplasia as, in the words of Markert (1978), 'an abnormal manifestation of biological phenomena within the purview of their particular disciplines'.

The historical growth of oncologic thought and practice, from the necessarily broad and diffuse foundations laid in ancient times, is the subject of the next two chapters.

2 HISTORICAL PERSPECTIVES: CONCEPTS

2.1 Introduction

A prejudiced history is useless; it is a record only of the mind of the writer. 'He who writes history has truth at his mercy' — this dictum of Shimkin (1977) has many supporters. Among these are Friedrich von Schlegel's 'A historian is a prophet in reverse'; Henry Ford's 'History is bunk'; Augustine Birrell's 'That great dust heap called history'; and Anatole France's 'History books which contain no lies are extemely tedious'. Discordant histories clutter the archives. Some examples are the histories of the Napoleonic Wars by French and British historians; of the Crusades by Muslim and Christian historians; and of the Reformation by Protestant and Catholic historians. In oncologic history, Sir Percival Pott's reputedly 'first' descriptions in 1775 of an environmental association with human cancer is belied by John Hill's report in 1761 of an association between nasal cancer and snuff, and by Paracelsus' report in 1531 of one between lung cancer and mining dust. The worst of Anatole France's 'lies' must be a truth fragmented and unbalanced, for this retains a semblance of authority. As aptly put by that most ubiquitous of authorities, Anonymous, 'truth has many faces, and any one of them alone is a lie'. The historical 'Columbus discovered America' exemplifies a 'bad intent', that he is not a 'discoverer' unless he is also my brother. In the words of William Blake:

A truth that's told with bad intent
Beats all the lies you can invent.

Only a scholarly history can provide a reliable record of the human legacy in an appropriate field. It can be an informative record of the triumphs, trials and tribulations of the indomitable human spirit, through which the complex structure of modern human culture and institutions has been built. This alone would justify the task of writing. Even more importantly, however, it can also provide a reliable background against which current and

32

future efforts in the field can be evaluated and placed in proper perspective.

In the face of such an ancient and vital but chronically intransigent problem as cancer is, it seems appropriate to pause and critically examine relevant past experiences. Hopefully we can learn anew from the triumphs and errors and find some clues as to whether and wherein the anti-cancer fight might have gone and may be going astray.

2.2 Approach and General Sources

The present approach to the history of cancer is in two chapters. This chapter attempts a broadly based chronological overview of those major concepts and trends which have shaped the growth of oncology from its simpler beginnings to its modern complex state. The next chapter traces the historical but not necessarily chronological growth of the major oncologic practices of today.

Except as otherwise indicated in the text, the major sources for these two chapters are the following history books by: Barnes (ed) (1965) on general culture; Garrison (1929), Major (1954), Castiglioni (1958), Singer and Underwood (1962), and Thorwald (1962) on medicine; Meade (1968) on surgery; Buschke (1958) on radiotherapy; Bernal (1975) on science; Long (1965) on pathology; and Braun (1977), Shimkin (1977), and Rather (1978) on oncology. This represents a list of further readings, and the source of those detailed references to the older literature which have been cited in the present text but which, in the interest of brevity, have been excluded from the present bibliography.

2.3 Pre-Grecian Contributions to Civilization

2.3.1 General Aspects

The basic foundations of human civilization were firmly laid down long before the advent of Greece as a cultural centre. Of these, the most important, the driving forces, have undoubtedly been language, writing, mathematics, and natural science (cf. Barnes, 1965).

The earliest writings were pictographic. Examples are the hieroglyphics on papyri of Egypt, the cuneiform on terra cotta of

Sumer, and the logographics on bone and bamboo of China. Some of these apparently gave rise to the modern alphabetic systems. The best known example of this is the pseudo alphabetic system of the 24 of their hieroglyphic signs selected by the Egyptians around 3000 BC to denote 24 consonantal sounds. This formed the basis of the Phoenician alphabet of 21 consonants, which was developed during the nineteenth century BC and to which, in turn, the Greeks later added the missing vowels through adaptation of some of the hieroglyphic signs. Thus arose the famous 'Greek' alphabet ('alphabet' denotes the first two Greek letters) which, with some further modifications mainly by the Byzantines and Romans in the Christian era, became the basis of the modern alphabets of the West. The origins of the other major alphabets, those of India, remain uncertain.

The other essentials of writing — paper, pen, and ink — were also pre-Grecian in origin. 'Paper' (from the Egyptian word 'papyrus') was made by the early Egyptians from papyrus reeds pasted together at right angles. The Babylonians used both papyrus and parchment, the latter chiefly from sheepskin. The Indians used cotton and other fabrics. True paper, as based upon wood, was first made by the Chinese around 200 BC, from the pulp of the mulberry tree. The first known pens, made from pieces of reed, as well as ink, from water, vegetable gum, and soot, were Egyptian in origin.

The printed word is probably the most revolutionary of civilization's instruments. Equally, one of the most unhistorical and unfounded of claims is the commonly encountered 'the invention of printing' with the arrival of the 'first printed book' the Gutenberg Bible in Germany during the fifteenth century AD. Printing, absolutely, is a child of writing and its associated arts which are, as discussed above, of pre-Grecian origin. In any event, at least seven centuries before the Gutenberg Bible, the Chinese were printing books from letters carved on wooden blocks, leading to the founding of their Imperial Academy of Printing in the eighth century AD. This Chinese 'block printing' art was handed down to Europe during the fourteenth century. Europe then developed the movable type that made printing the facile and highly practical art it has since become.

The oldest known mathematical treatise is the Ahmose papyrus of around 2200 BC. This shows that the Egyptians had already mastered the rudiments of arithmetic and mensuration, though not of multiplication, which they performed by repeated additions. Multiplication, and its tables, were developed by the Babylonians. The Egyptians also invented a crude abacus, as did the Chinese; and they also had a working knowledge of geometry and trigonometry (essentials for the construction of the pyramids, for instance), as well as of algebra (an Arabic word). In its more advanced forms, however, algebra reached Europe during the middle ages, through the Egyptians, Greeks, and Arabs, from India. India also contributed the so-called Arabic numerals.

Among the natural sciences, disciplines such as chemistry (alchemy), anatomy and pharmacology were developed in Egypt and India. The physiological basis of these pharmacologies, as well as that of Chinese pharmacology, acupuncture and pulsometry was holistic. These disciplines, with homeopathy, osteopathy, and chiropractice, now constitute the so-called fringe, alternative, or complementary medicine. China also introduced immunization, and India excelled in surgery. In astronomy, the most notable of the ancient practitioners were the Babylonians, who also developed an astrology relating the heavens to affairs of state and society. The individualization of Babylonian astronomy, e.g. as horoscopes, was mainly the work of the Greeks and then of the Romans, Muslims, and Christians.

This is but a partial list of the remarkable contributions of the pre-Grecian civilizations to the subsequent growth of human culture. It does not imply that the ancients represented the source of all wisdom to which any perplexed later generation must perforce turn for inspiration and guidance. Of necessity, the ancients built, at best, the cradle of civilization. This recalls J.H. Robinson's modern view of the growing human mind, and also the medieval aphorism, 'we are the ancients', that was so stressed by Roger Bacon (1561–1626). Historically, however, it has not been always true that each generation is culturally and/or intellectually superior to its predecessors. This is amply illustrated by features such as the cyclical declines of great civilizations; the various Dark Ages, e.g. of China and Europe, that followed periods of cultural brilliance; and the prostitution of antecedent or secular science in medieval Christendom (Section 2.4.1).

2.3.2 Oncology

It is untenable that the pre-Grecian ancients laid the foundations of oncology as a modern scientific discipline. However, they documented two important features of the human disease: its antiquity and the special difficulties in its management.

In one form or another, cancer was known in perhaps all of the ancient civilizations. Signs of cancers such as osteosarcomas and ovarian and nasopharyngeal carcinomas, as well as of other diseases, have been discovered in Egyptian mummies since 1893, by many paleopathologists, most notably Armand Ruffer, A.B. Granville, Elliot Smith, W.R. Dawson, W.A. Schmidt, A.B. Shaw, J.K. Mitchell, F.A. Boyle, and A.T. Sanderson. In Mesopotamia, as discovered by S.N. Kramer, J.L. Starkey, R. Labat, and others, various tumours were sometimes described in some of the over 20,000 cuneiform tablets that constituted the famous library assembled by King Assurbanipal (668–?626 BC) of the late Assyrian Empire. In India, at least fourteen distinct types of abdominal tumours alone have been described in the *Charaka Samhita*. From Peru of around the beginning of the first millennium BC, long before the reign of the Incas, have come down Mohican representations, e.g. in pitchers, of various diseases. Among the latter was a swelling over the right cheekbone, that has been interpreted as a malignant sarcoma (cf. Thorwald, 1962). In 1966, Urteaga and Pack described signs of malignant melanoma involving the skull and long bones in the fossilized remains of the pre-Columbian Incas of Peru.

Recognition of the special difficulties in cancer management is as old as is that of cancer occurrence itself. From Egypt, for instance, has come down the famous case 45, described in the Edwin Smith papyrus, of the 'bulging tumours' of the male breast. This case, according to the papyrus, represented 'an ailment with which I will attend. There is no treatment'. Another famous example is that of the 'tumour of the god Xensu', possibly a Kaposi sarcoma. This, according to the Ebers papyrus, 'is loathsome and suffers many pustules to come forth' and it 'calls with a loud voice to thee . . . Do thou nothing there against'. In Mesopotamia, failure to cure was sometimes a serious offence. Thus, paragraph 218 of the code of Hammurabi enacts: 'If the doctor has treated a man for a severe wound with a bronze instrument and the man dies . . . his hands are to be cut off'. The doctor would hence have been wise to leave cancer alone. One of the cuneiform tablets mentioned above, which came down from the nineteenth or eighteenth century BC and was dealing with the Babylonian practice of hepatoscopy (divination by inspection of the liver of animals) gave this prognosis: 'If a fleshy tumour is found at the bottom of the *na* [an unidentified part of the liver], the patient will get worse and he will die'.

As discussed below, available records show that cancer was sufficiently common by the sixth century BC to lead the Greeks to name and classify it, to speculate about its causation, and to attempt its treatment. It is highly unlikely that this commonness of the disease was a new phenomenon at that time, i.e. that it was not also a feature of pre-Grecian times.

2.4 Greece

2.4.1 The Greek Synthesis: Its Nature, and a Broad Appraisal of Its Mixed Influences down the Centuries

From around the sixth century BC, the gradual emergence of Greece as a cultural centre was marked by a period of decreasing parochialism and insularity, rising economic prosperity and political power and, above all, a brilliant synthesis of Oriental, Egyptian, and native cultures. So avidly did the Greeks collect and collate information from all the sources then available to them, 'with the vitality of bastards' according to one historian (cf. Thorwald, 1962), that Greece rapidly became the world's first international data bank and the focal point of antecedent and contemporary cultures. One illustration of this is the already discussed origins of the 'Greek' alphabet (Section 2.3.1). The overall result of the Greek synthesis was an unprecedented surge in civilization. This result, which has so impressed but variably influenced posterity ever since, remained unmatched until the peak of the Islamic culture that so dominated scholarship between the seventh and fourteenth centuries of the Christian era, i.e. until the flowering of the so-called Renaissance in Europe.

The beginnings of the cultural, commercial, and other interchanges which stimulated the synthesis are lost in antiquity. The pre-sixth-century Greeks such as the Helladians and exquisitely artistic Minoans, as well as the Archaeans and Dorians 'from the north' sometimes thought to have conquered Hellas, were apparently insular, primitive, and illiterate. However, as portrayed in the great Greek epics, the *Iliad* and particularly the *Odyssey* of the mysterious Homer, the Greeks, like the Phoenicians before and the Vikings after them, were compulsive wanderers and

explorers. The synthesis first became evident in their two successive centres of learning during Hellenic times (up to *c*.300 BC), i.e.
first at Miletus until its destruction in 494 BC, and then at the
more brilliant Athens. It gained momentum thereafter, i.e.
during Hellenistic times, reaching its peak at Alexandria (in
Egypt), which was founded as a port by Alexander the Great in
332 BC. Set up by the Ptolemies as the new hub of Greek
scholarship, the University of Alexandria boasted an expansive
botanical garden, a zoological collection, an anatomical museum,
and an astronomical observatory. It also contained an international library of over 750,000 volumes. The partial burning
down of the library which occurred when Julius Caesar was
besieged in the city was, according to different historians, either
accidental or deliberately perpetrated by the early Christians;
but, as once almost traditionally believed, it was not the work of
the caliph Omar. The scholars at the university represented a
polyglot, e.g. of Greeks, Romans, and Egyptians, as well as
Persians, Jews, Indians, and other Asians. It was not the world's
first university (cf. Thorwald, 1962) as is often claimed, but it was
the first with a truly international character — in its staff,
students, visitors, curricula, and ideologies. In this and its
liberalism, it had no known equal until the University of Paris in
the late Middle Ages.

The Greeks responsible for their civilization's intellectual
achievements represented but a handful of unusually gifted
emancipated thinkers who based their efforts primarily upon
philosophical deductions, not unusually from borrowed premises.
Among the Hellenic stalwarts were Anaximander, with his pre-
tentious notions of the infinite; and Xenophanes, a most remarkable and precocious proponent of non-anthropomorphic
monotheism. 'There is one god', declared Xenophanes in the
format of Islam centuries later, who is 'supreme among gods and
men; resembling mortals neither in form nor in mind'; and in
anticipation of Voltaire (1694–1778), 'if oxen and lions had
hands . . . they would make the pictures and images of their gods
in their own likeness'. There were also the mystical Pythagoreans
who became noted for their mathematics, both real and mystical,
and also for their Hinduistic philosophy of pre-existence. Later,
in the 'Idealism' of Plato (427–347 BC), as described in his
Timaeus, a mystical semi-poetic eulogy of imagination over
reason, this Pythagorean-Hinduistic philosophy was extended to

include the pre-existence and rebirth of ideas among selected souls. In his *Republic* Plato also reproduced the Hinduistic notions of caste. Plato's mentor was Socrates (*c.* 469–399 BC), and one of his students was Aristotle (384–322 BC), who was Greece's greatest logician and multi-specialist, and also the tutor of Alexander the Great. This celebrated trio of Socrates, Plato, and Aristotle believed in the existence of eternal truths that remain valid in all times, places and circumstances.

The leading Hellenic opponents of this latter belief were the Sophists. They were dedicated sceptics and agnostics, believing in the relativity, pragmatism, and non-absolutism of all knowledge. Among their leaders were Protagoras, Hippias, and Gorgias. Hippias, the most extreme of sceptics, followed in the footsteps of oriental ascetism and anticipated Rousseau (1712–1778) by advocating a return to nature as the only means to contentment.

This schism between the Hellenic philosophies of immutable eternal truths and of scepticism was continued and intensified, in various guises, at Alexandria in Hellenistic times by the Skeptics, Cynics, Cyrenaics, Stoics, Epicureans, Neoplatonists, and Eclectics. Of these, the Neoplatonists, who were led by Plotinus, an Egyptian, exerted a particularly lasting influence upon posterity, insofar as their principle of the superiority of faith over facts became enshrined as one of the central dogmas of Christianity.

Philosophical discussions in the market place and elsewhere, representing all shades of opinion, thus became a major preoccupation of the Greek scholars. This exercise engendered much freedom in thought and word and, as put by Professor Giddings, a 'legal-liberal' stage of civilization distinct from the 'religious-military' equivalent in previous times. However, this distinction was far from absolute, as the Greek masses, like the masses everywhere and even down to the present day, remained steeped in their traditions and superstitions. For instance, they believed in oracles, in a pantheism with gods indulging all the vices and virtues of men, in a future life spent in the realms of the dead ruled over by Hades (Pluto), and in the joys of Elysium and the sufferings of Tartarus. Church and State were considered indivisible. Priests were public officials. Religion and politics were intertwined, and piety and reverence were civic duties. Their principle of freedom in thought and word belied their encodement of atheism, heresy, and sacrilege as treasonable offences. Attesting to this were the poisoning of Socrates, and their fierce persecution of Anaxagoras who barely escaped their wrath by fleeing the city. Later, as their lives once again approached that of Hobbes's description of man in the state of nature — 'poor, nasty, brutish, and short' — they enthusiastically embraced Christianity and Mithraism, the two mysteries that held out the rosiest promises of eternal bliss in the hereafter. To Christianity, their neoplatonism gave the doctrine of salvation through faith; their rhetoric gave the model for preaching, as it is now for salesmanship and electioneering; and their common meal in the Eleusinian mysteries gave the eucharist. Even the great Aristotle reasoned that since the most godlike activity is pure thought, which only God can perform, God spends his time contemplating himself. In short, the legacy of superstition from preliterate times was as hard to shake off, even for the magnificent Greeks, as it has always been and still is.

The preoccupation of the Greek thinkers with philosophical conjecture at the expense of observational and experimental precision landed them in a large variety of intellectual mischief. Their rhetoric, according to Francis Bacon (1561–1626) in his *Novum Organon*, was central to his 'Idols of the Market' — i.e. it substituted 'well-said' for 'well-done' and made words 'force the understanding, throw everything into confusion, and lead mankind into vain and innumerable controversies and fallacies'. Their endless arguments about the 'ultimate reality', the primordial substance of all creation, centred upon their borrowed oriental notions of universal elements. Of these elements, Anaximenes championed air; Thales, water; Xenophanes, earth; and Heracleitus, fire. Aristotle declared the existence of a 'fifth element', the mysterious 'ether', which was absent from the earth but made up the heavens. Down through medieval times, it became widely believed that this element, the 'philosopher's stone' of the alchemists or the 'elixir' of life, could not only transmute base metals into gold but also rectify the faulty composition of the four earthly elements present in all individuals who would thereby be rejuvenated for ever. Aristotle also espoused the patently false notions of the 'primum mobile', the great heavenly sphere surrounding a Ptolemaic geocentric universe; of the superiority of the circular heavenly motions over the earthly rectilinear motions; of the speed of falling bodies being proportional to their weights; of the non-sexuality of plants; and of the heart being the seat of intelligence, brain function being to pump phlegm into the heart. Phlegm was one of the 'four body humours' which were also of ancient oriental origin and which, from Hippocrates (*c*.460–*c*.380 BC) to Galen (129–199 AD), were generally accepted by the Greek physicians as constituting the basis of pathophysiology. As discussed below (Section 2.4.2), the further Greek elaborations of this humoral theory can quite fairly be described as a futile exercise in the compounding of absurdity.

Many of the philosophical deductions were later adopted or adapted by Christendom in ways that effectively suppressed European secular science for over a thousand years after the Greeks. This fact is epitomized in the basic principles of the *City of God* (*Civitas Dei*) of St Augustine (354–430), which eulogized theology as 'the true queen of the sciences'; and in those of that even more colossal monument to intellectual futility known as 'scholasticism'. Scholasticism was produced, mainly through a revival of Aristotelian didacticism but with some contributions from Islam and the Jewish *Cabala*, by the church fathers from Peter Abelard (1079–1142) to Thomas Aquinas (1225–1274). The following is an illustrative extract from Aquinas's *Summa Theologiae*:

> This science [theology] does not argue to prove its principles, which are articles of Faith . . . faith rests on infallible truth, its contrary cannot be demonstrated; manifestly the proofs which are brought against it . . . are controvertible arguments. To argue from authority is most appropriate in this science; for its principles rest in [divine] revelation, and it is proper to credit the authority of those to whom the revelation is made.

The above extract would strain the credulity of any modern scientist, since science eschews any authority except fact. Its capacity to prostitute science to the extremes of absurdity is well illustrated by the following passage from Professor Preserved Smith's *History of Modern Culture* (1930–1934):

> The medievals cared not a whit to know anything about animals and plants for the sake of curiosity; they wanted to find in them something profitable to the soul . . . Besides including a large number of mythical beasts — dragons,

griffins, cockatrices, basilisk, mantichores, and phoenixes — in their menagerie, they had much to tell of the . . . lion born dead and coming to life after three days as a symbol of Christ, of the albatross feeding its young on its blood as a symbol of the eucharist, of the pelican that kills its young and then brings them to life with its blood as a symbol of redemption, and of the beaver that bites off its testicles when hard pressed by the hunter in order to give a practical lesson in the value of chastity to the sinner beset by that great hunter, the devil.

The following rather amusing quotation is one of several slavish medieval renditions of Aristotle, as compiled by John Langdon-Davies in his *Man and His Universe* (quoted in Barnes, 1965):

> The lioness whelpeth first five whelps, and afterwards four, and so each year less by one, and waxeth barren when she whelpeth one at last. And she whelpeth whelps evil shapen and small, in size of a weasel in the Beginning. And whelps of two months may hardly move. If a man shoot at him the lion chaseth him and throweth him down, and woundeth him not, nor hurteth him.

The corresponding quotation from Aristotle reads:

> The Syrian lion bears cubs five times: five cubs at the first litter, then four, then three, then two and lastly one; after this the lioness ceases to bear . . . If a hunter hit him, without hurting him, then if with a bound he gets hold of him, he will do him no harm . . . The cubs of the lioness when newly born are exceedingly small, and can scarcely walk when two months old.

Of course, the Greeks can hardly be blamed for any stultifying use made of their honestly derived albeit mistaken deductions, or for any undeserved adulation they received. To paraphrase J.H. Robinson (1924), the medieval scholars were so convinced that 'it had pleased God to permit Aristotle' whom they called 'The Philosopher' to have 'the last word upon each and every branch of knowledge that they humbly accepted him . . . as one of the unquestioned authorities . . . in every branch of science'.

In many ways, the Greeks adequately compensated for their deductive blemishes which, in the context of their time and approaches, were unavoidable. Their achievements in the arts and literature are legendary. So are the discoveries of Euclid (*c.* 300 BC) in geometry, of Archimedes (287–212 BC) in physics, and of Aristotle in botany and zoology. The mechanical inventions of Hero of Alexandria (*c.*100 BC) included the steam engine representing in design a true anticipation of the steam turbine, a more advanced conception than that of James Watt. Thales reputedly predicted the total solar eclipse of 585 BC. Aristarchus of Samos (*c.*275 BC) anticipated Copernicus by holding that the earth revolves daily on its axis and moves in a yearly orbit round the sun. Democritus of Abdera (460–361 BC) repudiated the doctrine of the four elements and proposed his atomic or mechanistic cosmology, i.e. that all natural objects including stars and living organisms are made up of numerous indivisible atoms. Alcmaeon (*c.*500 BC), a Pythagorean, and Herophilus of Chalcedon (*c.*300 BC) proposed the brain as the seat of intellectual life. Finally, the mysterious humoral doctrine of the equally mysterious Hippocrates was rejected chiefly by Erasistratos of Ceos (310–250 BC) and Asclepiades of Bithynia (128–50 BC).

Whatever their shortcomings, the Greeks instituted and maintained for a thousand years (from the sixth century BC to the fourth century AD) an intellectually most tolerant society. All types of human problem were tackled freely, intelligently, and from all conceivable angles, particularly at Alexandria where non-Greeks, largely Egyptians and Asians, far outnumbered Greeks, but mainly philosophically. Were the unrivalled talents of the time turned towards science and technology, these disciplines would almost certainly have been advanced by many centuries. That they were not, however, might have saved human civilization from an untimely end, particularly in view of the incessant warfares of later times and the latter's excommunications, inquisitions, witch-hunts, and other acts of barbarism perpetrated mostly in the cause of the Protestant Reformation and its Catholic countermeasures. As it was, the unrivalled culture and the advanced social institutions of the Greeks far outdistanced their science, machinery, and material wealth. It is a sobering thought that this situation has become increasingly reversed since the industrial and scientific revolutions of the eighteenth and nineteenth centuries, and there is now a 'cultural lag' which has already become the greatest threat to the survival of modern civilization or even of mankind.

Of special importance to the present discussion were the unprecedented attempts made by the Greeks to systematize contemporary oncologic knowledge, as discussed below.

2.4.2 Humoralism and the Origin of Tumours

To Hippocrates of Cos (*c*.460–*c*.380 BC) and Galen of Pergamus (129–199 AD) the origin of all tumours was atrabilis, or black bile. This mysterious substance, together with blood, phlegm, and yellow bile, constituted their four body humours. These humours were equated with the four universal elements or *stoicheia* (air, earth, fire and water) of Greek philosophy, and also with its four qualities or *dynameis* (hot, cold, moist and dry). Thus initially, black bile was dry, like the earth; blood was hot, like fire; phlegm was cold, like air; and yellow bile was moist, like water. Later, the four seasons were also brought into the scheme, and the elements mixed. Black bile then became associated with cold, dry, earth, and autumn; blood with hot, moist, air, and spring; phlegm with cold, moist, water and winter; and yellow bile with hot, dry, fire, and summer. To Galen, however, the four qualities were more important than the humours. Health depended upon the right balance (*eukrasis*) and various states of ill health upon imbalances (*dyskrasis*) of hot, moist, cold and dry. He recognized eight dyscrasias: four simple, with hot, moist, cold, or dry predominating; and four complex, with hot and moist, dry and hot, cold and moist, or moist and dry predominating. Food was digested first in the stomach and intestines, and the resulting chyle was then drawn into the liver where yellow bile (choler) was produced, and into the spleen where black bile formed. Phlegm was a waste product formed in the brain; and blood, formed in the heart, was the most important of the humours. However, the fluid in the veins and arteries, although called blood, was a mixture of all the humours and some of their breakdown products.

2.4.3 Classification and Treatment of Tumours

The Hippocratic writers classified tumours into *carcinos* (*karkinos*) and *carcinomas* (*karkinomas*). They distinguished these from *phyomas*, *oidemas*, and other kinds of growth and swellings. However, none of the distinctions was clear-cut in the modern sense. Galen classified tumours into three major groups, depending upon whether they were 'according to', 'above' or 'contrary to' nature. Here again, as discussed later, the classification was not clear-cut.

Both the Hippocratic and the Galenic views of cancer treatment were *primum non nocere* (first do no harm). If the cancer was 'occult' (concealed), it was best left alone. In other cases, various surgical, soothing, or escharotic remedies were used. One of these remedies, the salve of Archigenes of Apameia or the *medicamentum Archigenis ad cancros ulceratos*, remained in use up to the sixteenth century. Archigenes, a reputed pneumatist with extensive experience of cancers such as those of the uterus, and of the breast in both men and women, had come to recognize the futility of surgery and the necessity for palliative and other alternatives in cancer treatment.

2.4.4 Anatomy and Physiology

The anatomic knowledge of the Greeks was well summarized by Renouard (as translated by Comiegny) (cf. Long, 1965), as follows:

Piecing together all the fragments of the Hippocratic writers relative to the structure of the human body, it would be impossible to compose from them a regular or complete treatise on anatomy, for with the exception of the skeleton they possessed very limited and imperfect notions of any organic apparatus. They confounded under a common name nerves, ligaments and tendons; they distinguished very imperfectly the arteries and veins; and the muscles, in their eyes, were inert masses designed solely to cover bones, serving as an envelope or ornament. They possessed in short only gross and false ideas on the structure and functions of the brain, heart, liver, lungs, digestive and generative apparatus, for the reason that they had never been able to devote themselves to regular dissections. But this did not prevent them from adducing very decided opinions on the organs and their functions, which no one could verify or deny.

Erasistratos of Ceos (born *c.* 300 BC), a methodist, is widely regarded as one of the true founders of pathology. He believed in two circulations: one from the heart for blood, which provided nourishment; and the other from the lung for air (or *pneuma*, an aerial spirit), which provided energy. The arteries contained air which, in excess, caused fever; and any blood in the arteries was always pathologic. His pathology centred around *plethora* (fluids or air in excess ·or in the wrong place), such as plethora of the lung arteries in pleural inflammation, and of the joints in arthritis. Erasistratos, of course, could have known nothing about capillaries, the first recorded description of which postdated William Harvey; or about the natural elasticity of the walls of the arteries, driving the arterial blood into the capillaries after death and allowing replacement of the blood by air, an event inevitable in dissection.

Asclepiades of Bithynia (*c.* 128–43 BC) proposed a doctrine based upon the concept of *strictum et laxum*. This was the tonic constriction and relaxation of innumerable, hypothetical body pores through which the vital juices flowed. Disease, usually acute or chronic, resulted when, respectively, constriction or relaxation occurred unduly.

The pneumatists were championed by Athenaeus of Cicilia (*c.* 70 AD) and the eclectics by one of the then leaders in obstetrics and gynaecology, Soranus of Ephesus (*c.* 100 AD). They held that the pneuma governed the solids and liquids of the body in ways which were normal in health but aberrant in disease. Like humoralism, but at a lower pitch, pneumatism flourished on and off for centuries, showing up, for instance, in the vitalistic and iatrochemical mysticisms of Paracelsus, van Helmont, Recamier, and others. The eclectics subscribed generally to the hypothesis of constricted and relaxed pores. However, they believed that no single doctrine could alone explain health and disease. They thus remained free to select and combine elements from different doctrines.

A particularly interesting example of the early rebels was Herophilos of Chalcedon (*c.* 300 BC). A pupil of one of Hippocrates' most ardent followers, Praxagoras of Cos, he postulated four vital forces. These were a nourishing force, located in the liver and digestive tract; a warming force, in the heart; a neutral force, in the brain; and a sensitive force, in the nerves. According to Pliny, Herophilos was 'the first man who searched into the causes of disease through dissection of the human body'.

2.4.5 Galen and Galenism

History boasts no physician whose influence upon medical thought and practice was more lasting than that of Galen. As discussed above, the scene of his medical activities around the Mediterranean, particularly at Alexandria where he received his training, was a free-for-all of ideologies incapable of proof or disproof mainly because of the poor ground-work in human anatomy and physiology. Yet, out of this chaos, he created order, practically resurrecting Hippocratic humoralism which he endowed with his own conception of a guiding spirit or pneuma. He knew little about internal diseases, nothing about some such as metastases, and he never performed more than two or three dissections on human bodies. His stock in trade was a solid knowledge of the anatomy of apes and swine, a phenomenal understanding of external diseases, an apparently limitless energy, and an almost despotic authority. With this authority he so stamped his medical doctrines that they, inclusive of his own brands of humoralism (Section 2.4.3) with all their faults, dominated Mediterranean medicine for the next thirteen centuries.

Galen was not only a great medical figure, but also a wide traveller and a prolific medical writer. His travels took him to Pergamus, where he was born; Alexandria, where he received his medical training in the school developed by the anatomist Marinos, and where he subsequently spent most of his working life; to Rome, where as a physician and medical lecturer he spent five of his most illustrious years; and to Thrace, Macedonia, and other areas as medical adviser to the army of the Roman Emperor Marcus Aurelius Antoninus. It was during his career with the army that he barely escaped a visitation of the plague in 166 AD. Among his some 150 publications, the more important were *Seats of Disease*, a large treatise on local pathology and diagnosis; *Abnormal Tumours*, a brief but important work on the subject; *Therapeutic Method — Addressed to Glaucon*, a textbook on pathology and therapeutics; *Natural Faculties*, a treatise on physiology, with allusions to pathology; and *Parts Affected*, a textbook on special pathology and pathological physiology.

As described in these works, much of Galen's pathology was

based upon his conception of 'presentation' and 'adhesion'. This is exemplified by food presented to the intestines and undergoing normal adhesion when its absorption and digestion were also normal, but impaired adhesion when these were abnormal and vomiting resulted; and by absorption of bile into blood to produce jaundice. Tumours resulted from the adherence or abnormal concentration of black bile to produce melancholy. Galen claimed to have repeatedly observed a peculiar proneness of melancholy women to develop carcinoma, particularly in regions such as the face, lips and breast where black bile thickened. An acrid bile produced an ulcerating tumour, but a milder bile produced *cancer occultus*, i.e. non-ulcerated cancer.

In 1567, Thomas Gayle, in his *The Institution of Chyrurgerie*, gave the following summary of Galenic tumour pathology:

> Of blacke color, without boylying (that is to say melancholic) cometh cancers, and if the humor be sharpe, it maketh ulceration, and for this cause, these tumours are more blacker in colour, than those that cometh of inflammation, and these be not hote, but the veines in these, are both more fuller, and more distended forth than those whiche be in inflammations. For lesse matter goeth out of the veines, into the fleshy partes, whiche compasseth them about, through the grosseness of the humor, which breadeth the Cancers, neither yet are the veines so reade as they be in inflammations, but sheweth themselves accordyng to the humor, that they be filed with.

2.5 Islam

2.5.1 The Rise of Islamic Culture

From the seventh to the fifteenth centuries it devolved upon Islam to carry aloft the torch of learning lit in the ancient Orient and refuelled in Greece. Unlike medieval Christianity, Islam encouraged and eagerly sought useful cultural exchanges and secular scholarship, probably because of Islam's lack of a priestly hierarchy and the prosperity of its vast empire. At its peak, this empire sprawled across the Mediterranean and the Orient from Spain to India. Its major centres of learning included Córdoba, Meraga, Baghdad and Damascus.

2.5.2 Science

Islamic science represented a synthesis of Egyptian, Indian, Greek and other elements reinforced by many home-grown contributions. Among its features were the introduction of 'Arabic' numerals from India, and notable advances in arithmetic, algebra, geometry and trigonometry. In astronomy, Islamic scientists established good observatories at Baghdad and elsewhere, and they manufactured the best astrolabe and quadrant before the sixteenth-century Danish astronomer Tycho Brahe. They also calculated the precise latitude and longitude of their cities, edited the famous Toledo planetary tables, and made notable advances in chronology and the calendar. In physics, they made original contributions to the principles of the lever, pulley, the triangle of forces, specific gravity, and optics. Ibn al-Haitham was hailed by George Sarton as 'the greatest of Muslim physicists and one of the greatest students of optics of all time'. Their contributions to optics formed the basis of the later inventions of the telescope, the microscope, the prism and the other optical instruments on which the progress of modern science has so depended. Islamic scientists advanced ancient alchemy to the borders of modern chemistry. One of the ablest of Islamic alchemists, Abu Bakr al-Razi, or Rhazes (d. 924 AD), constructed elaborate chemical apparatus, worked out an extensive classification of minerals and other chemicals, and applied chemistry to medicine. Among their geographical contributions was the representation, by Idrisi (1099–1154) over three centuries before Columbus, of the earth as a sphere, on which Idrisi located the chief climatic zones.

In botany and zoology, the Islamic scientists made no original contributions. In fact, they propagated a debased form of Indian and Greek biology. They also shared with medieval Christian writers the habit of compiling strange bestiaries and other works of 'wonders' (cf. Section 2.4.1), though not the latters' motivation 'to drive home Christian truths'.

2.5.3 Oncology and Medicine

Islamic medicine, though extensive and sometimes original, was essentially a compilation of Greek, Indian and Persian medicine. In his *Paradise of Wisdom*, Ali-al-Tabari synthesized Islamic medical treatises such as *The Comprehensive Book* of Rhazes, who was the greatest clinical physician of the Middle Ages; and

The Canon of Avicenna drew heavily upon Hippocrates, Dioscorides and, in particular, Galen. Rhazes gave excellent descriptions of measles, smallpox and surgery of the eye. He also extended knowledge of gynecology and obstetrics, and suggested new ways in which chemistry might aid medicine. Existing knowledge of drugs and materia medica was extended by Abu Mansur Muwaffak and Masawaili al-Mardini. One of the leading Islamic surgeons was Abulcasis of Córdoba who, among other achievements, was one of the first to pay special attention to antisepsis during surgery.

Islamic contributions to oncology, though essentially Galenic, were considerable. Aetius of Amidia, who was physician to the emperor Justinian, gave an excellent description of uterine carcinoma, which he considered incurable. He also distinguished the cervical from the corpus and the ulcerated from the non-ulcerated forms of the disease. Rufus of Ephesus described skin cancers, some melanotic. Soranus dealt well with schirrous tumours, 'scleromata', and uterine inflammations; and Archigenes described various cancers including breast cancer in both men and women. Esophageal and gastric cancers were well described by Avenzoar, a Jewish physician of the western caliphate in Córdoba.

The greatest medical figure of the Middle Ages was Ibn Sina, or Avicenna (980–1037). His million-word encyclopedia, *The Canon*, summarized all existing medical knowledge. This quickly became the most authoritative medical work of the time in the Islamic world, and it competed with Galen elsewhere. It continued to influence oncologic and other medical thought and practice well into the fifteenth century.

An important feature of these developments in oncology was that, even as early as the latter half of the seventh century, internal cancers of many types had become well known. This led to the belief that cancer can involve any of the body's tissues. Thus, Paul of Aegina (625–690), a Persian, recorded in his *Epitome* that 'in omni corporis parte cancer nasci solet'.

2.5.4 Islamic Contributions to Western Culture

Curiously, wars and preparations for war, the supreme follies of mankind, can sometimes produce unexpected spin-offs even for the loser, e.g. getting to know and profiting from the enemy. Significant cultural contacts between the Islamic and Christian countries around the Mediterranean occurred during the Crusades of the eleventh, twelfth and thirteenth centuries. They were facilitated by the proximity of Islamic Sicily and southern Spain to Christendom, and by the ready availability of Latin translations of Islamic scholarly works due to the efforts of Gerard of Cremona and others from the twelfth century.

The resulting Islamic influence upon Western culture was aptly summarized in 1931 by the Baron Carra de Vaux thus:

> The Arabs kept alive the higher intellectual life and the study of science in a period when the Christian West was fighting desperately with barbarism. From the twelfth century anyone in the West who had any taste for science, some desire for light, turned to the East or to the Moorish West . . . The Arabs thus formed a bond . . . between ancient culture and modern civilisation. When at the Renaissance the spirit of man was once again filled with zest for knowledge . . . if it was able to set promptly to work, to produce and to invent, it was because the Arabs had preserved and perfected various branches of knowledge, kept the spirit of research alive and eager, and maintained it pliant and ready for future discoveries.

2.6 The Modern West

2.6.1 Historical Background

It is traditional to regard the cultural upsurge which began in Italy from around 1450 and thence spread to most parts of Europe and beyond as a distinct historical period, that of the Renaissance. However, this period simply marked the re-emergence of European culture, since its decline in Greece a millennium before, to make Western Europe a major contributor to the global material and intellectual cultures of today.

This modern phenomenon was the inevitable outcome of a convergence of powerful antecedent and continuing trends. Among these were the steady decline of, and the mounting dissatisfaction with, both medievalism and the Roman Catholic Church from the twelfth century. Feudalism with its attributes of fealty and serfdom had become, in the hands of greedy landlords, a ready means for suppression and exploitation of the masses by the few, including the Church. The latter, as the Vatican, had become the richest and the most powerful and oppressive of States in all of Christendom. It subjugated secular science through scholasticism (Section 2.4.1), as well as kings and subjects alike through skilful instillation of fear of God in this world and of the devil in the next, with appropriate backing by military and other forces. This trend was the real power behind the so-called Protestant Reformation traditionally accredited to Luther, Zwingli, Calvin and Knox in the sixteenth and seventeenth centuries. The overall attribute of this trend was the reign of that disastrous medieval principle of the 'right of might', the principle behind the then prevalent features such as the trials by combat, the duels to the death, the divine rights of conquest by force, and the greatest shame of all, the 'cowardice' of the non-violent. It was a trend that fed the prevalent fear, oppression, poverty, and even the resort to the occult 'sciences' of magic, witchcraft and sorcery. Such 'sciences', as popular responses to the inquisitions, excommunications, tortures, burnings, and other acts of barbarism perpetrated in the names of the Protestant Reformation and the Catholic Counter-Reformation, reached their peak in the witchcraft epidemics and countermeasures of the sixteenth and seventeenth centuries in Europe and the New England colonies. This long experience in the arts and crafts of violence made the empire-builders of Western Europe invincible, except among themselves, when, after Columbus, they turned their attentions overseas, Bible in the left hand and sword in the right, to 'civilize' the non-European world by giving it the gospel and taking away everything else.

This empire-building enterprise introduces the second of the major trends, the gradual submergence of Europe's traditional parochialism and insularity and the parallel rise of secularism and an international outlook. From as early as the twelfth century, European and Muslim explorers such as Piano Carpino, William of Rubruquis, John of Monte Corvino, Ibn Battuta, and the most famous of them all, Marco Polo, had brought back dazzling reports of the fabulous wealth and advanced cultures of China, India and Persia. These reports, together with her new ship-building skills and navigational aids, set Europe off into her age of great explorations, marked by the exploits of the likes of Diaz, Columbus, and Magellan. In consequence, Europe's trade and outlook became increasingly international; her new trading guilds such as the Levantine and the British and Dutch East India Companies were established; her colonial empires proliferated and flourished for over three centuries; and every aspect of her economic and cultural life became transformed. This prosperity, together with the steady growth of useful inventions, towns, and the middle class, brought on the industrial revolutions of the eighteenth and nineteenth centuries. Europe thus became beneficiaries not only of the wealth of 'Ind and Cathay' and of the Incas and others but also of the ancient cultures of the orient and elsewhere.

These cultural benefits, however, represented the culmination of a trend which began with revival of interest in the classics, an interest which, by the time of the Renaissance, had already become a 'fad'. From as early as the seventh century, the Persian and the Muslim wars, as well as the Iconoclastic controversy of the eighth century and the fall of Constantinople to the Turks in 1453, had forced Greek scholars to seek refuge in southern Italy. During the fourteenth and fifteenth centuries, Petrarch and others such as Giovanni da Ravenna and Gasparino de Barzizza had revived interest in Latin literature. Indeed, the revival of classicism, called 'humanism', was so great that it became not uncommon for scholars of the time to freely classicize their names. For instance, Hiero Fabrizio, the anatomist and tutor of William Harvey, became Hieronymus Fabricus da Aquapendente; Johannes Jaeger, the humanist, became Crotus Rubianus; Johann Müller, the astronomer, became Regiomontanus; and Schwarzerd, a German family name meaning 'black earth', became the Greek equivalent, Melancthon.

Such a new-found freedom, however, did not readily extend to civil liberties. This represented another major trend, a struggle which, despite the Magna Carta of 1215, had to be waged relentlessly until the famous Bill of Rights of 1689 in England, the Declaration of American Independence in 1776, and the clarion call of the French Revolution of 1789–95.

In terms of overall economic wealth and intellectual motivation, Western Europe, from the time of the Renaissance, gradually became a match for the golden ages of antecedent civilizations. Indeed, it certainly surpassed them in terms of the cultural legacy it inherited, built, and passed on. Anatomy flourished in Italy from the sixteenth century when, also, Girolamo Frascatoro, in his *De Contagione* of 1546, named syphilis and theorized about infections and contagious diseases. This was also the century of Copernicus, Galileo, and the first printed book in Europe, the Gutenberg Bible. The seventeenth century, the century of physics and mathematics, was graced by stalwarts such as Descartes, Leibnitz, Fermat, Pascal, Huygens, Kepler and Newton. In the eighteenth century, the process of conversion of alchemy into modern chemistry begun earlier by the Arabs and others such as Paracelsus, Sydenham and Boerhaave was extended by Priestley, Scheele, Cavendish, Lavoisier, Prout, Berthollet, Dalton, Gay-Lussac, Avogadro, and many others. The nineteenth century saw biology becoming the science first of tissues and then of cells. Towards the end of the century, the microbiology mooted by Frascatoro over three centuries earlier had become a reality. Analogously, the laws of heredity of Gregor Mendel and the natural selection of Charles Darwin, both elaborated around the middle of the century, began to acquire a basis in molecular genetics.

The above roughly sketches only some of the highlights of the remarkable European period from the middle of the fifteenth century to the close of the nineteenth. It was a period of enlightenment marked by a gradual dispersal of the dark clouds cast by scholasticism and other features of medievalism upon the brilliance of classical Greece and its predecessors. The achievements of this period in science and medicine, as they relate to oncology, are discussed below.

2.6.2 Anatomy and Surgery

With Antonio Beniveni (1443?–1502) began, at Padua in Italy, the longest continuous line of eminent anatomists the world has ever known. This line included Andreas Vesalius (1514–1564). At the age of 29 years, he published his *De Humanis Corporis Fabrica*, which has marked him as one of the great anatomists of all time. In the artistry of his dissections, Vesalius had no peer, except the phenomenal Leonardo da Vinci (1452–1519), who surpassed even Aristotle in terms of overall versatility and genius. Despite his vast knowledge of the body's structure, Vesalius' physiological theories remained essentially those of Hippocrates and Galen. This line ended with the celebrated Bernardino Morgagni (1682–1771) (see below).

Among the other notable anatomists of the period were Michael Servetus (1511–1553), Bartolomeo Eustachi (1520–

1574), Gabriello Fallopio (1523–1562), and Fabricus da Aquapendente (1537–1619). Servetus, who was burnt at the stake for daring to disagree with Calvin about the nature of the Trinity, discovered blood circulation between the heart and lungs. Fabricus, among whose students at Padua was William Harvey, discovered the valves of the veins. Eustachi discovered the tube connecting the inner ear and throat, and Fallopio the oviducts.

The example of Padua inspired other parts of Western Europe and as far afield as the United States. The famous anatomists and surgeons then included Marco Aurelio Severino (1580–1652) in Switzerland, and Wilhelm Fabry or Fabricius Hildanus (1560–1634) and Johannes Schultes (1595–1645) in Germany.

Schultes was one of the first surgeons to use radical mastectomy in breast cancer. Over the ensuing centuries, this procedure became widely followed, extended and refined. Among the more important surgeons involved were Lorenz Heister (1683–1758) and Christian Billroth (1829–1894) in Germany, Henri Francois Le Dran (1685–1770) in France, John Hunter (1728–1793) in Britain, and William Halsted (1852–1922) in the United States. This procedure eventually came to mean removal of the affected breast *en bloc* with the pectoral muscles and the adjacent axillary lymph nodes. In recent decades, it has been losing popularity in surgical practice because of its resulting unacceptable disfigurement.

As stated above, the Paduan dynasty of anatomists ended with Morgagni. In his great classic, *The Seats and Causes of Disease*, Morgagni dealt with practically all the then known aspects of pathologic anatomy based upon naked-eye observations. Among the malignancies forming part of his subject were those of the esophagus, stomach, rectum, pancreas, adrenal, prostate, ovary, and liver. Among the other stalwarts in oncology who also worked in Italy during this period were the already-mentioned Schultes (from Ulm) and Ramazzini, with the latter describing, in addition to nuns' breast cancer, an association between lung disease and dusty trades.

2.6.3 Tulp and Others: The 'Contagiousness' of Cancer

From Italy, the centres of scientific progress moved to other parts of Europe. In Holland, for instance, Frederick Ruysch (1683–1731) described chronic bone inflamations, calculi, and, among other tumours, stenosing tumours of the rectum, gastric tumours, and a papillary tumour of the urinary bladder. In Holland also, Nicolas Tulp (1593–1674), Zacutus Lucitanus (1575–1642), a Jewish physician originally from Portugal, and others believed in the contagiousness of mammary and other cancers. This belief evoked much controversy during the late nineteenth century, the heyday of microbiology.

2.6.4 Gendron: Cancer as a Degenerative Growth

In France, Claude Deshais Gendron (1663–1750) made a clean break from the then still prevalent time-honoured humoralistic views of cancer genesis from body fluids. In his little book of 1700, *Recherches sur la Nature et la Guérison des Cancers*, he proposed that cancers were not due to fluxed humours or ferments, or to the corrosive acids whose very existence he had come to doubt (*a douter de l'existence de cet acide corrosif*). For what could be their source? Surely not the blood, since cancer starts in healthy people; nor a lymphatic humour at the site of its extravasation (*où il se sera extravasé quelque humeur lymphatique*), since extravasations due to blows or compression occur commonly and resolve spontaneously. To Gendron, cancers are degenerative growths. Their actual masses represent the 'transformation of nervous, glandular and lymphatic-vascular parts into a uniform, hard, compact, insoluble substance capable of growth and ulceration'. Some benign lesions such as scirrhous, scrofulous tumours (écrouelles) polyps (*polyps*), and soft-tissue tumours (*sarcomes*), which lack filaments and dispersal in neighbouring parts, are not truly carcinomatous (*véritablement carcinomateuse*). They can grow into cancers but, strictly, through degeneration of the involved part rather than of the lesion itself. Scirrhous and scrofulous tumours represent 'simple excesses of humours coagulated in the vessels of the part'. These can readily be cured by extirpation, but true cancers have 'many filaments . . . which are imperceptible to the touch but form part of the cancer. Being capable of growth and ulceration, and dispersed as they are in the neighbouring parts, it is not surprising that they would come together after the extirpation and seem to form a new cancer, more dangerous than the one that was undertaken to be extirpated'.

One of Gendron's pronouncements shows that the tendency of shady practitioners to profit from the plight of patients with incurable disease is certainly not new. 'The cure of disease', he wrote in 1700, 'labelled incurable by those who master the Art of Healing, is not the privilege of those who excel in the practice of deception.'

2.6.5 Spagyric Theory: A Second Version of Humoralism

Following the example of the alchemists of Islam, those of Western Europe from the early sixteenth century began to free chemistry from its old mysticism. This began with Paracelsus (1493–1541), who substituted the three basic elements (mercury, sulphur and salt) of 'spagyric' theory for the four universal elements and the four body humours of the Greeks. Paracelsus also instituted 'iatrochemistry', the treatment of disease with defined chemicals and drugs. The best of these early alchemist-spagyricist-iatrochemists were Valerius Cordus (1515–1544), who prepared ether from sulphuric acid and ethanol; Andreas Libavius (1540–1616), whose *Alchemia* became a standard chemical textbook; and François Dubois (1614–1672), who distinguished between acids and alkalis.

During the seventeenth century, the spagyric theory received considerable support and criticism. Van Helmont accorded credit to Paracelsus for being the first to openly ridicule the humours of the Greeks and Arabs. However, he considered that Paracelsus had been insufficiently fixed in his views and had been too prone to lapse into humoral categories (*ad humores labitur, et complexiones, nondum sat in suis thesibus funditus*). According to van Helmont, the Galenists and Arabists 'often observe the supernatant water [of the blood] and call it yellow bile or gall . . . they call the sediment at the bottom, where it is heavier and darker, the black bile. And in the intervening space they observe red blood wherein they detect whitish fibers, the matrices of coagulation. These, they say, are phlegm (*pituitan*)'.

Sennert, who was professor of medicine at Wittenberg and author of *De Chymicorum cum Aristotelicis et Galenicis Consensu at Dissensu*, stated that no one can be an accomplished physician without being skilled in chemistry. However, his departure from classical Galenism was hardly significant, as indicated by his view of 'adust' as a degenerated form of melancholy humour capable of causing scirrhous tumours but being the same as black bile (*adusta seu atra bile*). To Horst, the spagyrical principles were 'philosophical'. Salt, sulphur, and mercury for instance, were, respectively, the principles of solidity, tempering, and liquidity.

Elements such as those of acidity, acridity, effervescence, volatility, and fermentation were the hardware of the iatrochemists.

2.6.6 Astruc's Biochemical Disproof of Atrabilism and Spagyricism

To Jean Astruc (1684–1776), the French anatomist, the humoral theory of the Greeks and Arabs and the spagyric theory of Paracelsus and his followers were, literally, equally distasteful. As recorded in the second volume of his *Traité des Tumeurs et des Ulceres* of 1759, he incinerated a piece of prime beefsteak and a piece of cancerous breast. He then tasted the burnt remains and, finding no difference, he concluded that this result 'disproved' both theories.

The first report of a biochemical difference between any cancer and its normal tissue counterpart was that of Henry Bence-Jones (1814–1873), a London physician. He described an abnormal 'hydrated deutoxide of albumen' (now known to be monoclonal immunoglobulin light chain dimers) in the urine of patients with 'mollities ossium' (multiple myeloma). He found the initially water-soluble protein to precipitate on heating at around 55°C, to redissolve on further heating, and to re-precipitate on subsequent cooling.

2.6.7 The Lymphatics and a Third Version of Humoralism

A third version of humoralism centred around the role of the lymphatic system in oncogenesis. This, which constituted a major oncologic precoccupation of the so-called Renaissance period, had a long antecedent history that spanned the discoveries of the circulatory systems of the body.

The early Egyptians reported that 'there are vessels in it [the heart] leading to every part of the body'. They did not clarify whether the pulsation they felt everywhere in the body signified the flow of blood or whether the flow was one-way or two-way. From the days of Aristotle, Erasistratos, and Galen, movement of the body fluids had been traditionally regarded as a mainly one-way traffic. This involved supply of blood to the body parts by the veins, originating in the liver, and of 'pneuma' (an 'airy spirit') by the arteries, originating in the heart. The pneuma, rather than the heart, was held responsible for the pulsation of the arteries, since the heart was envisaged more as a stove than a pump, i.e. as a site for 'cooking' and distribution of body heat. To Erasistratos, the terminal branches of the arteries contained small passages or anastomoses ('synanastomoseis') which opened only under abnormal conditions. This allowed interchange between pneuma and blood, thus interfering with the proper distribution of heat and pneuma, and providing one of the ancient rationales for the efficacy of blood-letting in the treatment of fever.

Towards the close of the sixteenth century, just before William Harvey's arrival at Padua, where he was a student of Fabricus da Aquapendente, Andreas Caesalpinus of Pisa had, in 1583, introduced the term 'circulation' ('circulatio'). He had also stated that the veins and arteries transmitted blood, respectively, to and from the heart. Harvey, in his elucidation of blood circulation theory (in his *De Motu Cordis et Sanguinis in Animalibus*), had denied the existence of the anastomoses (capillaries) between arteries and veins; but these were demonstrated microscopically by Marcello Malpighi in 1661, four years after Harvey's death. Earlier, in 1622, Gasparo Anselli had discovered certain milky vessels ('vasa lactea' or 'venae lacteae') in canine and other mesenterias; and, in 1651, Jean Pecquet had described the 'cisterna chyli' and its continuation, the thoracic duct, which emptied into the great veins of the neck.

Thus was discovered the new circulatory or 'lymphatic' system, which, during the 1650s, was called the 'vasa glandularum serosa' by Olaus Rudbeck, and the 'vasa lymphatica', 'vasa aquosa', and 'vasa crystallina' by Thomas Bartholin. This discovery gave a new meaning to the classical humoralistic theory of tumour origin. Georg Ernst Stahl regarded the circulating fluid as composed of three major elements. These were true blood with its 'ruddy globules' ('globulos rubicundos') or blood corpuscles ('corpuscula sanguinea'); useful nutritious lymph ('lympha utilis, nutritia'), a 'gelatinous' fluid derived from the chyle and containing corpuscles in proportions suitable for combination with the various solid parts of the body; and serum, a watery mixture of excrementitious saline, mucilaginous, oleaginous, and similar matter. There was general agreement between Stahl, his colleagues at the University of Halle, Friedrich Hoffman, and their more famous contemporary, Hermann Boerhaave, in regarding cancer as, simply, the most unfavourable outcome of inflammation which, in turn, was due initially to stasis of the circulatory humours, particularly of the lymph. That spontaneous coagulation of lymph could produce cancer was suggested by René Descartes during the seventeenth century. This concept was made more exact by John Hunter's late-eighteenth-century description of 'coagulating lymph', later named 'fibrin', as that component of the blood which can be coagulated by heat, alcohol, and other agents and, more importantly, which can undergo spontaneous coagulation in extravascularized blood. Other related, notable eighteenth-century developments were those of Jean-Louis Petit, who drew attention to regional lymph node enlargement in cancer; Antoine Louis, who distinguished cancer types according to the manner of lymph coagulation; and Henri François Le Dran, who regarded the tendency of cancer to recur in spite of its surgical excision as good evidence of an intrinsic lymph abnormality.

2.6.8 Tissues: Bichat and Laënnec

In the field of biology, the opening thrust of the nineteenth century was in histopathology. This was due largely to the efforts of two young French pathologists, Marie-François-Xavier Bichat (1771–1802) and one of Bichat's students, René-Théophile-Hyacinthe Laënnec (1781–1826). Although their combined lifespan was but 76 years, they laid the foundations of histophysiology and histopathology prior to the assumption by these disciplines, from the fourth decade of the century on, of the fundamental cellular aspects of today. In their time, as before them, the term 'cell', as in von Haller's 'tela cellulosa' or Bichat's 'tissu cellulaire', meant, simply, any macroscopically visible enclosed space within the body's tissues.

Shunning the unreliable microscope of his time, and relying only upon naked-eye observation, the knife, and a few simple stains, Bichat, in his *Anatomie Générale Appliquée à la Physiologie et la Médecine* of 1801, categorized 21 tissue systems of the body. To each of these he ascribed its own 'vital force' (e.g. toxicity, sensibility, and capacity for growth and reproduction), that is, the 'vita propia' previously ascribed by others only to separate organs or to the body as a whole. Harmony relative to the vital forces produced health, but disharmony produced disease. His 21 systems were: (1) cellular; (2) and (3) nervous, governing 'animal' or 'organic' life; (4) arterial; (5) venous; (6) exhalant; (7) absorbent; (8) medullary; (9) cartilaginous; (10)

osseous; (11) fibrous; (12) fibro-cartilaginous; (13) and (14) muscular, governing 'animal' or 'organic' life; (15) mucous; (16) serous; (17) synovial; (18) glandular; (19) dermoid; (20) epidermoid; and (21) pilous. This categorization has several notable features. In its resemblance to the 'similar parts', and omission of the 'fluid parts' of older lists, it is more reminiscent of Galen than Aristotle. In its ascription of autonomy to tissues, it came nearer than previously to the concept of cells as the fundamental units of biology. In its divisions, it essentially recognized the four categories generally accepted by contemporary histologists: epithelium (systems 15,16,17, and 20), connective tissue (systems 1,9,10,11,12, and 19), muscle (systems 13 and 14), and nerve (systems 2 and 3). Its distinction between 'animal' and 'organic' in the nervous systems would correspond to that between the voluntary and involuntary nervous systems. However, Bichat's medullary system has no known modern counterpart, and his exhalants and absorbents (which he regarded as open-ended vessels) either are unmatched or have been replaced by the lymphatics.

Laënnec is generally remembered nowadays as a clinician and as the inventor of the stethoscope, but he was also a specialist lung pathologist. He followed Bichat in regarding 'maladies nerveuses' as distinct from 'maladies organiques', the former being those disorders that, simply, are not characterized by any visible (organic) lesion. However, in disagreement with Bichat but in agreement with today's opinion, Laënnec contended that any type of lesion might develop in any organ or tissue; and, further, that a lesion of a single (e.g. inflammatory) type might present different clinical features in the same tissue.

The efforts of Bichat and Laënnec, as extensions of Paduan pathophysiological anatomy from Beneveni to Morgagni, were soon extended further. In 1809, for instance, Karl Rudolphi followed Bichat's procedure and divided the tissues, along structural, functional, and chemical lines, into eight systems: tela cellulosa, tela ossea, tela cartilaginea, fibra v. tela tendinea, tela v. fibra cornea, fibra arteriosa, fibra muscularis and fibra nervea. In 1821, he distinguished 'similar parts' as structures present throughout the body, from 'simple parts' as simple but not ubiquitous tissues. In this same year, Montfalcon, after reviewing several tissue classifications, e.g. Richerand's and Depuytren's eleven tissue systems (cellular, vascular, nervous, osseous, fibrous, muscular, erectile, mucous, serous, epidermoid, and parenchymatous) and Cloquet's twelve tissue systems (cellular, membranous, vascular, osseous, cartilaginous, fibrocartilaginous, ligamentous muscular tendinous, aponeurotic, nervous, and glandular), proposed his own list of three 'fundamental' (i.e. cellular, vascular, and nervous) tissue systems.

2.6.9 Cells: Schleiden and Schwann

The seeds of the next major stage in the growth of pathophysiological anatomy and other branches of oncology and general biology were sown during the 1820s in the form of two important improvements: in microscopy and in histologic staining techniques. From the fourth decade of the century onwards, these improvements have led to the growth of biology, for the first time, along modern cellular rather than the old macroscopic lines. Much of this was due initially to the efforts of Mathias Jacob Schleiden (1804–1881); and then, in particular, to those of Johannes Mueller (1801–1858), his long line of illustrious students including Theodor Schwann (1810–1882), Jacob Henle (1809–1885), Adolph Hannover (1814–1894), and Rudolph Virchow (1821–1892) and, in turn, their students. Among the latter were two of Virchow's students: Julius Conheim (see below) who is famous particularly for his 'cell rest' theory of oncogenesis; and Katsusaburo Yamagiwa (1863–1930). With his associate Koichi Ichikawa (1888–1948), Yamagiwa initiated the modern era of experimental chemical oncogenesis. Among the many such landmarks in cancer history which emanated directly or indirectly from the hierarchy of illustrious oncologists established by Mueller was Hannover's introduction of chromium-based solutions for fixation of histologic specimens. This can be regarded as the forerunner of today's great arsenal of histologic stains, e.g. Garlach's ammoniated carmine, discovered in 1847; Bohmer's alum hematoxylin (1865); Flemming's chrom-osmium-acetic acid (1882); Blum's formaldehyde (1893); and Zenker's potassium dichromate-mercuric chloride or 'Zenker's fluid' (1894). The histologic classifications developed by Henle with the aid of the new staining and microscopic techniques have been described by Garrison to 'take rank with the anatomical discoveries of Vesalius'.

Schleiden is sometimes regarded as the father of cellular biology. In 1838, he described plants as aggregates of cells

(*Zellern*) which were more-or-less autonomous living units that contained a nucleus (*Kern*) and were visible only under the microscope. This concept of plant cells, however, was not new in 1838. As microscopically visible, relatively autonomous units, they had already become well-known to botanists by the end of the first quarter of the nineteenth century. Also, during the early 1830s, the English botanist Robert Brown had described the cell nucleus in orchids and *Aesclepiadae*. What was new in 1838 was Schleiden's description of the way in which 'that peculiar, small organism, the cell' reproduced itself. The already small nucleus, he said, contained one or more smaller bodies, the corpuscles or nucleoli (*kernkoerperchen*). During cell reproduction, a vesicle or blister, sitting on the surface of the nucleus like a watchglass (*Uhrglas*) on a watch, appeared and gradually expanded. After persisting for some time in the cell wall, the nucleus began to be absorbed. Finally, both the nucleus and the mother cell disappeared. Schleiden was clearly describing the type of endosporulation which occurs in some fungi.

Not unexpectedly, these findings in plants were quickly extended to animal systems, first by Schwann and then by Mueller and others. In a series of three papers published in 1838, Schwann investigated the relationship between the cellular phenomena described by Schleiden in plants and those he observed in animals. He came to the conclusion that 'all these phenomena can be demonstrated in animal structures', and that 'all animal tissues might be referable in origin to cell formation of an analogous kind'.

With this second conclusion, Schwann introduced the concept of cells as the ultimate source of cells and tissues of similar kinds. He regarded adult tissues as cellular transformations from embryonic sources. He concluded further that the origins of even those tissues, such as muscular and nervous tissues which appear noncellular in adults, were traceable to clearly recognizable cells in components of the embryonic primary tissue (*Urgewebe*). The ultimate source of this tissue was the germinal vesicle (*Keimblaeschen*). This was a single cell that contained nucleus and nucleolus and that gave rise to the germinal membrane (*Keimhaut*) and its various layers, or leaves. He established the principle of the cell as the fundamental unit of ontogenesis, embryogenesis, and histogenesis in animals. In 1839, he made his famous generalization that 'cellular formation is a principle of development common to the most different elementary parts of the organism'.

Schwann discarded Schleiden's 'Uhrglas' theory as an exclusive mechanism of cell reproduction, as did Schleiden himself eventually. However, the concept of both plants and animals as structural aggregates of autonomous living subunits (i.e. cells) contained in tissues derived ultimately from germinal vesicles became firmly entrenched as one of the major principles of modern biology.

2.6.10 Cancer Cells and Cancer 'Seeds': Mueller

The idea that pathological tissues, like their normal counterparts, may be composed of cells was also being mooted during the 1830s. In 1836, Mueller had used the term 'cell' (*Zelle*) in his descriptions of the fine structure of tumours. However, as he then conceived it, this term had deviated little in meaning from that of standard pre-nineteenth-century usage, i.e. any macroscopically visible enclosed space within a tissue. As early as 1830, Everard Home, in England, had published microscopic pictures of neoplastic tissues, which showed some rounded bodies that were clearly cells, but Home saw no such thing. What he saw were 'lymph granules', of size equal to that of 'blood globules deprived of their colouring matter'.

In 1838, largely in the light of the new developments, Mueller began a re-assessment of his own results. This was to determine whether the 'new discoveries of Schleiden concerning the development of young plant cells from the nuclei of mother cells, and those of Schwann concerning the structural correspondence between plants and animals, the composition of all embryonic tissues from cells . . . and, finally, the subsequent transformation of cells into tissues' were applicable to tumours. This passage occurs in his paper of 1838 entitled *Ueber den Feinern Bau und die Formen der Krankhaften Geschwuelste*, in which he concluded that Schwann's cellular concepts are largely applicable to tumours also. Mueller thus placed the cancer cell at the centre of oncologic interest. However, he could not quite dismiss the concept of at least some cancer cells or cancer tissues representing *neo*-formations, rather than *trans*-formations from their pre-existing normal counterparts. For example, he also concluded that: 'The germinal cells of carcinomas arise not from already present fibres but independently from a true *seminium morbi* which develops between the tissue components of an organ'. He did not make himself clear on the point, but it seems difficult to conclude other than that he retained, at least partly, the old belief in cellular formation from an acellular substance, or blastema.

2.6.11 The Blastema Hypothesis: A Fourth Version of Humoralism

Belief in the old blastema hypothesis of tumour genesis was widely held during most of Mueller's lifetime. Formally, the hypothesis states that all the formed body elements (e.g. cells and tissues, whether normal or pathologic) arise from a primitive body fluid (blastema or cytoblastema), by a kind of intracorporeal spontaneous generation or crystallization around a nucleus (*Kern*) or nucleolus (*Kernkoerperchen*). It began to decline significantly from 1855, just three years before Mueller's death, when Virchow, Mueller's star pupil, coined his immortal aphorism: *omnis cellula a cellula* (every cell arises from a pre-existing cell). Throughout the 1840s, however, even Virchow had remained a blastema adherent. In 1847, for instance, he had written: 'All organic formation takes place from an amorphous substance; nutrition and new formation, embryonal and pathologic, are in essence the differentiation of a formless, solid, or fluid substance'. This substance was microscopically visible as a 'gelatinous mass' tinged yellow, brown, or red; it contained few if any formed elements; it was particularly evident in 'colloid' cancers; and it was also abundant, in a more solid form, between the cells and fibres of bone cancers; but its chemical nature was unknown.

Among Mueller's contemporaries, other notable believers in the theory included Karl von Rokitansky, Julius Vogel, and Schwann himself. Rokitansky, an acknowledged leader in the gross pathological anatomy of his time, in the first volume of his *Handbuch der Pathologischen Anatomie* of 1846, wrote that, in the case of pathological new formations, 'a native anomaly in the blastema' was 'practically demonstrable'; and that the blastemas responsible for such formations contained 'protein compounds . . . in various states of oxydation'. Like Julius Vogel, who had supported the blastema theory (cf. his treatment of the subject in Volume 1 of Rudolph Wagner's *Handwoerterbuch der Physiologie mit Ruecksicht auf Physiologische*

Pathologie of 1842), Rokitansky supported the old concept of heterology of heteroplasia, claiming that the cells, fibres, and tissues in many malignant new growths are morphologically and chemically different from normal ('homologous') structures.

Schwann also shared the belief in blastema. His above-mentioned view of the cell as the ultimate source of major biological processes might suggest otherwise, even that he had anticipated Virchow's aphorism by almost two decades. This is highly unlikely, however. For instance, according to Schwann, during some later stage of embryonic development, cells arise *de novo* from 'the gelatinous, structureless mass' constituting the bulk of embryonic connective tissue.

Belief in the formed from the formless was both time-honoured and persistent. For instance, the doctrine of spontaneous generation, whose most famous adherent was Aristotle, persisted for about 2,000 years before it was disproved, over a period of two centuries — by Francesco Redi (1626–1697), Lazarro Spallanzani (1729–1799) and, finally, Louis Pasteur (1822–1895). The ancient and bizarre doctrine of pangenesis, which was based upon inheritance transmission through invisible replicas (or 'gemmules') of various body substructures in blood, had commanded, even during the late nineteenth century, the adherence of no less a master than Charles Darwin. Analogously, the concept of formation of tumours from acellular body elements had persisted from the time of the Hippocratic writers, Aristotle, and Galen to the middle of the nineteenth century. By the seventeenth century, the black bile of the ancient Greeks (Section 2.4.2) had become the various (e.g. fermentative, putrefactive, and acidic) 'juices' of the iatrochemists such as Paracelsus, van Helmont, Sylvius, and Willis; or the fluxed humours or 'cancer seeds' of Stahl and Hoffmann, a concept which was developed later by Mueller. By the eighteenth century, it had become the 'plastic' lymph, e.g. the 'coagulable' lymph of Descartes, Hunter, Harvey, and Hewson, and the 'solidistic' lymph of Gendron. The plastic lymph, during the eighteenth century and up to the first half of the nineteenth, had become the general amorphous 'blastema' or its cellular-exudative analogue, the 'cytoblastema', composed mainly of albumin and fibrin. In one form or another, the blastema theory had been championed by stalwarts such as Chomel, Lobstein, Liebig, Vogel, Schwann, Mueller, Rokitansky, Hodgkin, and even the younger Virchow. Among others, Andral had regarded the source of cancer as disturbed nutritional and secretive processes, and Hodgkin as generative membranes.

Indeed, it would seem that the concept of the formed from the formless, inclusive of the animate from the inanimate and the cellular from the acellular, is as old, and as durable, as is the mind of man.'In the beginning, God created heaven and earth. And the earth was without form, and void' is the start of Genesis, for instance, as perhaps every Sunday School child knows; and analogous views are commonplace among the Holy Writs of man's religions. Lest it be concluded that such views are just mystical and are not held by the modern scientific die-hard, the most popular of biogenetic concepts held by modern evolutionary biologists might be considered. This envisages the derivation of the first cellular organisms, representing the ultimate live ancestors of man and all living creatures, from inanimate, 'formless' chemical components of the primeval soup of some three thousand million years ago. The principle involved has become more 'scientific' and more restricted, but it has not changed.

2.6.12 Cellular Pathology: Virchow

Virchow's celebrated aphorism ('every cell from a cell') is, of course, a developmental, not an evolutionary concept. It says as little about the evolutionary origin of cells as does its modification, 'omnis cellula a [or e] cellula ejusdem naturae [or generis]', due to Louis Bard exactly three decades later, about the developmental origin of all the body's phenotypes from a single cell (the zygote) or of more than one phenotype from a partly differentiated progeny of this cell.

Though formally announced in 1855, Virchow's aphorism was the result of a gradual realization rather than a sudden inspiration. It was a consequence of his studies initially with the 'tubercle' (*Tuberkel*), the nodular proliferative lesion which is characteristic of tuberculosis. As early as 1850, these studies had led to his misgivings about the blastema theory which he had supported during the 1840s. In this year, for instance, he had reported to the Wuerzberg Physical-Medical Society that 'tubercle arises . . . from a *metamorphosis of organized elements* and in no way from an exudate'. However, even by 1854, he did not quite believe in an *exclusive* cellular histogenesis. In this year, for instance, after reconsideration of the four possible ways of cytogenesis (division, budding, free formation and formation within 'brood spaces'), he had concluded that: 'A great, indeed perhaps the predominating, part of new-formations is therefore to be derived from the progressive development of pre-existing tissue components'. The exclusivity of his aphorism of a year later then became the basis of his new 'cellularpathologie' (a term, apparently, of his own coinage) enshrined, for all time, in his now classic *Die Cellularpathologie in ihrer Begruendung auf Physiologische und Pathologische Gewebelehre* of 1858. This work ran into several editions inclusive of the fourth German edition of 1871 which has been translated and retranslated, e.g. into English by Frank Chance in 1971. This book has continued to occupy the same top shelf in the library of oncology as has the venerable *Archiv für Pathologische Anatomie und für Klinische Medizin* which he and Benno Reinhardt had launched in 1847. The latter, as a tribute to Virchow's greatness but, sadly, with a submergence of Reinhardt's contribution, has become known simply as *Virchow's Archiv*.

Under the banner of *omnis cellula a cellula*, Virchow dealt with all the then known aspects of tumour pathology. Among his new-formations (*Neubildungen*) are heteroplasias (atypical growths) which, to him, include tubercles, 'true cancer', and miscellaneous tumours such as cancroids, dermoids, and sarcomas. Among the now common terms he introduced on the basis of his investigations are 'leukemia', 'osteoid tissue', 'thrombosis', 'embolus', 'parenchymatous inflammation', and 'amyloidosis' (previously termed 'lardaceous degeneration').

Virchow distinguished 'homologous' neoplasms, such as the common uterine fibroid with its muscles resembling those of the normal uterus, from the 'heterologous' counterparts. Among the latter he included malignant neoplasms as well as the tubercle and some inflammations. The former were due to 'hypertrophy', i.e. increase in size and number of cells already present; and the latter to metaplasia, i.e. change in the intrinsic character of such cells. The nature of the change, however, was not foreign to the body's histophysiology. Thus, in Lecture 3 of his *Cellular-pathologie*, he stressed that:

there is no other kind of heterology in morbid structures than in the abnormal manner in which they arise . . . this abnormality consists either in the production of a structure at a point where it has no business, or at a time when it ought not to be produced, or to an extent which is at variance with the typical formation of the body. So then, to speak with greater precision, there is either a *Heterotopia*, an aberratio loci, or an aberratio temporis, a *Heterochromia*, or lastly, a mere variation in quantity.

In similar vein, in the same Lecture, he also wrote: 'Throughout the whole range of pathological growths, no structure of an absolutely new form is to be found, but . . . we everywhere meet with structures which may in one way or another be regarded as reproduction of physiological tissues'.

The great importance of Virchow's aphorism is that it placed the cell at the dead centre of *all* biological processes, normal or pathologic; and that it thenceforth directed oncologic research and debate along cellular lines. According to Virchow, it permitted reconciliation of the ancient and opposing doctrines of 'humoral and solidary pathology' (*Humoral- und Solidar- pathologie*) while, at the same time, threatening the then pre- valent dogma of free formation of cells, just as the parallel dictum, 'omne vivum ex ovo', was threatening the persistent dogma of spontaneous generation (*generatio aequivoca*). How- ever, as this dictum suggests, the basic notion behind Virchow's dogma had been 'floating about' some years before its for- malization in 1855, e.g. in Remak's stated view of 1852 that the origin of all cells during embryogenesis is pre-existing cells. Also, Virchow's *Cellularpathologie* was not the first of the treatises on pathology to be written under the guidance of *omnis cellula a cellula*. This distinction belongs to the *Handbuch* of August Foerster, published in two volumes in 1855, who openly admitted his indebtedness to Virchow.

Virchow's *Cellularpathologie* has remained, to this day, one of the greatest expositions of the subject of cancer as a disease of cells. However, from his experiences with 'tibial cancroid', a rare tumour, and the 'early tumour' (*tumeur perlée*) of Cruveilhier, among others, he arrived at two highly controversial conclusions. First, he proposed a connective tissue-origin for even epithelial tumours. 'The vast majority of new-formations,' he wrote in 1858 'arise from the connective tissue (*Bindegewebe*) and its equivalent . . . One can therefore with a few *restrictions actually substitute the connective tissue and its equivalents for the earlier*

*blastema and the later exudate, and for the original plastic-lymph of
the older writers, as the common germinal stock (Keimstock) of the
body.*' Second, although he introduced both the term and the
concept of 'embolism', he believed that metastases are due to
some 'harmful fluid', 'juice' (*succus*), or 'humour' which was produced by the primary tumour cells or was provocative of the
primary growth in the first place, rather than to migrating tumour
cells or emboli. He viewed the propagation as a consequence of
the spread of the harmful agent via the blood, lymph, and other
body fluids, 'precisely as with the propagation of many inflammatory processes'; and the action of the fluid as being upon
the undifferentiated cells of the ubiquitous connective tissue, at
the site of metastasis. He based this belief largely upon his observations of the somewhat random spread of metastases, which
often occurs with skipping of organs lying in the direct line of
spread and with localization at far removed sites.

In summary, the continuing impact of Virchow upon biology is
in his view of the body as an ordered society of cells subject, in the
course of development, to natural laws which, when disturbed,
may give rise to disease.

As a man, he was no less impressive than he was as a scientist.
Son of a Pomeranian farmer, he graduated from the Friedrich
Wilhelm Institute in Berlin in 1843, with a thesis on a phase of
inflammation, one of the many topics which occupied his subsequent long career. Among his many accomplishments, he was an
ardent humanitarian. His efforts against the mid-nineteenth
century anti-Semitism of his country, for instance, earned him,
during 1849, an official threat of instant dismissal from his pros-
ectorship at the Charite Hospital in Berlin. He later became director of Berlin's newly-founded Institute of Pathology. Among his
worldwide distinctions were the French Legion of Honour
awarded in 1896, and the English Croonian (in 1893) and Huxley
(in 1898) lectureships. His passing, in 1902, was mourned in all
Germany as the loss of her greatest pathologist, anthropologist,
sanitarian, and liberal. It was also mourned in many other
countries, from Japan, through other parts of Asia, to Europe and
North America, each for its own reasons.

2.6.13 Histogenetic Specificity in Normal and Neoplastic Development: Waldeyer, Bard, and Others

For any theory to be truly great, it must do at least three things:

systematize extant, even jumbled knowledge; make testable predictions; and encourage debate and further research. Virchow's *omnis cellula a cellula* did all of these things. That Virchow himself, in application of his aphorism, came to the two controversial conclusions mentioned above, both of which were subsequently discredited, adds strength rather than weakness to both the man and the theory. The former is because the proven error encourages lesser mortals, since even a Virchow can be wrong; and the latter because the proving itself spurred on debate and research, and thus the march of oncology.

The proving process was due to the efforts of several of Virchow's contemporaries including Robert Remak, Carl Thiersch, Theodor Billroth, who had previously accepted Virchow's connective tissue hypothesis, and, in particular, Wilhelm Waldeyer and Louis Bard.

In 1867, in a remarkably reasoned paper in *Virchow's Archiv*, Waldeyer reviewed available evidence including his own, and advanced strong arguments in favour of a purely epithelial origin for epithelial cancer, whether external or internal, primary or metastatic. He reached the following implicit conclusions, which have since become standard textbook dogma down to this day: (1) normal epithelium, embryologically derived from the two epithelial germ layers, is the *sole* source of epithelial cells contained in a given carcinoma; (2) neoplastic transformation of normal epithelium does not involve cell dissolution, e.g. into a blastema or any other presumptive cancer cell-generating noncellular substance; (3) all the epithelial cancer cells present in a given carcinoma are the progenies of, with or without contribution from, the original epithelial cancer cells formed by transformation of the normal epithelium and then undergoing division to an extent capable of inhibiting further neoplastic transformation of the normal epithelium; (4) the sole mechanism of local spread is movement, active or passive, of the cancer cells into adjacent tissues; (5) the sole mechanism of metastatic spread is through transport of cancer cells to the metastatic sites via blood, lymph, or other body fluids; (6) connective tissues or their cells are never transformed into the epithelial cancer analogues; (7) two forms of connective tissue proliferation are incited or accompanied by cancer cell multiplication: a small-cell accompanying (*begleitende*) proliferation, and a more fibrocellular introductory (*enleitende*) proliferation, the latter constituting the newly-formed stroma of the tumour; and (8) fibrous, fatty, cartilaginous, and/or other forms of the stroma can be present in breast and other carcinomas.

These conclusions would apply, *mutatis mutandis*, to sarcomas as well as to carcinomas. Waldeyer steered clear of speculations regarding cause(s) of the neoplastic transformation or of the antisocial behaviour of the transformed cells. However, in a second paper, published in 1872, he rejected the so-called infectious theory of carcinogenesis based upon any infectious agent, such as 'the virus as the basis of carcinoma' described by Wilhelm Mueller to be capable of transforming neighbouring connective tissue cells, endothelial cells, or 'wandering cells' into epithelial cancer cells. What kind of agent is this infective virus, Waldeyer asked, and where does it come from? Why does its presumed contagiousness allow handling of a carcinoma with impunity, and how is it able to change the form of the cell it infects? Does not this theory 'smuggle the hardly banned specific cells [of cancer] back into tumour doctrine'? These objections by Waldeyer became all but universally overruled later in the nineteenth century, the heyday of microbiology, and indeed during this century until the 1960s; since when, however, an infective etiology for many types of animal neoplasms and for any type of human neoplasm has been becoming increasingly unlikely. His objections, at least insofar as human neoplasia is concerned, are more germane today than ever they were.

During 1885–88, Bard, a pathological anatomist at Lyons, rejected Virchow's 'notion of an undifferentiated tissue, capable of almost unlimited metaplasia' in favour of the 'notion of *the absolute specificity of differentiated anatomical elements*'. The 'tissue' in question is Virchow's connective tissue; and 'metaplasia' is a term Virchow had coined to signify transformation of one kind of tissue into another. Bard stressed the 'specificity of cellular elements', by which he meant that 'the various cell types constitute so many families, genera and species, which, like the families, genera and species of animals, may well be traced through an ancestral series to a common stock, but which have pursued their collateral courses of evolution and have become incapable of transformation into each other'. Essentially, Bard was stressing no more than the tumour histogenesis of Waldeyer, Thiersch, and others. However, he also advanced the concept of an origin for composite tumours in mixed cell types, a 'bouquet cellulaire', undergoing the initial neoplastic transformation. He ruled out of hand any recourse to 'differentiations', 'adaptations', 'metaplasias', 'dedifferentiations' (*retours des élements nobles a l'état indifferent*), and 'redifferentiations' in attempts to define mechanisms of tumour histogenesis; and any notion that 'everything is in everything, and everything can come from something else'. Virchow's aphorism, he maintained, must yield to *omnis cellula a cellula ejusdem naturae* (every cell from a cell of the same kind). As indicated earlier, this latter aphorism may be too restricted in certain instances, e.g. those associated with early embryogenesis and with the increasing demonstrations of tumours expressing alternative (including ectopic) modes of differentiation, reflective of the embryonic nature of many cancer cells.

2.6.14 Embryology and 'Cell Rests': Remak and Conheim

During the 1830s and 1840s, workers such as von Baer and Rusconi had described cleavage of the egg yolk rather than of the nucleus or whole egg cell during embryogenesis in frogs and other lower animals; and as indicated above, even Schwann, while stressing that cells alone were the ultimate elements of all animal tissues, believed in the intermediation of a cell-forming blastema at some stage in the process. However, by the 1850s, embryologists such as Reichart and Koelliker began to reject the concept of free formation of cells during embryogenesis. During the 1850s, Remak went even further. He announced that all cells, whether embryonal or adult, or normal or abnormal, arise from pre-existing cells only. No tumour, not even a cancer, is, properly speaking, a 'new-formation' (*Neubildung*) of pathological tissue from an amorphous blastema, but always a result of a 'transformation of normal tissue' (*Umbildung normaler Gewebe*) through nuclear and cell division. In 1854, while discussing Virchow's statement that epidermal cells of cancroids could originate in bone marrow, Remak stated that: 'Since the penetration of epithelioma into bone has so often been observed, the derivation of aggregates of epidermal cells found within bones from similar detachments (*Abschnuerungen*) seems likely; these have perhaps taken place at an early developmental stage of the human embryo'. With this statement, Remak at once introduced the concept of the developmental potency of cells and tissues into tumour histogenesis, and foreshadowed Conheim's 'cell rest' theory. This theory, which Conheim first advanced in 1875, states that extra (i.e. unused) 'quanta of cells' produced during normal embryogenesis, because of the persisting embryonic nature and high proliferative capacity of these cells, eventually develop into tumours. Some experimental support for the theory was obtained, notably by Zahn in 1877 and Leopold in 1881, who found that bits of tissues (including those from a human euchondroma) transplanted into the anterior chamber of the rabbit's eye or other sites grew better when the tissue source was embryonal or neoplastic than normal adult. Zahn reached the precocious conclusion that 'embryonal tissues are more closely related to neoplasms than to normal adult tissues'.

The cell rest theory, based as it was upon embryonal cells retaining both their multidevelopmental and their high growth capacities, has survived mainly as a histogenetic hypothesis for teratomas from aberrant germ cells.

2.6.15 The Problem of Etiology and Histogenesis in Neoplasia

The question of ultimate origins in Nature is one of the great bugbears in the mind of man. This applies also to tumour etiology, which, according to Conheim, is a dark chapter, if there ever was one, in the science of pathology. He recognized that tumour etiology involves multiple factors, e.g. age, sex, social position, infection, previous harmful ailments, emotional and nervous disturbance, local irritation, and trauma, none of which correlates with neoplasia. He stressed that: 'Never has a surgeon been "infected" while operating on a tumour; never has a man acquired a cancroid of the penis from the uterine cancer of his wife'; and that 'through trauma of various kinds certain products of hypertrophy and inflammation, but no *true tumours*, arise'. Such products would include today's well-known 'acute phase' proteins. These considerations led Conheim to seek tumour etiology within the natural developmental capabilities of germ cells. However, the dark chapter he described would even include what should be a much simpler question, that of the histogenetic classification of tumours. This, however, in the words of MacCallum, in the sixth (i.e. 1936) edition of his authoritative *Textbook of Pathology* is 'rather a tissue of assumptions than one formed on a true histogenetic basis'. This well-put 'tissue of assumptions' situation has not changed, as evidenced by two of Fould's statements in his no less authoritative *Neoplastic Development* of 1969. Foulds wrote: 'The undertones of retrospection inherent in histogenetic classifications of tumours are distasteful to myself; if strictly applied the classification can be misleading or worse . . . when used moderately, as by Willis for example, they are less objectionable although, in my view, not particularly helpful'. He also wrote: 'Identification of the parent cells of a tumour, as attempted in histogenetic classifications, is not the only problem in early neoplastic development. The point of origin is often inferred, more or less plausibly, but it is scarcely ever seen, and the validity of inferences about histogenesis is rarely subjected to crucial tests.'

Irrespective of the body's tissue in which a neoplasm is found, the time lag between the latter's origin and its clinical detection spans not only many years, usually between two and four decades, but also many events, and many stages. Currently therefore, considerable uncertainty surrounds practically every feature of the origin, whether in relation to the nature or existence of the inciting event; the timing of this event, if it exists; or the identity or embryologic derivation of the originating cell, cell type, or tissue.

2.6.16 Foreshadowing of Molecular Genetics With its DNA Constancy Rule

It has become practically impossible to treat adequately any aspect of the biology of normal or neoplastic processes without drawing heavily upon the molecular aspects of nuclear phenomena. There can be no doubt that molecular genetics has become a modern discipline in its own right only since the 1950s with the elucidation of the double-helical structure and the coding properties of DNA. Equally, there can be no doubt that the germinal notions of the discipline were developed during the nineteenth century. This is suggested by some of the above-discussed features of this remarkable period, e.g. its cells (*Zellen*), its nucleus (*Kern*) and nucleolus (*Kern koerperchen*), and its germinal vesicle (*Keimblaeschen*). Related features would include the principle of heredity adduced by Gregor Mendel from his studies of pea seedlings, and those of natural selection adduced by Charles Darwin from his studies of species in their natural environments.

Neither Mendel nor Darwin could have known about genes in

the modern sense. However, the closing decades of the nineteenth century were graced by geneticists such as Friedrich Miescher, Carl Wilhelm Naegeli, Moritz Nussbaum, August Weissmann, Wilhelm Waldeyer, and Rudolf Koelliker. During the 1870s, Miescher and others independently isolated various nucleoproteins, collectively termed 'nuclein' by Miescher, from digests of nuclear material prepared from sources such as brain tissue, leukocytes, and fish sperm. Nuclein became Waldeyer's 'chromatin' corresponding to the 'idioplasm' postulated by Naegeli during the 1880s to be capable of underpinning a common molecular basis for biological phenomena as diverse as cell function, embryonic development, and heredity transmission.

This period knew little about the chemical structure of the heredity material. However, it witnessed a most fascinating controversy about the relative conservation of the material in germ cells and somatic cells. It was a controversy that remained central to all molecular theories of normal and neoplastic development. In 1880, Nussbaum reported the extra-embryonic origin of primordial germ cells or sex cells and their later amoeboid migration into the middle germ-layer rudiment wherein, up to then, they had been believed to originate. Between 1883 and 1892, Weismann extended Nussbaum's finding and advanced his famous postulates. These were: (1) that germ cells and somatic cells had separate identities; (2) that germ cells, which were the archives, guardians, and transmitters of the heredity of individuals and species, were inviolate; (3) that the heredity-specifying particles (*bestimmenden Thielchen*) were preserved intact in the germ plasm; and (4) that these particles were differentially doled out to specific somatic cell types during embryonic development.

It was this fourth postulate in particular that was the main bone of contention. It had to be. It addressed the crucial questions regarding the molecular basis of two sets of differences: those differences which are so obvious between the normal cell types of the body; and, because of Mueller's principle of cancer as cellular structures (Section 2.6.10) and Virchow's principle of *omnis cellula a cellula* (Section 2.6.12), those which are so indefinable but which must exist between a normal cell and its neoplastic derivative.

One of the chief dissidents was Koelliker. In 1886, Koelliker backed up with much reviewed evidence his claims that there was no sharp difference between germ cells and somatic cells; and, more importantly, that the idioplasms of the fertilized egg and of all of its embryonic descendants, whether germinal or somatic, were structurally identical. Koelliker was only reiterating what the Grand Master of the time, Naegeli, had said two years earlier. In 1884, Naegeli had conceived of the idioplasm of the zygote not only as being reproduced intact in all of this cell's descendants, but also as a self-reproducing 'proteinaceous' substance arranged in linear strands consisting of differently arrayed 'crystalline molecular groups or micelles'. During mitosis, he had maintained, these strands assumed microscopic visibility as threadlike bodies, i.e. the metaphase bodies which, in 1888, were christened 'chromosomes' by Waldeyer. Naegeli had also proposed that 'the form, size, and arrangement of the idioplasmic micelles yield innumerable combinations of effective powers and, thereby, also innumerable chemical and formative processes in living substance, which bring about just so many differences in growth, inner organization, external form, and function'.

Within the context of his time, Naegeli was enunciating that modern rule, the first principle from which all modern molecular theories of normal development must start. The rule states that this development is the specifically staged and phased differentiational expression of a zygotic genome that is replicated and transmitted structurally intact to all of the nucleated cells of the organism. Among the ultimate proofs of the validity of the rule which have already been obtained are the well-known capacities of suitable roots, shoots, buds, leaves, and even single cells to grow into normal plants true to type, and the increasing demonstrations of cloning in animal systems. Analogous proofs in relation to neoplasia also exist; and these, as appropriate, are discussed in later chapters of this work.

Its modern name is 'the DNA constancy rule'. With rare exceptions, it appears to be of universal applicability in the known biosphere.

2.7 Summary and Outlook: The Non-originality, Interdependence, and Continuity of Concepts

It is almost an arrogance of histories that a discovery is meritorious only when it is made by a member of a particular ethnic or other group. The commonly encountered 'Columbus discovered America' is every whit as outrageous as the unthinkable 'Marco Polo discovered China'. Not so long ago, the roots of modern culture were traced no further back than to the Romans or, sometimes even nowadays, to the Greeks.

As the discussion in this chapter shows, the roots of modern culture reach back to prehistoric times, many millennia before the Greeks or Romans. It is inconceivable that the civilizations of Egypt, China, India, Babylonia, Greece, Rome, Islam, and Western Europe or elsewhere in the modern world could have developed as they did independently of their legacy from their antecedent cultures. All literate civilizations including the present ones owe to preliterate civilizations the foundations of such features as material culture, language, and religious and moral codes. The cultural contributions of pre-Grecian civilizations included the very foundations of any literate civilization, namely those of writing, whether pictographic or alphabetic, and of printing and natural science (cf. Section 2.3.1).

It is patently true that many of the notions of ancient times have later been proved erroneous. However, so also have many of the more recent ones, even in science, and it is almost certain that many currently cherished dogmas await the same fate.

In the historical saga, even some of the most fanciful notions have engendered new knowledge, through the controversy and experimentation they stimulated. The roots of chemistry are traceable to ancient Egypt; and the ancient alchemists, in their feverish search for the mysterious philosopher's stone, slowly converted chemistry into an exact science. As another example, the many attempts at disproof of the ancient Orient-derived Greek humoral theory of oncogenesis, particularly from the fifteenth century, led to the discovery of iatrochemistry (the chemical treatment of disease), of the lymphatics, and eventually, of tissues and cells. Hence, some of civilization's growth has been like the unintended tillage of virgin ground through digging for a nonexistent but fervently believed-in buried treasure. The real worth of an idea is less in its truth or falsity than in its capacity to stimulate useful controversy and experimentation.

All of civilization's growth has been dependent upon one overriding principle: that of continuity and interdependence from the remotest reaches of human history. Thus, it is conceivable that the real origin of the pictographic writings from which modern alphabets were derived antedated even 4000 BC, the generally accepted start of the historical period. For instance, the origin might have been the cave drawings of prehistoric times. As a more recent example, the discovery of the solar system as heliocentric, which is traditionally accredited to Copernicus in the sixteenth century, was anticipated by Aristarchus of Samos in classical Greece (Section 2.4.1). Similarly, the Dutch 'inventions' of the compound microscope, by Zacharias Jansen in 1590, and of the telescope, by Hans Lippershey in 1608, had their antecedents in the advanced optics of Islam (cf. Section 2.5.2). Again, that famous law of inverse squares or universal gravitation of Isaac Newton (1642–1727) had antecedents in Islamic astronomy (Section 2.5.2). Moreover, it represented a synthesis of the law of falling bodies of Galileo (1564–1642) and the third law of Johann Kepler (1571–1630). Even the evolutionary theory of Charles Darwin (1809–1882) was foreshadowed many times — from Aristotle in Grecian times, who believed in an ascending scale of complexity for organic life; through Francis Bacon and Leibnitz in the Middle Ages; to Erasmus Darwin (1731–1802), Wolfgang von Goethe (1749–1832) and Jean Lamarck (1744–1829) in later times. These pre-Darwinian contributions to the theory have been reviewed by Robert Chambers in his *Vestiges of the Natural History of Creation* of 1844. Among the many other examples supporting the principle (cf. Thorwald, 1962) are those centred upon immunization (developed in China); obstetrics and medical schools (in Egypt and India); anatomy, plastic surgery, lithotomy, hospitals, and the 'Hippocratic' oath (in India); and 'Arabic' numerals and 'alternative' medicine (Section 2.3.1).

The principle is well illustrated by the growth of oncologic concepts up to the end of the nineteenth century. By the year 1900, practically the whole framework of today's oncology had been laid down. There was general agreement about the tissular and cellular nature and origins of neoplasms, about their major types and classification, about their association with the environment, and about their metastatic and other features. Thus true neoplasms were distinguished from inflammatory lesions of both specific and nonspecific types, and from retention cysts, parasitic cysts, and tubercles, and the many other swellings with which they had been grouped together for well over two thousand years. The cellular nature of tumours was recognized, as were their origin from normal cells and tissues of corresponding types, their retention of many features of their originating structures and their composition of essentially tumour cells multiplying mainly by mitotic division. The tumours were known to be supported in most instances by a stroma of blood vessels and connective tissue, and nourished in all instances by the blood of the host organism to whose economy and well-being they contributed nothing at best, and to whom, at worst, they were lethal. 'Malignant' neoplasms were named and recognized, through their capacity for both invasive and metastatic growth, the former by tumour cells thrusting themselves aggressively and selfishly into crab-like projective growths into peritumoral tissues including basement membranes, and the latter by colonization of distant body sites after transport largely as emboli in blood and lymph streams. These were distinguished from 'benign' neoplasms, the localized, circumscribed growths derived from epithelial or connective tissue but failing to invade or metastasize. Whether malignant or benign, the neoplasms were classified according to their derivation from the three embryonic germ layers (ectoderm, mesoderm, and endoderm), or from the epithelial and non-epithelial cells. The latter cells were designated 'endothelial' when they were the flattened cells that line the blood and lymph vessels, and 'mesothelial' when they were the similar cells that line the body cavities. The malignant epithelial neoplasms were termed 'carcinomas', and the non-epithelial analogues 'sarcomas' or 'carcinosarcomas'. The benign neoplasms were given names such as 'lipomas', 'chondromas', and 'myomas', in accordance with their histologic derivation, e.g. from fat, cartilage, and muscle, respectively. There were debates about the holistic and mechanistic approaches to cancer management; and about the role of various factors and principles in tumorigenesis, e.g. embryonic rests, the lymphoid system, acrid and acid substances, dedifferentiation, redifferentiation, adaptation, stress, and, as discussed in the next chapter, environmental agents or habitual practices. Cancer genetics was already born, as discussed above or, as discussed in later chapters, familial cancers were recognized and the foundations of the somatic mutation hypothesis as later enunciated by Boveri were laid. In the treatment of cancer, surgical concepts were well advanced as were those based upon the use of chemicals in the form of soothing and escharotic ointments and salves; and hormonal concepts were introduced when Beatson used ovariectomy for the treatment of breast cancer.

Perhaps the achievements of nineteenth century oncologic concepts are best epitomized in two quotations, respectively from Rudolph Virchow and from Thomas Denman and others of the medical committee of the British Institution for Investigating the Nature and Cure of Cancer. Under the banner of his celebrated aphorism (*omnis cellula a cellula*),Virchow, in his *Cellular Pathology* of 1858, recorded that 'there is no other kind of heterology in morbid structures than the abnormal manner in which they arise . . . there is either a *Heterotopia*, an aberratio loci, or an aberratio temporis, a *Heterochromia*, or lastly, a mere variation in quantity'. Even more so in recent than in Virchow's time, the major features of neoplastic cells or tissues have been found to be those of the normal counterparts, but representing aberrations (whether structural or functional) in space, time, or quantity, rather than in quality. These features are thus less anomalous than are the terms '*neo*plasia' and '*neo*plastic' themselves. No tumour is ever a 'new' growth, in the sense of its being independent of its normal cellular or tissular progenitor for its origin, existence, and characteristics.

The committee headed by Denman and others posed, in 1802, the following 13 questions which, with some obvious exceptions (mainly questions nos. 10, 11, and 12), still pinpoint the areas of cancer's continuing mystery:

1. What are the diagnostic signs of cancer? 2. Does any alteration take place in the structure of a part, preceding that more obvious change which is called cancer? If there does, what is the nature of that alteration? 3. Is cancer always an original and primary disease, or may other diseases degenerate into cancer? 4. Are there any proofs of cancer being an hereditary disease? 5. Are there proofs of cancer being a contagious disease? 6. Is there any well-marked relation between cancer and other diseases? If there be, what are those diseases to which it bears the nearest resemblance, in its origin, progress, and termination? 7. May cancer be regarded at any period, or under any circumstances, merely as a local disease? Or, does the existence of cancer in one part, afford a presumption, that there is a tendency to a similar morbid alteration, in other parts of the animal system? 8. Has climate, or local situation, any influence in rendering the human constitution more or less liable to cancer, under any form, or in any part? 9. Is there a tempera-

ment of body more liable to be affected with cancer than others, and if there be, what is that temperament? 10. Are brute-creatures subject to any disease, resembling cancer in the human subject? 11. Is there any period of life absolutely exempt from the attack of this disease? 12. Are the lymphatic glands ever affected primarily in cancer? 13. Is cancer under any circumstances susceptible of a natural cure?

The principle of non-originality, interdependence, and continuity is also applicable to practices in oncology. This is considered in the next chapter.

3 HISTORICAL PERSPECTIVES: PRACTICES

3.1 Introduction

This century has already seen an unprecedented growth in practical attempts to understand and manage cancer. From its humble beginnings oncology has become not just a biological discipline in its own right but also a major international growth industry. The anecdotal reports from Paracelsus in 1531 to Rehn in 1895, and the cancer statistics of Tanchou in France and Rigoni-Stern in Italy during the 1840s, have grown into the sophisticated cancer epidemiology of today. This has been revealing an ever-growing compendium of physical, chemical, biological, and psychosomatic environmental associations in cancer genesis and development. For the proper testing of such associations, diverse experimental systems of animal, plant and human origins have been developed. At the human level, there have been notable advances in the classification, detection, treatment, and biology of cancer, and in public counselling and patient after-care. At the biospheric level, cancer has become recognized as a common affliction of all species of the *Metazoa* and *Metaphyta*, most probably from the early stages of their evolution. Overall, the ancient mysticisms and philosophizings about cancer have been slowly, over the centuries, becoming transformed into the practical approaches of today.

3.2 Antiquity and Ubiquity of Neoplasia

3.2.1 Neoplasms in Fossils and Animals

As discussed above (Chapter Two, Section 2.3.2) human neoplasia appears to be as old as mankind. There is also suggestive evidence that the disease is as old and as ubiquitous as are the multicellular species of organisms. Thus direct and indirect evidence for neoplasms of bone and soft tissues respectively have been unearthed in the petrified remains of reptiles and other animals of remote geological times (Moodie, 1923; Brothwell, 1967;

Jenssens, 1970). Examples are vertebral osteomas and hemangiomas found in Cretaceous dinosaurs that became extinct over 60 million years ago, and a femoral osteogenic sarcoma in a Pleistocene cave bear. Among poikilothermic animals, a skeletal tumour was found in the remains of a corallite from a coral colony (*Madrepora kauaiensis*), an epithelioma of the mantle in a Sydney rock oyster (*Crassostrea commercialis*), and a melanoma with multiple subcutaneous, renal, and bronchial metastases in a sea lamprey (*Petromyzon marinus*). Neoplasms of many types have been found in insects, and in reptiles, amphibians, and fish.

Widespread recongition of the natural occurrence of neoplasms in animals began in the sixteenth century. Skin cancer in the carp was described by Gessner in 1553; and, by the mid-eighteenth century, neoplasms of several types had become well known in domestic and wild animals. By the first half of the nineteenth century, animal neoplasms had become sufficiently available to have formed a major part of the course material used by Johannes Mueller in his now classic microscopic studies of the cellular nature of neoplasms (Chapter Two, Section 2.6.10). In 1854, Crisp is reputed to have observed a mammary tumour in a mouse caught in a trap. In 1902, Sticker described over one thousand carcinomas of larger domestic animals, mainly from abattoir and veterinary sources, through records kept in Germany between 1858 and 1900.

Some of the more thorough studies of neoplasms of common laboratory animals have been conducted in the United States from around the turn of the present century, particularly by Harry Gideon Wells, Maude Slye, Ernest Edward Tyzzer, Clarence C. Little, and Harriet F. Holmes. One long series of articles in particular, that published between 1914 and 1941 by Slye, Wells, and Holmes, remains unmatched for the completeness and thoroughness with which neoplasms of practically every organ and tissue, from a study of 143,132 mice, have been meticulously observed, recorded, and described.

3.2.2 Neoplasms in Plants

Plant neoplasms were first reported in 1907. Smith and Townsend then described crown gall tumours occurring in association with the gram-negative soil bacterium *Agrobacterium tumefaciens*. This association has since been observed in many species of dicotyledonous plants. As reviewed by Braun (1977), plant tumours of various types and of widespread natural occurrence tend to mimic, but in plant-specific ways, some of the basic properties of their animal counterparts. For instance, the development of the tumours is stimulated by various chemical, physical, and biological factors. The tumours show a dependency upon normal growth-promoting factors, such as the auxins, gibberelins, and a cell-division-promoting factor; and they progress towards autonomy as the tumour cells themselves synthesize such factors. They tend also to retain structurally-unaltered, multipotential genomes capable of reproducing their parent organisms and of undergoing spontaneous regression to normal phenotypes.

In the plant-bacterium system mentioned above, the actual tumour-stimulating agent is not the bacterium itself. Rather, it is some segment of the DNA of a group of 'tumour-inducing' ('Ti') plasmids collectively called the 'tumour-inducing principle' ('TIP'). TIP is carried by certain strains of *A. tumefaciens*; and its plasmid DNA is large, varying in size between strains from about 150 to over 200 kilobase pairs. Thus, the oncologic activity is not expressed by TIP-negative or TIP-deprived strains of the bacterium, but it is expressed by such strains into which TIP has been subsequently introduced. By use of cloning, restriction enzymatic, kinetic, blot hybridization, nucleotide sequencing and other modern recombinant-DNA techniques it has been becoming increasingly apparent that the active agent is, as indicated above, one or more parts, termed transferred DNA (T-DNA), of the Ti plasmid which alone (not the bacterium itself) enters the cell. Once inside the cell, TIP may proceed to incorporate its T-DNA into the host cell's genome, as happens analogously in the case of oncogenic animal viruses. Within the genome, the incorporated T-DNA may then be repeated in tandem, involving direct or inverted repeats (Zambryski *et al.*, 1980). Presumably through expression of the integrated T-DNA in association with some unknown alteration of the normal gene controls of the host cell, the infected cell is induced to produce one or more of those basic amino acid-derivatives ('opines') by which the Ti plasmids are nowadays classified. The opines, exemplified by nopaline (a di-carboxypropyl arginine) and octopine (a carboxyethyl arginine), are utilizable (as sources of carbon and nitrogen) by the agrobacterium but not by the infected plant cell, i.e. in a newly-discovered but most likely very ancient type of parasitism that has been dubbed 'genetic colonization'. Despite the increasing array of the specificities (e.g. for conjugative transfer between bacteria, sensitivity to antibiotics, exclusion of bacteriophage Ap1, and opine biosynthesis and catabolism) which are being elucidated to be encoded by the Ti plasmids, there are several indications that their oncogenic encodements are highly dependent for their expressions upon intrinsic host-cell capacities and specificities of very ancient establishment. Among these indications are the host-cell specificities themselves, e.g. relative to infectivity and to susceptibility to the neoplastic transformation, as well as the capacity of the infected cells to participate in tissue regeneration following injury. For instance, induction of crown-gall disease by *A. tumefaciens* is highly dependent upon infection of susceptible plant cells during the specific period of about 24 hours that is marked by active cell division but is just about 20 per cent of the total wound-healing cycle of about 120 hours. As recently discussed by Braun (1977), this situation has its counterparts in other neoplastic diseases of plants as well, e.g. in the Black's wound-tumour disease that is associated with an oncornavirus, and the Kostoff genetic tumours which occur in certain hybrids within the genus *Nicotiana*.

3.3 Tumour Classification

3.3.1 The Pre-Hippocratic Era

At any historical stage in oncology, as in any discipline, classification, like definition, reflects and essentially summarizes basic knowledge and understanding at that stage. The simplistic 'bulging tumours of the breast' and the tumours of gods of ancient Egypt (Chapter Two, Section 2.3.2) for instance, are a long way from the elaborations of modern times, e.g. relative to tumour classes, subclasses, grades, and stages. Between these two extremes lies a period of progressive growth in concepts surrounding the elaborations, e.g. in those of benign and malignant; carcinomas and sarcomas; histologic, embryologic, and cellular types and origins; and morphologic, cytogenetic, behavioural, and functional features. Between just the Egyptian priest-physicians and the Hippocratic physicians, for instance, was Archilocus (719–633 BC), whose archaic 'phymata' had already included true neoplasms, but also pathologic growths such as abscesses, carbuncles, and the dreaded tubercle that so fascinated and even confounded the incomparable Virchow some 2,500 years later

(Chapter Two, Section 2.6.12). Not inconceivably, forward extrapolation of this progression would render today's sophisticated classifiers tomorrow's mystical Egyptians and archaic Archilocuses.

3.3.2 Hippocrates and Galen

During the Grecian period the two notable attempts made to classify tumours were those based upon, respectively, gross appearance and relationship to nature (Chapter Two, Section 2.4.3). The first attempt was due to the Hippocratic writers. Noting the highly localized, almost symmetrical appearance of some abnormal growths, and the crab-like appearance with tentacular infiltrations of others, these writers dubbed the former carcinos (*karkinos*) and the latter carcinomas (*karkinomas*). However, these were hardly exclusive terms. They were confused with some of the non-carcinomatous phymata of Archilocus, with the suppurating growths (*phymata empya*) seen more commonly in children than in adults; with the hard growths (*phymata sklera*) seen mainly in breast that do not suppurate but increasingly harden (*aiei sklerotera*) and eventually develop into occult cancers (*karkinoi kryptoi*); and with others including the soft swellings (*oidemata*) and, especially, the occult and deeply seated cancers (*karkinoi hypobrychthoi*) of mature adulthood. To the Hippocratic writers, the *kryptoi* and *hypobrychthoi* cancers were especially the ones that were best left untreated (Section 3.5, below).

The second attempt was due to Galen. Having derived the term 'tumour' from the Latin *tumere* (to swell) and the Greek *tymbos* (a sepulchral mound), he distinguished three types of tumour. The *tumores secundum naturam* designated all physiological swellings such as the gravid uterus and the breasts at and following puberty. Productive growths following tissue injury such as callus after fracture and scar after wound were *tumores supra naturam*. The third class, the *tumores contra* (or *praeter*) naturam, included abnormal growths which would now be called neoplasms, but also no less than 61 varieties of swelling, inflammation, local edema, cyst, gangrene, and other non-neoplastic but, to Galen, 'praeternatural' tumours. To him, a distinguishing feature of malignancy was ulceration, but he could not avoid the older terms such as *karkinos*, *karkinomas*, and *oidemata*. He agreed with the Hippocratic writers that the occult cancers were the ones that were best left untreated, for, 'so to speak, to cut out and extirpate the roots' (*ut sic loquer, radicibus exscindere et exstirpare*) was possible only in the case of superficial cancers.

3.3.3 Ingrassia and Fallopio

Galen's system of tumour classification, like most of his oncology and medicine, persisted, though not without extensions and/or modifications, up to the end of the eighteenth century, i.e. until Bichat introduced his tissue theory (Chapter Two, Section 2.6.8). During the sixteenth century, for instance, the list of Galen's praeternatural tumours had grown, as recorded by Giovanni Fillippo Ingrassia (1510–1580), to 287 varieties of ulcers, gangrene, carbuncles, erysipelas, furuncles, leprosy, tubercles, scabies, and others including aneurysms, hernias, varices, and buboes. Attempts were also made to subclassify the praeternatural tumours, e.g. by Gabriele Fallopio, in accordance with their mode of genesis from black bile concocted with other humours:

> The material cause of a cancerous tumour (*cancerosi tumoris*) is an atrabiliary juice (*atrabiliaris succus*) which is either a melancholy humour and mild sediment (*faex mitis*), whereby the cancer itself is mild (*mitis*), or it is a true and adust atrabiliary matter (*atrabiliaris materia vera et adusta*) which, since it is malignant, gives rise also to malignant cancers; or it is black bile mixed with phlegm, a benign matter from which comes a mild cancer; or it is black bile admixed with blood, thus giving rise to inflammatory cancer (*cancer phlegmonodes*); or it is mixed with (yellow) bile, and becomes erysipeloid. All of these matters may be with or without putrefaction. If the matter putrefies it produces an ulcerated cancer. (Cf. Foerster, 1855.)

Fallopio went on to distinguish cancers, caused mainly by intrinsic factors (black bile and its concoctions), from scirrhous tumours, caused mainly by external injury but capable of developing into cancer. He also distinguished between benign and malignant (*benignos et malignos*) forms of cancer, the former characterized by colour (black or bluish), temperature (cool to touch), and surrounding veins (often, but not always, blackish and swollen). The malignant tumours had eight distinguishing features. They were large; hard to touch; irregular in shape; and adherent due to their extended roots. They also had swollen veins 'resembling the legs of a crab' and causing the cancer to be called *noli me tangere* ('touch me not'); had blackish-ashen-lustrous texture; produced lancinating pain; and, in extreme cases, were associated with 'some heat, sharp and piercing, perceptible to the touch of the physician or patient'.

3.3.4 Morgagni, Bichat and Others

Fallopio's subclassification of praeternatural tumours was based upon various concoctions of atrabiliary humours collecting in body parts and undergoing various alterations to produce cancers and their closely-related scirrhous tumours. The subsequent development of the growths was determined by their chemical constitution, but each was an essentially uniform mass. His views thus diverged little from those of classical Galenism, and were unrelated to the concept of similar and dissimilar parts that led up to Bichat's tissue classes at the beginning of the nineteenth century. Like his predecessors, Fallopio made no distinction between inflammatory lesions and true neoplasms. This distinction was, in fact, first made late in the nineteenth century, some 60 years after Bichat's tissue theory (Chapter Two, Section 2.6.8) and some 25 years after Schwann's cell theory (Chapter Two, Section 2.6.9).

The combined efforts of the Paduan anatomists, which culminated in Morgagni's comprehensive treatment of cancer types known up to the eighteenth century (Chapter Two, Section 2.9.2) and of Bichat and the Muellerian school of cellular histologists and pathologists (Chapter Two, Sections 2.6.9 and 2.6.10) led up to several attempts, during the latter half of the nineteenth century at modern-style cancer classifications. The first of these was a joint attempt, made in 1853, by William Farr of England and Jacob Marc d'Epine of Switzerland. Two later attempts deserve special mention: one in 1855, made by August Foerster, and the other in 1899, by Adolphe Louis Jacques Bertillon of France.

3.3.5 Foerster

Foerster regarded inflammatory and tuberculous new-formations as special cases, from which he distinguished tumours of ten provisional categories. These were: (1) lipoma, consisting of fat tissue; (2) fibroid (connective tissue); (3) enchondroma (cartilage); (4) osteoma (bone tissue); (5) angioma (vascular tissue); (6) adenoma (glandular tissue); (7) cystic tumour (closed sac or sacs); (8) papilloma (papillary tissue); (9) sarcoma (underdeveloped connective tissue); and (10) carcinoma. Carcinoma consisted of indifferent cells growing without restraint (*in-differenten, schrankenlos wuchernden Zellen*).

3.3.6 Bertillon

The Bertillon classification dealt with various causes of death, but it also recognized the following seven histological categories of cancer: (1) *Cancers of the mouth*, included cancer of the lip, tongue, roof of mouth, velum palati, or jaw; epithelioma, carcinoma, or cancroid of those parts; and smokers' cancer. (2) *Cancer of the stomach and liver*, included cancer of the esophagus, cardiac stomach, or pylorus; carcinoma, scirrhous or encephaloid tumour of those parts; gastrocarcinoma; and tumour of the stomach, but not hematernesis or organic lesion of the stomach. (3) *Cancer of the intestines and rectum*, included cancer of the colon or anus; carcinoma, scirrhous, encephaloid, cancroid or epithelioma of those parts. (4) *Cancer of the female genital organs*, included cancer of the womb, ovary, vagina, or vulva; carcinoma, scirrhous, encephaloid, colloid, heteromorphous or neoplastic tumour, sarcoma or epithelioma of those organs. (5) *Cancer of the breast*, included carcinoma, scirrhous, encephaloid, colloid, heteromorphous or neoplastic tumour, cancroid, and epithelioma of the breast or mammary gland. (6) *Cancer of the skin*, included cancroid (without epithet), epithelioma or epithelial tumour (without epithet), cancer of the face or cervico-facial cancer, and noli-me-tangere; but not lupus, or estiomene. (7) *Cancer of other organs*, included cancer of the peritoneum, cancerous peritonitis; cancer of the pelvis, kidney, bladder, or prostate; cancerous goitre; thyreo-sarcoma; sarco-hydrocele; cancer of the bone; osteosarcoma; cancerous tumour or sarcoma of the neck; carcinoma, scirrhous, encephaloid, cancerous ulcer, malignant tumour, sarcoma, or malignant fungus of these parts or of an un-specified part of the body. This category excluded cancer of the esophagus, anus, ovary, vagina or vulva.

3.3.7 The Twentieth Century

By the turn of the present century, tumour classification had thus developed considerably since the time of the Egyptians and Greeks. It has remained a developing discipline, becoming in-creasingly sophisticated since the 1950s, a period marked by an unprecedented growth in understanding of the body's phenotypes and their cellular and subcellular structure, function, and general biochemistry. A most notable development is the increasing recognition that the phenotypic heterogeneity of tumours may actually exceed that of the body's normal substructures. This is because neoplasia is already known not only to involve practically any of the normal tissue phenotypes but also to introduce further heterogeneity in the latter due to clonal proliferation with aberrant differentiation of specific transformed phenotypes during tumour development. For instance, in the 1950s, non-Hodgkin lymphomas were first divided into reticulum cell sarcoma, lymphosarcoma, and follicular lymphomas, and then into lymphocytic, histiocytic, and mixed disorders with subtypes based upon whether the disorders were nodular or diffuse. During the subsequent decades, with the growth of knowledge about the various (B, T, null, and histiocyte-macrophage) cell types of the immune system, the lymphomas and lymphatic leukemias became classified according to their derivation from these cell types. These latter groups are now even further subdivided, e.g. through use of specific heteroantisera and monoclonal antibodies to lymphocyte differentiation antigens. Thus the B-cell disorders now include Burkitt lymphomas, most non-Hodgkin lymphomas, and most chronic and some acute lymphatic leukemias. Analogously, the T-cell disorders include some acute and some chronic lymphomas, Sezary syndrome, and mycosis fungoides. The entire classification process is a continuing one, and further subdivisions are already indicated. (For detailed discussions, see Madler *et al.*, 1980; Vianna and Strauss, 1983; Linch *et al.*, 1984.)

3.4 Cancer and the Environment

3.4.1 Introduction

Current notions about the role of environmental factors in the genesis and/or development of human cancers are a far cry away from the mystical equivalents of ancient times (Chapter Two). Today, the implicated factors are numerous, involving practically every aspect of human life and thus necessitating their proper evaluation and grading (cf. Chapter Nine, Sections 9.3 and 9.4). The historical development of this state of affairs is outlined below.

3.4.2 The Chemical Environment

3.4.2.1 Miners' 'Mala Metallorum': Paracelsus and Agricola. In 1531, Paracelsus described 'mala metallorum', a lung disease which had, for centuries, been plaguing miners of the Black Forest regions of Schneeberg and Joachimstahl. This finding was later confirmed in 1556 by Gregorius Agricola in his *De Re Metallica*, and extended in 1879 by G.H. Harting and W. Hesse in their article *Der Lungenkrebs, die Bergkrankheit in den Schneeberger Gruben*. These later studies showed that mala metallorum, long regarded as mediastinal lymphosarcoma with infiltration to the lung, was mainly bronchogenic carcinoma induced by radioactivity from the uranium, or by this in combination with one or more of the other metals (mainly arsenic, silver and cobalt), which had been mined at the two towns for over 500 years.

3.4.2.2 Nuns' Breast Cancer: Ramazzini. In 1700 and 1713, Ramazzini reported unusually high frequencies of breast cancer among Italian nuns. In his *De Morbis Artificum* of 1700, Ramazzini wrote:

> As a consequence of disturbances in the uterus, cancerous tumours are very often generated in the woman's breast, and tumours of this sort are found in nuns more often than in any other woman. Now these are not caused by suppression of the menses but rather, in my opinion, by their celibate life . . . Every city in Italy has several religious communities of nuns, and you seldom can find a convent that does not harbour this accursed pest, cancer, within its walls.

Today, increased risk of breast cancer is more strongly associated with factors such as familial predisposition, childlessness, and late first delivery than with celibacy itself; but the distinction between celibacy and childlessness, at least among nuns, is a fine one.

3.4.2.3 Chimney Sweepers' Scrotal Cancer: Pott. In 1775, Pott reported an apparent association between scrotal cancer and chimney soot among British chimney sweepers. He gave no numerical values, which were given over a century later, by Henry Butlin in 1892.

There are indications that these 'soot cancers' were well known around 1775. To the young sweepers, for example, 'the trade call is the soot wart', entailing a 'singularly hard life' and poor hygienic conditions as described in the line: 'So your chimneys I sweep, and in soot I sleep', from William Blake's 'The Chimney Sweeper'.

3.4.2.4 Dyestuff Workers' Bladder Cancer: Rehn. The discovery of 'aniline' (arylamino-type) dyestuffs by William Henry Perkin in 1856 initiated the era of the aniline dyestuff industry in Europe. In 1895, Rehn reported the occurrence of bladder cancers, which he called 'aniline' cancers among dyestuff workers in Germany. Similar reports soon came from England, Switzerland, Holland, the United States, and other countries. The association between bladder cancer and exposure to the dyestuffs or their inter-mediates thus became well-established. Subsequent reports from various sources have identified the causative agents not as aniline itself but as naphthylamines, benzidine, and magenta, among others.

3.4.2.5 Arsenicals and Iatrogenic Cancers: Hutchinson, Neubauer, and Paris. The first example of today's well-known phenomenon of the double-edged cancer chemotherapeutics was reported by Hutchinson in 1888. He reported upon six patients treated with Fowler's solution for many years: four patients for psoriasis, one patient for pemphigus and another for tonsillar cancer. Three of the psoriatic patients developed skin cancer,and the other three patients developed keratosis.

Arsenic-based escharotic and soothing ointments had been used in cancer therapy from ancient times. By Victorian times, potassium arsenite in the form of Fowler's solution had become a universal tonic. In more recent times, arsenic and certain arsenicals have been associated with lung cancer.

Suspicion that arsenic might pose a cancer risk is older than Hutchinson's report. In 1822, Paris noted hoof loss and 'a cancerous affection of their rumps' among horses and cows exposed to arsenical fumes from the copper-smelting works of Wales and Cornwall. Among the smelters, he found occasional, 'cancerous disease in the scrotum, similar to that which infest chimney sweepers'.

3.4.2.6 Tobacco Cancers: From Von Soemmering and Hill to Doll and Others.

3.4.2.6.1 The 'Origins' of Tobacco. The origin of smoking of various materials, like that of drinking intoxicating brews, is lost in antiquity.

Pliny the Elder, Herodotus, Pomponius Mela, and other ancient writers have recorded the smoking of various herbs for diverse reasons, and even the smoking of cow dung, reputedly for the cure of melancholy!

Tobacco smoking is sometimes thought to have originated with the Amerindians. From these ancient people, the European invaders and settlers of their continent, perhaps as a fair exchange for the European whisky-drinking habit, acquired the smoking habit and then proceeded to introduce it, via Europe, eventually to all parts of the world. Despite history, the true origins of the tobacco-smoking habit are unknown. An old legend describes the tobacco plant, with corn and potato, as a gift from the Great Spirit responding to the prayers, during a long, dry famine, of the Hurons. The Great Spirit sent a young naked maiden who sat down and placed both her hands upon the parched earth. Her right hand marked the spot where corn sprang, her left hand where potato sprang, and her seat where tobacco sprang. However, despite the simple charm of this legend, tobacco was well known outside the American continent long before Europe even suspected its existence. It was known to the Turks, for instance, who introduced it into Egypt in the fourteenth century.

The first introductions of tobacco to Europe from America were apparently by Juan Ponce de Leon of Portugal in 1558 and by Sir Walter Raleigh of England in 1565. Tobacco adulation, in many languages, soon followed, e.g. as the 'Herba Panacea', the 'Sacra Herbea', and the 'Indianisch Wunderkraut'. But so also did widespread condemnation. In 1604, for instance, in his famous *A Counterblaste to Tobacco*, James I of England, the 'wisest fool in Christendom', lambasted tobacco as being devoid of all medicinal properties but as an emitter of a black, smelly smoke that resembles 'the horrible vapours that exhale from hell'. A year later, the king organized an Oxford debate during which he exhibited, openly for all to see, several brains and viscera, all blackened, allegedly through the habitual smoking practices of their owners during the latters' lifetimes. The desired effect, however, was lost upon at least one participant in the debate, who was, perhaps significantly, himself a physician. While contentedly and defiantly puffing away at his brim-filled pipe, the physician, a Dr Chaynell, mounted the podium only to deliver, between puffs, a most impassioned eulogy on the miraculous herb.

Nearly 400 years later, the debate still rages unabated.

3.4.2.6.2 Snuff Cancer: Hill. The first of the various tobacco preparations reported to be associated with cancer was snuff, i.e. various aromatized preparations of powdered tobacco. The taking of snuff, or snuffing, was initiated in England during the seventeenth century, as an almost ritualistic habit of pushing a 'pinch of snuff' up the nostrils, to induce sneezing. The habit is still in vogue, though not as much as before, especially during the eighteenth century when the British had all but given up smoking for snuffing (Russell *et al.*, 1980).

The story of sneezing, whether induced by snuff or some other means, is as curious and amusing as it is old. Sneezing was recommended by Hippocrates as a cure for hiccups; and it has long been regarded by some African tribes as a good omen, an overflow of the life spirit. Sneezing releases high-velocity droplets which might have been partly responsible for spreading the influenza epidemic of 1918 and even the Black Death of the Middle Ages. Its enforced suppression or holding of the nose while sneezing, can cause nosebleed, fraction of nasal bones, dislocation of one of the middle-ear bones, and/or forcing of bacteria up into the sinuses which then become infected. In nineteenth-century Britain, some robbers known as 'sneeze-lurkers' threw snuff in the faces of their victims, who were robbed during the resulting fit of sneezing. Whatever the humour associated with snuffing and sneezing, it becomes quite wry in the face of the health hazards posed by snuff. Over 200 years ago, in 1761, John Hill reported six cases of snuff users' 'polypusses', one of which was a hard nasal swelling. It later developed 'all the frightful symptoms of an open cancer'.

3.4.2.6.3 Smokers' Cancers: Von Soemmering, Doll, and Others. Tobacco smoking was first reported to be associated with cancer in 1795. In this year, von Soemmering described labial cancer, particularly of the lower lip, among long-term pipe smokers. However, over 150 years elapsed before the now notorious association between cigarette smoking and lung cancer was first reported, i.e. in 1950, by Richard Doll (now Sir Richard) and A. Bradford Hill in England, and by Wynder and his colleagues (Wynder and Graham, 1950; Wynder and Hoffmann, 1976) in the United States. Neither these latter reports nor the many others, whether regional, national, or international, which have since followed have exonerated the pipe or cigar; they have merely shown that, comparatively, the cigarette is the worst offender.

3.4.2.6.4 'Chutta' and 'Supari' Cancers: Khanolkar. In 1958, V.R. Khanolkar reported 'chutta' cancer, a cancer of the buccal mucosa, occurring in association with the type of 'reverse' smoking practised in Andhra Pradesh. In India, this practice involves re-traction, into the mouth, of the burning end of a small cigar or chutta, analogously to the reverse smoking of cigarettes practised by Panamanian washerwomen.

In India, Malaysia, and certain other parts of Southeast Asia, buccal cancer is also associated with the ancient habit of chewing 'supari' or betel-quid. Supari refers to various concoctions of crushed nut of the betel palm (*Areca catechu L.*), mixed usually with tobacco, slaked lime, and flavourings, and wrapped in a betel leaf. Among its many components are the potent hallucinogenic and narcotic alkaloid ester, arecoline, and its free acid, arecaidine, both derived from the Areca nut. To most of its millions of devotees, the habit is a panacea for all ills, including boredom. Often lifelong, it is sometimes indulged continuously, with re-tention of the chew between teeth and cheek even during sleep.

Both of these practices are associated with an excess of oral cancer.

Like alcohol (discussed below), tobacco can exert its harmful effects from before birth. Retardation of growth and development of fetuses of smoking mothers is well documented. Several reports have suggested that this effect is due to smoking-mediated maternal undernourishment — for a discussion see Haworth *et al.* (1980). These authors concluded that the factors responsible for the growth retardation of infants of smoking mothers are inde-pendent of those behind the growth enhancement of infants of obese non-smoking mothers, and that neither of the two effects is related to maternal dietary intake. They demonstrated a similar degree of fetal growth retardation in infants of overweight smokers as in infants of smokers in general.

Thus, the biochemical mechanisms by which tobacco abuse ex-erts its biological effects, whether in the enhancement of neoplas-tic development or the retardation of fetal growth, remain to be elucidated.

3.4.2.7 Alcohol Cancers: Schwartz, Tuyns, and Others. The known historical age of man's abuse of tobacco is a babe-in-arms compared with that of his abuse of ethanol-based intoxicating be-verages. Almost continuously and universally, he has been resorting to the Bacchic cup for at least 50,000 years, ever since he first learnt to produce the various brews from berries, cactuses, flowers, fruits, grain, milk, tree saps, tubers, and any other suitable source of sugars or more complex carbohydrates. Within caves and adobes, temples and monasteries, or bodegas and chateaux, he has kept his brewing skills and equipment numbered among his most precious and most jealously guarded of 'top secret' treasures.

Like tobacco in public and private affairs and economies, alcohol has been the source of much revenue and employment, but also the butt of much disapproval and banning, through awareness of the attendant dangers to health and home. To health, for instance, the dangers of alcohol starting from life *in utero* have been recognized at least from Biblical times. 'Behold', says Judges 13:7, 'thou shalt conceive and bear a son: and now drink no wine or strong drink'. Alcohol drinking on the wedding night was prohibited in early Carthage, for fear of producing a defective child. In ancient Greece, Aristotle recorded: 'Foolish, drunken and harebrained women most often bring forth children like unto themselves, morose and languid'. According to Warner and Rosett (1975), in 1834, a report to the British House of Commons said that infants of alcoholic mothers often have a starved, shrivelled, and imperfect look. In 1899, Sullivan ascribed fetal damage to 'maternal intoxication' in Liverpool. In more recent times, it has become only too well recognized that alcohol, like thalidomide, diethylstilbestrol (Chapter Four, Section 4.2.3), and other substances of low molecular weight, can cross the placenta and enter the pregnant uterus from the maternal circulation, and thus affect fetal development. Today, it is well established that alcohol abuse by pregnant mothers can produce the fetal alcohol syndrome, characterized by low birth weight, mental retardation, and other developmental abnormalities in offspring (cf. Clarren and Smith, 1978; Streissquth *et al.*, 1980).

The dangers to health posed by alcohol abuse are not restricted to the developing fetus. In chronic alcoholics, serious brain damage can result, e.g. lessening of the advantage of the dominant over the non-dominant hemisphere (Golden *et al.*, 1981). Cancer can also result, suggesting that alcohol-associated cancers are as ancient as chronic alcoholism.

Discovery of the alcohol–cancer association, however, is of relatively recent origin. Since 1962 there have been increasing reports of an association between alcohol and cancers of the larynx, pharynx, and other parts of the upper digestive tract. After establishment of the International Agency for Research on Cancer (IARC), in 1971, 'to determine the role of the environment in all forms of human cancer', large-scale epidemiology of alcohol-associated cancers was instituted. During and after 1971, Tuyns of the IARC and his associates, notably Pequignot of the French National Institute of Health and Medical Research, traced an association between excessive consumption of alcoholic beverages, particularly the local apple brandy, and the remarkably high incidence (30–60 cases per 100,000 local inhabitants reported during 1971, as compared with the usual 3–4 cases in most other parts of the world) of esophageal cancer in parts of Brittany and Normandy. Alcohol abuse is a growing problem in many countries; and extensive epidemiological studies have already associated it with cancer of many body sites including the tongue, mouth, hypopharynx, oropharynx, larynx, esophagus, and liver (Tuyns, 1979), and also the stomach (Williams *et al.*, 1981).

To date, the mechanism by which alcohol exerts its harmful effects is unknown. There is no convincing evidence that these effects are due to carcinogenic residues or contaminants in the common alcoholic brews. However, the usual co-indulgence of alcohol and tobacco would seem to represent a particularly hazardous combination.

3.4.2.8 Asbestos Cancers: Lynch, Wagner, and Others. In 1935, observations at autopsy led Lynch and Smith to propose an association between asbestosis and lung cancer. This was later (1955) confirmed by Doll and extended by others to include the associations of asbestosis with pleural and peritoneal mesotheliomas and with gastronintestinal and laryngeal cancer. Other epidemiological studies have shown these associations to have complex relationships with type and physical properties of asbestos, individual genetics, and, in particular, cigarette smoking (Selikoff *et al.*, 1968). Recently, crysotile asbestos has been implicated as a cofactor in the etiology of cancers of the lung and nasal sinus among nickel-processing workers (Langer *et al.*, 1980).

The asbestos cancers belong to a large group of 'foreign body' (FB) cancers, mainly sarcomas, which are also associated with various other (e.g. plastic, glass, and stainless steel) fibres. In general, the physical or physicochemical rather than purely chemical nature of the fibres appear to be important in FB tumorigenesis (Stanton *et al.*, 1977; Wagner *et al.*, 1984).

3.4.2.9 Vinyl Chloride and Liver Angiosarcoma: Creech and Johnson. Among the astute observations not previously mentioned are those of Foulds and Steward in 1956, who observed an association between arsenic and/or hematite and lung cancer, and, in particular, of Creech and Johnson in 1974, between vinyl chloride monomer and liver angiosarcoma. This effect of the monomer might have been suspected from the observations of experimental tumorigenesis by the monomer and by the somewhat structurally related bischloromethylether. (For references and fuller discussions see Maltoni and Lefemine, 1975; Shimkin, 1977.)

3.4.3 The Physical Environment

3.4.3.1 Radiation Cancers: From Paracelsus to Hiroshima and Nagasaki. As discussed above (Section 3.4.2.1), Paracelsus' description of miners' lung cancer implicated several chemicals as the culprits, among which were radioactive chemicals. Uranium, one of the metals mined at Schneeberg and Joachimstahl during and long before the time of Paracelsus, has been later implicated as a cause of the high incidence of lung cancer among uranium miners and millers, e.g. on the Colorado plateaus (Wagoner *et al.*, 1964).

Radiation cancers are now known to be of several types. Malignant epitheliomas (as well as skin burns) were observed on the hands of radiologists and other users of X-ray devices and radium within a few years of their discovery in 1895 and 1898. By 1915, 104 such cases had been collected and analysed by Feygin of France. Also, during the 1920s in Orange, New Jersey, some 800 young women employees habitually pointed brushes with their tongue while painting watch dials with a luminous preparation containing radium and mesothorium. In this group the true mortality from radioactive poisoning remains unknown, but Martland in 1925 showed that 9 of 41 recorded deaths were due to osteogenic sarcoma. That ionizing radiation is also associated with leukemia was first shown in 1944, by Henshaw and Hawkins, among physicians, and by March, among radiologists.

The radiation–leukemia association achieved prominence after the atomic bomb explosions over Hiroshima and Nagasaki in 1945. Long-term survivors of the explosions have been kept under surveillance by the Atomic Bomb Casualty Commission, which was set up in 1948, and which, under the joint auspices of the US National Academy of Sciences and the Japanese National Institute of Health, became, in 1975, the Radiation Effects Research Foundation. The survivors have been observed to develop several forms of leukemia, though rarely of the chronic lymphocytic variety, as well as other types of cancer, notably of bone and thyroid. Also, it was first shown by Alice Stewart, in Britain, that children of mothers exposed during pregnancy to diagnostic radiation run an increased risk of early death from cancer, particularly leukemia (Stewart *et al.*, 1958; review by Stewart, 1971). Various types of radiation have thus now been associated mainly with leukemias and sarcomas, but also with carcinomas, e.g. of the skin and thyroid gland.

3.4.3.2 'Kangri' Cancers: Neve and Neve.

Cancer has been known for centuries to develop sometimes from old burns and scars, e.g. 'from a hot abscess or wound' as described by Theodoric in the thirteenth century (Section 3.5.1).

A well-known example of such cancers is the 'Kangri' cancer, the type of abdominal epithelioma first described, in 1900, by Arthur Neve (1858–1919) of the Kashmir Mission Hospital. According to Neve, the cause of Kangri cancer 'is not far to seek. During the severe winters and indeed for a great part of the year, every Kashmiri man, woman or child carries a portable charcoal brazier (a Kangri) under the loose gown which constitutes his or her only garment . . . Slight burns frequently occur. . . .' By 1923, Neve's brother, Ernest F. Neve (1861–1946), was able to report upon 2,491 operations for epithelioma carried out in Kashmir. Of these, some 2,000 were for Kangri cancer. He considered the cause of the Kangri cancers to have been the heat and recurrent burns, 'but it is possible that the volatile substances resulting from the combustion of the wood play a secondary part'.

3.4.3.3 Mechanistic Speculations.

Very little is known about the mechanism(s) by which radiation in its various forms induces neoplasia in man and animals. Ionizing radiation alone, whether in the form of photons, electrons, neutrons, mesons, or heavy ions, produce the same primary alterations (ionization and excitation) in roughly the same number of alterations per unit energy imparted; but the different forms, even at equal absorbed doses, do not have the same 'relative biological effectiveness' (RBE). The RBE differences are due less to differences in primary radiation products than to those in microscopic distribution of ionization and excitation in charged particle tracks. For example, more cellular damage per unit of absorbed dose is produced by radiations such as α particles or the heavy recoils of neutrons, which produce ionization closely spaced along their tracks, than by sparsely ionizing radiation. Also, whatever the mechanisms, they do not operate independently of host factors, e.g. host genetics. This is indicated by features such as the differential species-specific or individual-specific responses to the same dose of the same radiation; the higher sensitivity of some human (e.g. those with xeroderma pigmentosum) than others to the same type of (e.g. ultra violet) radiation; the high spontaneous incidence of some types of neoplasm (e.g. thymic lymphoma in AKR mice) which are particularly associated with radiation (Gross, 1970); and the highly variable (from non-existent to very high) incidences of spontaneous leukemia in F_1 hybrids produced by crossing AKR mice with mice of various low-leukemia inbred strains (Gross, 1970). In such mice, but apparently not in man, the oncologic effects of radiation may be associated with one virus or another (e.g. the murine leukemia viruses). In various systems, other variable effects of radition include immunosuppression, cytotoxicity, hormonal changes, and subcellular damage, e.g. to nucleic acids and proteins, inclusive of pyrimidine dimerizations in some instances (e.g. UV radiation) but not others (e.g. X-rays). Chromosome anomalies of various types (e.g. chromatid breaks in Japanese survivors of the atomic bomb explosions, trisomy 21 in Down's syndrome, and chromosome fragility in Bloom's and Fanconi's syndromes) are common to persons at high risk of leukemia induced by radiation or various 'radiomimetic' agents. However, as will be discussed later, the relationship between such anomalies and the associated cancers or predispositions to the latter does not appear causal.

In the face of such a paucity of definitive information it is perhaps not surprising that there is no dearth of mechanistic speculations. Some of the more common of these are the hypotheses centred around radiation induction of somatic mutation, activation of an endogenous oncogenic virus, depression of immunocompetence, epigenetic changes resulting in permanent changes in gene expression, various types of cellular disorganization or damage, and hormonal imbalance and/or stimulation (for a review, see Bustad *et al.*, 1976). In this review, Bustad *et al.* listed 12 major features of radiation oncogenesis in man and animals. These included the similarities in dose–response curves for various radionuclides, the non-linearity of the curves over wide dose ranges; the confinement of the neoplastic response mainly to the irradiated tissues; the importance of a minimal degree of induced tissue injury to the subsequent development of neoplasia, which may take, in man, anything between 6 and 56 years; the dependence of the neoplastic response upon the subsequent tissue-regeneration process effected, presumably, by population of pluripotential cells in the injured tissue; and the possible appearance of the neoplasms independently of virus(es) or changes in immune competence.

3.4.4 The Biological Environment

3.4.4.1 Non-viral Parasites. Parasites Galore, Inclusive of Schistosomes, Cysticercus, and Spiroptera: Fibiger and Others. The last quarter of the nineteenth century was the heyday of parasitology and general microbiology. These disciplines flourished, as never before, in the hands of Pasteur, Koch and others. Microbes and other parasites had become well-known causes of a sufficient number of non-neoplastic diseases to make almost inevitable a widespread and almost unquestionable belief in a parasitic etiology for most if not all neoplasms of man and animals. Thus, Rappin in France, Sanfelice in Italy, and Gaylord in the United States argued their respective cases for the cause of cancer being a bacillus, a blastomycete, and a protozoan or spirochete. The point of disagreement was not the parasitic etiology itself; it was only the nature and identity of the parasite. The concept of oncogenic parasites of every description became the order of the day. In 1907, Ewing competently reviewed the situation and listed 38 representative papers all making claims for such parasites that ranged from bacteria and coccidea to sporozoa, blastomycetes, mycetozoa, and spirochetes.

Such claims were by no means new to the late-nineteenth-century scientists. In 1806, for instance, the French dermatologist, Jean-Louis Alibert had described 'une eruption furfuracée'. This, in 1832, he had renamed 'mycosis fungoides', a name which has persisted to describe a cutaneous form of malignant lymphoma. However, it is now known that the mycosis fungoides of Alibert or of more recent times has no mycotic etiology, and that fungation of the lesions can be prevented by treatment with radiation and chemicals.

By the turn of the twentieth century, the nineteenth century theory of cancer being a nonviral parasitic disease was already in its final death throes. However, some doubts still lingered, as rare examples of such a disease remained known or suspected in plants, animals, and even man.

In plants, crown-gall disease was reported by Smith and Townsend in 1907 to be inducible by a bacterium (Section 3.2.2).

In man, the prime example is bilharzia. This is a form of hematuria due to chronic cystitis, a condition which has been plaguing the Nile Valley since the time of the Pharoahs. In 1851, the German parasitologist, Theodor Maximillian Bilharz (1825–1862) showed the condition, which became named after him, to be caused by a flatworm. The latter, *Schistosoma haematobium*, has a complex life cycle spent partly in certain species of the freshwater snail, *Bulinus*. Bilharzia is widely associated with human urinary bladder cancer, e.g. in Egypt and certain other parts of Africa and elsewhere. In 1972, Kuntz *et al.* in the United States reported induction of bladder cancer in a telapoin monkey and a capuchin monkey infected with the schistosome. However, the exact nature of the inducing agent, e.g. whether it is the schistosome itself, a schistosomal toxin, or a viral-type agent carried by the schistosome, remains problematical. Since the building of the Aswan dam, the relative prominence of the schistosome and the related *Schistosoma mansoni*, the latter being associated with intestinal rather than urothelial pathology, has altered in favour of the latter, resulting in a corresponding predominance of the intestinal disorders (for a review, see Caldwell, 1983).

In animals, two famous examples are cysticercus sarcoma and 'cockroach cancer', both in rats. The sarcoma was first shown, in 1924, by two Americans, Frederick D. Bullock (1878–1937) and Maynie R. Curtis (1880–1971), to be due to larvae of the common tapeworm, *Cysticercus fasciolaris*, of the domestic cat. These workers investigated this problem extensively and, in 1933, in collaboration with Wilhelmina F. Dunning, they studiously collected and analyzed the then available published data which involved a total of 3,669 rats. Their analysis showed that the oncogenic response to the parasitic infection was determined by the genetic suscepticibility of the infected rats to the parasitic disease and by their general resistance to common laboratory diseases.

The tale of cockroach cancer has added a new dimension, with an implied warning, to the complexity of host-parasite oncologic relationships illustrated in the above examples. In 1907, Johannes Andreas Grib Fibiger (1867–1928) began his now notorious investigations of 'stomach tumours' which were common among rats infesting a Danish sugar refinery. His conclusions that the tumours were papillomas and carcinomas caused by a nematode, which he named '*Spiroptera neoplasticum*', passed on to the rats through the common cockroach earned him the Nobel Prize in 1925. However, more careful subsequent investigations (cf. Hitchcock and Bell, 1952) failed to confirm his conclusions but, instead, showed the 'stomach tumours' to have been gastric hyperplasia caused apparently by avitaminosis A and chronic irritation.

3.4.4.2 Viruses: from Pasteur, Ivanowski, and Borrell to Burkitt, Epstein, and Barr. The use of the term 'virus' in association with disease is of untraceable antiquity, but the concept of a virus being a 'filterable agent' smaller than microorganisms belongs to the nineteenth century. In 1884, Pasteur suggested that an 'infinitesimally small' microorganism was the cause of hydrophobia. This suggestion has since been proved correct when rabies was found to be transmitted by a virus from dog to man. However, it still remains problematical whether or not viruses are true organisms of any kind, since they are neither cellular nor capable of performing any cellular function independently of the cells they infect.

The first virus to be purified and identified, however, was not the rabies virus, but the tobacco mosaic virus (TMV). In 1892, the Russian botanist, Dmitri Alexievich Ivanowski (1864–1920), presented evidence before the St Petersburg Academy of Sciences to show that tobacco mosaic disease was transmissible to the healthy plant by the filtered sap from the diseased plant. This finding was confirmed in 1898 by the Dutch botanist, Martinus Willem Beijerinck (1851–1931), who described the filterable factor as a 'contagium vivum fluidum'.

It was not until 1935, however, that this contagious living fluid, or its active principle, was isolated, purified by crystallization, and partly characterized. This remarkable feat was performed by the American chemist, Wendel Meredith Stanley (1905–1871). He thereby showed for the first time that tobacco mosaic virus and, by implication, other viruses, resemble common laboratory chemicals in some ways.

With the development of the electron microscope in the 1930s, it became possible to visualize viruses and other small particles beyond resolution by the wavelengths of visible light. From around 1947, electron microscopic examination of tumour viruses, even as components of intact tumour cells, became a growing art. This innovation was due most notably to the efforts of the Polish-born American, Leon L. Dmochowski.

3.4.4.2.1 Viruses in Cancer Etiology. The concept of a viral etiology for cancer was born at the University of Strasbourg, where it was championed by Amedee Borrell (1861–1936) in a series of papers he published from 1907 onwards. Charles C. Oberling (1895–1960) became an ardent convert to Borrell's views; and, in 1943, he published his now classic *Le Cancer* which, in 1952, was translated and published by W.H. Woglom as *The Riddle of Cancer*.

A concept proposed is not a concept proved. The first *clear* proof of Borrell's concept came from Denmark where, in 1909, Wilhelm Ellerman (1871–1924) and Oluf Bang (1881–1937) introduced a cell-free filtrate from chicken erythromyeloblastic leukemia into healthy chickens, which later developed the disease.

A related earlier experiment with rabbit myxomatosis is as noteworthy as is the disease itself. In the wild South American rabbit, the disease is common, mild, and temporary, probably due to a long period of this rabbit's (perhaps immunological) adaptation to the causative virus; but it is fatal to previously myxomatosis-unexposed rabbits such as the European domestic rabbit. During the 1950s, myxomatosis was introduced into Australia to control the over-multiplying European rabbits which, earlier, had been introduced by the country's farmers to aid control of crop-pests. In consequence, myxomatosis threatened extinction of Australia's and even some other countries' entire population of domestic rabbits until the fittest rabbits that survived, bred, and became adapted towards the milder disease. This episode explains the mildness of the myxomatosis reported to be virally caused, by G. Sanarelli in Montevideo, in 1898, i.e. preceding by over a decade the report of Ellerman and Bang.

Thus, Sanarelli deserves credit for the first reported causal association between a virus and a cancer-like disease, a credit which might easily have supplanted that accorded to Ellerman and Bang, had it not been for two rather minor omissions. First, myxomatosis is hardly a true neoplasm, although it can develop into one. Thus, in 1935, in the United States, Peyton Rous and J. W. Berd showed that subcutaneous transplant of the papillomas from wild rabbits into domestic rabbits sometimes develop into invasive squamous cell carcinomas. These workers had been pursuing an earlier observation, made in 1933, by Richard Edwin Shope (1901–1966) in the United States, that cell-free filtrates from the papillomas of wild but not domestic rabbits can transmit the papillomatous disease (now known as 'Shope papilloma') to wild as well as domestic rabbits. Second, Sanarelli had not, in 1898, reported any filtration experiments, which were, in fact, reported in 1911, the year in which Rous also reported transmission of chicken sarcoma to healthy chickens by a cell-free filtrate of the tumour.

3.4.4.2.2 Two Chemical Classes of Oncovirus. The modern era of molecular genetics, from the 1950s onwards, saw the division of all known viruses into two chemical classes according to whether their component nucleic acids are RNA (RNA viruses) or DNA (DNA viruses), and analogously for the oncoviruses (onco*rna* viruses and onco*dna*viruses). The essential viral components also became recognized to be DNA or RNA together with viral-specific proteins. One of the latter, RNA-directed DNA polymerase or 'reverse transcriptase', was discovered in 1971 simultaneously by Temin and Mizutani and by Baltimore, and was later found to be an obligatory component of all oncornaviruses.

Despite its lack of such knowledge, the first half of the twentieth century had witnessed the discovery of some of the important viruses of modern experimental oncology. Among these were some of the oncorna viruses of chickens, and the papilloma virus of rabbits which, though strictly not an oncovirus, is a DNA virus.

A true oncodnavirus discovered before the era of molecular genetics is the 'Lucké virus'. This herpesvirus, which is endogenous to the North American leopard frog in which it produces renal carcinoma, was discovered by the American pathologist, Baldwin Lucké (1889–1954) during the 1930s. Lucké described the carcinoma in 1934; and he deduced its viral etiology in 1938, from observation of the capacity of the desiccated or glycerinated tumour tissue to increase the frequency of the frog tumour. In 1956, D.W. Fawcett showed the causative agent to be a DNA virus.

Thus, by the 1950s, an important principle of animal viral oncology was beginning to emerge. The oncodnaviruses show a tendency to produce epithelial tumours, and the oncornaviruses to produce nonepithelial tumours (leukemias, lymphomas, and sarcomas). The former is exemplified by the Lucké frog renal carcinoma and, for this purpose, by the above-mentioned demonstration by Rous and Beard of the rare capacity of the Shope rabbit papilloma to grow into invasive carcinoma. The latter is exemplified by the virally-induced leukemias and lymphomas of chickens, mice, cats, monkeys, and several other non-human species.

3.4.4.2.3 Host-virus-response: A Complex System of Variables in Neoplasia. In all nonhuman species of animals (and plants) which have so far been sufficiently investigated, complex systems involving the host organism, its natural infective oncoviruses, and the nature of the oncogenic response have been discovered.

Of these systems, that involving the domestic chicken has been particularly well-investigated. As noted above, oncogenic viruses were first detected in chickens which are now known to be naturally infected with several species of oncornaviruses including the Rous sarcoma virus (RSV), the Rous-associated virus, type O (RAV-O), and the groups of lymphoid leukosis viruses (LL viruses) and the reticuloendotheliosis viruses (RE viruses). Of these, RAV-O is an infectious endogenous virus whose proviral form is thought to be carried intact in the genome of all chickens, though rarely with small deletions in some genetically distinct chickens. Chickens are also naturally infected with a herpesvirus, the Marek's disease virus (MDV), the associated disease (MD) being an acute lymphoid neoplasia which was first described in 1907, by Joseph Marek of Hungary. MDV itself has been investigated since the 1960s, first by Peter M. Biggs in England and Ben Roy Burmester in the United States, and then by many others (e.g. notably, R.L. Witter, H.G. Purchase, and L.B. Crittenden) in various countries. The subject has been extensively reviewed (e.g. Nazerian *et al.*, 1976; Hofstad *et al.*, 1978).

The chicken has been selected for this discussion because it illustrates the complex system of variables which is known to operate in animal neoplasia. Thus, the same animal species (the domestic chicken in this case) can become infected with member(s) of both chemical classes of oncoviruses and yet develop its characteristic (epithelial or nonepithelial) type of neoplasm. For instance, the chick, in common with most domestic animals and laboratory rodents, is significantly more prone to the nonepithelial than the epithelial type of neoplasms, and this situation is reflected in its neoplasms induced by either class of its oncoviruses. Further, any of the natural neoplasms of the species can apparently occur in the absence of infection with any of its known oncogenic viruses. This has been demonstrated in chickens by Crittenden *et al.* (1979) for lymphoid neoplasms, and by Hemboldt and Fredrickson (1978) for carcinomas such as those of the oviduct and ovary. Crittenden *et al.* also found evidence to suggest that the endogenous RAV-O, whose spontaneous full or partial expression is controlled by at least four single dominant genes, did not participate in the production of the lymphoid neoplasms. Finally, virally-induced neoplasms are potentially preventable by appropriate immunization. In chickens, this has been achieved by use of at least three different viral antigens: an attenuated form of MDV, a naturally apathogenic field MDV, and a turkey herpesvirus antigenically related to MDV.

These considerations support what may be a general principle of oncology: viruses and/or other suitable environmental factors can enhance the rate of overt expression (e.g. by shortening the latency and/or increasing the age-adjusted incidence) of a tumour to which the host organisms are innately susceptible, but they cannot cause that tumour in non-susceptible hosts. Thus, in the report of Crittenden *et al.*, qualitatively identical tumours were observed in the presence as in the absence of the viral agents, but the tumours were more frequent in the presence of the agents. Analogously, in the report of Hemboldt and Fredrickson, the tumours appeared in old chickens.

3.4.4.2.4 Species-specificity. A recurrent theme in oncology, that of species-specific differences in spontaneous or induced neoplasia, is well illustrated by experiences in viral oncology. In 1932, for instance, Christopher Howard Andrewes, a British pathologist, used filtrates of chicken sarcoma to transmit the disease to adult pheasants. One decade later, Francisco Duran-Reynals, a Spaniard at Yale University, repeated this experiment, but used newborn poultry (ducks, turkeys and fowls) as recipients of the filtrates. He found the types of lesion produced in the recipients to differ considerably among themselves (some were bone sarcomas, or hemorrhagic lesions, for instance) and also from the donor chicken sarcoma.

Duran-Reynals's results constituted a landmark in experimental viral oncology. In addition to their demonstration of species differences in response to the same virus (RSV), they raised the possibility of alteration of the viral genome as a cause of the altered viral activities in the young animals. They also introduced the use of newborn recipients, a technique which was destined to become standard in such experiments.

Another historic example came later from studies initiated in the United States by the great Polish virologist, Ludwik Gross, between 1951 and 1953, and later extended by others, notably Sarah Elizabeth Stewart and Bernice Elaine Eddy. These studies identified the murine 'polyoma' virus, an oncodnavirus, specifically from mouse parotid and adrenal tumours. Stewart, Eddy, and their colleagues propagated the virus by cultivating the minced tumours on monkey kidney cells and on chick chorioallantoic membranes. In rabbit, rat, hamster, guinea pig, and other animals, the virus was found to induce a great variety of tumours including mesotheliomas, endotheliomas, and tumours of adrenal, bone, breast, hair follicle, kidney, and parotid, but in different combinations and relative extents.

A new dimension was added to the species-specificity of the tumorigenic response in 1962. In the United States, John J. Trentin, Yoshiro Yabe, and Grant Taylor reported the capacity of human adenovirus, type 12 (but not any of the eight other types of the virus tested) to produce 'a very high incidence of malignant tumours at the site of injection in from 1 to 3 months' in hamsters 'injected intrapulmonarily with tissue culture fluid within 24 hours after birth'. Infection with adenoviruses, including adenovirus type 12, is common among humans who may, in consequence, suffer mild to severe upper respiratory tract disorders, but never cancer. Man is also almost ubiquitously subject to infections from a large variety of herpesviruses, among them cytomegalovirus (CMV), the Epstein-Barr virus (EBV), herpes simplex virus (HSV), and the varicella-zoster virus (VZV). Generally, CMV and EBV are innocuous, although the latter has been associated with some types of Burkitt's lymphoma, particularly among

African children. One type of HSV, HSV-1, may cause usually mild cold sores; while another type, HSV-2, can cause serious genital disorders such as venereal disease; and VZV may re-emerge many years after chicken pox to cause shingles. (For a review, see Darby, 1980.)

The capacity of human viruses which display no oncogenicity in man to do so in susceptible nonhuman animals is not restricted to the adenoviruses. Two additional examples of such viruses are the JC virus (Padgett *et al.*, 1977), a polyoma virus, and the BK virus (Uchida *et al.*, 1979), a papova virus.

3.4.4.2.5 Viruses and Human Cancer. The classic and still the preferred candidate for a virally caused human cancer is the lymphoma first described in 1958 by the Irish pathologist, Dennis P. Burkitt, to be endemic in certain parts of Africa. In most of Kenya, Tanzania, and Uganda, up to 3 of every 1,000 children under 15 years of age can develop the disease, which is now known as Burkitt's lymphoma or BL.

Extensive later studies have revealed some other unusual features of BL which suggest its causation by a local environmental factor, possibly a virus. BL, which commonly involves the jaw, shows a degree of response to chemotherapy which, within the annals of clinical cancer therapy, is matched only by that shown by choriocarcinoma, a disease which undoubtedly contains (paternal) genes that are different from those of its human host. Also, BL is as rare in a 200-square-mile area within the countries mentioned as it is in most other countries of the world. Finally, in 1964, two virologists at London's Middlesex Hospital, Tony Epstein and Yvonne Barr, identified an infectious virus (now known as the Epstein-Barr virus or EBV) in cells from some of the Ugandan patients with the disease. The conclusion that EBV is a virally-caused infective disease thus seemed wholly justified.

Other studies, however, have cast serious doubts upon the validity of this conclusion. These studies have shown that EBV commonly infects most African children by the age of two years, including those in the above-mentioned area of low BL incidence; that it also commonly infects most humans worldwide; and that it is absent from some American, European and other extra-African cases of BL. Although it is commonly associated with most cases of African BL, it is similarly associated with nasopharyngeal carcinoma among the Cantonese and Tunisians, but with infectious mononucleosis among Jews and Europeans. Further, EBV does not seem to be transmissible among humans, not even from one individual who is highly EBV-seropositive to another who is EBV-seronegative (Chang and Le, 1984). In the EBV-BL association, such indications of a host genetic-viral specificity are further complicated by the reported involvements of other factors such as the malarial plasmodium, immune deficiency, trans-placental or neonatal infections, and chromosomal defects. If, as indicated above, EBV infection is widespread among humans, it might also have been so from as ancient a time as malaria has been, i.e. from time immemorial as one of the most ubiquitous of tropical diseases. Finally, EBV has also been associated with dis-eases other than those already mentioned, e.g. leukemias, and Hodgkin as well as non-Hodgkin lymphomas. (For discussions or reviews, see Zur Hausen, 1980; Gallo and Gelman, 1981; Caldwell, 1983; Chang and Le, 1984).

At present, definitive proof of any human oncogenic virus re-mains restricted to the Ciuffo's wart virus (Bayon, 1927). Despite this, virology has an important role in human oncology, specifically in the study of the molecular genetics of interindividual inherited cancer susceptibility differences and their expressions during carcinogenesis. As discussed in Chapter Nine (Sections 9.2.6, 9.6.3, and 9.8.4), this role is well exemplified by the recently discovered 'oncogenes'.

3.4.5 Socioeconomic Status: Weinberg and Others

Socioeconomic status has implications of differing standards of nutrition, medical care, personal hygiene, and perhaps other lifestyle components such as exercise, psychosomatic stress, and sexual practices. It has been associated with cancer risk since 1912, when Weinberg reported a higher incidence of uterine cancer among some of the poorer than wealthier women in Germany. Similar findings were made in the United States in 1959 by Dorn and Culter, and also in Denmark in 1965 by Clemmeson, with both studies showing higher incidences, among the poor, also of cancers of the mouth, esophagus, and stomach. Clemmeson, in particular, made a detailed study of the subject, and also of cancer epidemiology in general, including its historical development. Be-tween 1965 and 1974, he published his findings in a landmark 4-volumed work. This also described the activities of the Danish Cancer Registry, the first national organization of its kind, which he himself founded in 1942 and directed ever since until his retirement.

3.4.6 Cancer Statistics: Tanchou and Rigoni-Stern

Modern type analysis of cancer incidence and mortality in specific populations, as based upon histologic types of cancer in men and women and upon temporal changes, was instituted during the nineteenth century by Tanchou in France and Rigoni-Stern in Italy.

Tanchou gathered data on a total of 382,851 deaths occurring around Paris between 1830 and 1840, of which 194,735 were in males and the remainder in females. Cancer accounted for 9,118 of the total: 2,161 in males and 6,957 in females. Of these, the five most frequent causes, by body site from among over 20 sites considered, were, in decreasing order: uterus, stomach, breast, liver, and rectum. His analysis showed a number of interesting features: an approximately 3:1 female-to-male ratio; a preponderance of female-type cancers, i.e. of uterus and breast; a low incidence of lung cancer, i.e. at a time antedating the prominence of the smoking habit; a very high incidence of uterine cancer, which is associated with poor feminine hygiene, and which occurred before the Pap-smear era; and an increasing trend in cancer mortality over the decade, i.e. from 1.96 to 2.40 per cent of the total deaths.

Rigoni-Stern collected data on a total of 150,673 deaths occurring around Verona between 1760 and 1839. Of these 76,489 were in males, and the remainder in females. Cancer accounted for 1,142 deaths: 142 in males and 994 in females. Like Tanchou, Rigoni-Stern found a preponderance of uterine (365 cases) and breast (319 cases) cancers, although uterine cancer was less frequent around Verona than Paris. By elaborate analysis of the data in almost modern terms (age, sex, occupation, and other variables), he came to several conclusions, including: overall cancer incidence was higher in females than males, in the unmarried than married, and in urban than rural areas. The incidence increased with age, particularly for uterine cancer and for breast cancer among women 10–15 years post-menopausally.

Rigoni-Stern published his findings in 1842, Tanchou in 1843. In 1946, Tanchou's findings were used by Walshe in England and by LeConte in the United States. Those of Rigoni-Stern were forgotten for over a century, but they afterwards attracted much deserved attention, especially from Clemmeson in 1951, Mustacchi in 1961, and Scotto and Bailor in 1969.

Cancer of the breast is the classical cancer described in the surgical annals of history, but uterine cancer was probably commoner, at least since the days of Paul of Aegina in seventh-century Alexandria. In nineteenth-century Germany uterine cancer was well described by Adam Elias von Siebold (1775–1826) in 1824 and by Ernst Leberecht Wagner (1829–1888) in 1858.

3.5 Treatment

3.5.1 'Incurability'

From its remotest recorded history, cancer has been regarded as incurable at least in the more responsible quarters. This designation became extended to the multiple forms of the disease as they became increasingly recognized.

The incurability of cancer was first recorded in the medical papyri of ancient Egypt of approximately 4,000 years ago. For instance (cf. Chapter Two, Section 2.3.2), the therapeutic approach of the physicians of the Pharoahs to 'a tumour of the god Xensu' was 'do thou nothing there against'; and to 'bulging tumours of the breast', it was 'there is no treatment'. At best, some benign superficial growths, such as polyps and lipomas, were cauterized or excised by the priest-surgeons, but the more serious neoplasms were either untouched or treated palliatively with various concoctions from plant, animal, and/or chemical sources. A possible stomach cancer, for example, was treated with a mixture of boiled barley and dates, and a possible uterine cancer with a vaginal suppository concocted from fresh dates and pig's brain (cf. Shimkin, 1977).

The ancient Greeks promulgated this preferential 'untouchability' of cancer. For instance, Hippocrates' celebrated aphorism no. 38 reads: 'It is better not to apply any treatment in cases of occult cancer; for if treated, the patients die quickly; but if not treated, they hold out for a long time.' By the subsequent authority of Galen himself, the law of the incurability and preferential untouchability of deep-seated cancers became entrenched for well over 1,000 years. The rare older claims of 'cancer cures' thus invite scepticism. One such claim, as recounted by Herodotus, was that Atossa, the wife of Darius the Great, was cured of breast cancer by a captive Greek physician, Democedes. Even today, it is not always easy to distinguish benign from malignant lesions of the breast, or those from certain inflammatory and dysplastic lesions. This, together with the ancient Greeks' awareness of the poor prognosis of breast cancer, the readiness with which Democedes promised a cure, and the ease with which he affected it, would suggest that Atossa did not have breast cancer by modern or even Democedes' standards.

The state of the art up to the seventh century was well summarized by Paul of Aegina. In Book VI of his *Seven Books*, Paul wrote:

> Cancer is an uneven swelling, rough, unseemly, darkish, painful, and sometimes without ulceration (which Hippocrates called also concealed cancer), and if operated upon, it becomes worse, and sometimes with ulceration, for it derives its origin from black bile, and spreads by erosion; forming in most parts of the body, but more especially in the female uterus and breasts. It has its veins stretched on all sides as the animal the crab (cancer) has its feet, whence it derives its name.

Paul also described the circumstances in which surgery, cauterization, and evacuation by 'purging the melancholic humour' were feasible, and the details of the procedures. In Book IV, he commented extensively upon Hippocrates and other authorities, and included this statement from Archigenes concerning palliative treatment of 'carcinomatous and malignant ulcers': 'Levigate equal parts of burnt river crabs and calamine, and sprinkle or apply the ashes of crabs with cerate; or apply the seed of hedge mustard triturated with honey'.

This situation had changed little by the thirteenth century. Thus in Book III of his *Surgery*, Teodorico Borgogni (Theodoric) of thirteenth-century Salerno dealt with classification and treatment of tumours. He distinguished two classes. Those 'arising from a hot abscess or wound' were wide round ulcers of shell-like hardness, 'proceeding from external causes, i.e. a wound or an ulcer improperly treated', and included 'nolimetangere', 'lupus', and 'cancer'. A second class, 'the melancholic abscess', occurred in any part of the body, but mainly in the breasts of women. 'The signs of this are that a hot abscess begins at the size of a hazel nut or smaller, and then increases in size little by little, with notable hardness, darkness of colouring, round shape, and some warmth to the touch. When it begins to grow larger, green veins appear in it, and it has roots penetrating into the body.'

Treatment, according to Theodoric depended upon several variables:

> The older a cancer is, the worse it is. And the more it is involved with muscles, veins and nutrifying arteries, the worse it is, and the more difficult to treat. For in such places incisions, cauteries and sharp medications are to be feared.
>
> But if the cancer should be in fleshy places where one need not fear for veins and muscles, incise it as far as the sound flesh and burn it away afterwards, to treat it just as was said in the case of fistulas.
>
> Or employ the treatment which we ourselves always use, and have proved times without number: Mortify the cancer with arsenic sublimate according to our teaching, for it kills fistula, cancer, herpes estiomenus (or lupus), 'nolimetangere' (or formix), and all similar affections, on the first day. Thereafter, see to it that the dead flesh is sloughed off, and then treat as has been stated.

The incurability of deep-seated cancers was repeatedly stressed. In the fourteenth century, for instance, John of Arderne, who was the first of the great British surgeons, wrote this in his *Of Bubo (Cancer) Within the Rectum and the Impossibility or Great Difficulty of the Cure of It*: 'I never saw or heard of any man that was cured of the bubo of the rectum but I have known many that died of the foresaid sickness'. In sixteenth-century Italy, Fallopio summarised the situation thus: 'quiescente cancro, medico quiescendam'.

Today, over four thousand years after the heyday of the priest-physician-surgeons of the Pharoahs, the principle of the incurability of cancer has not changed: no cancer is treated at its root cause, which is not known. What has changed is the post-treatment survival prospects of some cancer patients, based upon surgery and cytotoxic therapy, i.e. upon treatment of symptomatology after cancer has become firmly established. These prospects have been extended to about five years on average, for about one-third of cancer cases overall, excluding cases of non-melanoma skin cancer and carcinoma in situ of the uterine cervix. The best results are obtained with the use of combination therapy, involving surgery (which is becoming progressively less radical), radiotherapy, and chemotherapy, of which radiotherapy has fewer and less harmful side-effects than chemotherapy. Among the cancers showing improved prognosis in some patients are acute lymphocytic leukemia, Burkitt's lymphoma, and Wilm's tumour in children; and choriocarcinoma, uterine (cervical and endometrial) cancer, Hodgkin's disease, malignant melanoma, testicular carcinoma, and leukemias in adults mainly. Among most of the commoner cancers, five-year survival rates are dismal. For instance, 80–85 per cent of women with breast cancer die of the disease, even though only about 75 per cent present with metastatic disease. Prognosis improves with early stages of the disease at presentation. For some cancers, clinical presentation is practically synonymous with impending death. These include cancers of the lung, colon, rectum, or pancreas in both sexes, and of the prostate in men or ovary in women. Even where some improvements have been effected the survival rates have been levelling off, most notably for uterine and oral cancers. Overall, prognosis in most cancers has changed little since around 1960. (For a review, see McWhirter and Siskind, 1984; see also Chapter Nine, Section 9.2.2.)

3.5.2 Surgery

'Whenever feasible, incise it [the cancer] . . . and burn it away afterwards' wrote Theodoric in the thirteenth century. During the seventeenth-century reign of morbid anatomy in Padua (Chapter Two, Section 2.6.2), total mastectomy (removal of the whole breast with its underlying pectoral muscles) became a widespread treatment for breast cancer, as described by its chief proponent at the time, Johann Schultes (1595–1645), or Scultetus, of Padua and Ulm, in his *Armamentarium Chirurgicum* of 1645. This excruciating operation was performed without the use of anesthesia, which was first introduced into clinical surgery in 1846, when John Collins Warren, a founder of the *Boston Medical and Surgical Journal* (today's *New England Journal of Medicine*), removed a neck tumour from a patient anesthetized with ether. Since then, but perhaps not before, the unfortunate patients with this vicious disease began to escape at least the pain of the surgeon's knife or of the hot iron (or, nowadays also, the laser beam) of the cauterer.

From around the mid-nineteenth century, surgery under anesthesia, as well as surgery and anesthetics, began to make significant advances. Among others, Christian Albert Billroth (1829–1894) of Germany excelled in gastrointestinal surgery; William Stewart Halsted (1852–1922) of the United States in radical mastectomy; Richard von Volkman (1830–1889) of Germany, Theodor Kocher (1841–1917) of Switzerland, and William Ernest Miles (1869–1947) of England in abdominal surgery; Ernst Wertheim (1864–1920) of Austria and Joe Vincent Meigs (1892–1963) of the United States in gynecological surgery; and Evarts Ambrose Graham (1883–1957) and Hugh Hampton Young (1870–1945) of the United States in thoracic and urological surgeries respectively.

An important departure from established protocol occurred in 1948. In this year, Robert McWhirter of Scotland showed that, in breast cancer treatment, the type of mastectomy developed by Halsted 54 years earlier (removal of the breast *en bloc* with its pectoral muscles) was, when combined with radiotherapy, as effective as Halsted's mastectomy combined with resection of the internal mammary lymph nodes. Even today, however, results from large, randomized and controlled trials are still inconclusive as to whether (Urban and Marjani, 1971) or not (Veronesi and Valagussa, 1981) Halsted mastectomy with or without radiotherapy but with node resection is more effective than the mastectomy alone. (For other discussions of this controversial topic, see Lacour *et al.*, 1976; Fisher and Gebhardt, 1978.)

3.5.3 Radiotherapy

Cancer radiotherapy was a logical development from the discoveries in the 1890s of X-rays by Röntgen, of radium by the Curies, and of the capacity of these agents to produce skin damage. In 1903, George Parthes (1869–1927) of Germany, following upon some exploratory work by Grubbe of the United States, showed a correlation between the radiosensitivity of cells and their rate of reproduction. In 1906, in France, Jean Alban Bergonie (1857–1925) and L. Tribondeau (1872–1914) advanced three principles which are still basic to cancer radiotherapy. The effects of radiation of living cells, they said, were directly proportional to the extent of the cells' proliferative activity, the duration of their mitotic activity, and the state of their morphological and/or functional undifferentiation. These findings were soon greatly extended, by two other Frenchmen in particular, Claudius Regaud (1870–1940) and Henri Coutard (1876–1950). Thus was laid the foundations upon which the theoretical fabric of modern cancer-radiotherapy is being built and applied clinically, with its realization of the critical importance of factors such as dose and dosage, dose fractionation and timing, oxygenation, radio-sensitizers, and cell kinetics. The birth of the modern era of radiotherapy of clinical cancer can be dated to 1922, when Regaud and Coutard with A. Houtant, demonstrated the efficacy of radiotherapy of advanced laryngeal cancer. Nowadays, the usual use of radiotherapy is as an adjunct to chemotherapy and surgery.

3.5.4 Chemotherapy

In its earliest forms, at least from the days of ancient Egypt, cancer chemotherapy involved topical application of various concoctions (from plant, animal, bacterial, and inorganic sources) to super-ficial growths to produce escharotic and soothing rather than curative effects. Some examples already given (Section 3.5.1) are the mixtures of 'boiled barley and dates', or of 'fresh dates and pig's brains', described in the Egyptian papyri; and the con-coctions of 'burnt river crabs and calamine' with sprinklings of 'the ashes of crabs with cerate', and 'the seeds of hedge mustard triturated with honey', described in the Greek writings. A persistent ancient remedy was the salve of Archigenes (cf. Chapter Two, Section 2.4.3).

The favourite chemical concoctions appear to have been arsenic-based. One of these, the potassium arsenite-based Fowler's solution, came to be used systemically, apparently for the first time, in 1865 by the little-known Lissauer of Bendorff for the treatment of leukemia. Also, about three decades later, in 1893, William B. Coley (1862–1936) of New York introduced the use of 'Coley's toxin' (a mixture of streptococci and *Bacillus prodigiosus*) for the treatment of lymphosarcoma. Retrospectively, this venture also represents the forerunner of today's nonspecific 'adjuvant' cancer-immunotherapy protocols based upon vaccines from microorganisms such as Bacillus Calmette Guérin (BCG), or *Mycobacterium tuberculosis, M. phlei, Corynebacterium parvum*, and even certain viruses (cf. the Ciba Foundation's *Immunopotentiation* of 1973).

Like all other branches of oncology, cancer chemotherapy, as discussed above, has its roots in remote antiquity. Hence, the modern practice of designating the 'fathers' of this and that can hardly be other than tongue-in-cheek. Yet, if any one man can be called the father of modern chemotherapy, inclusive of clinical cancer chemotherapy, that man must be Paul Ehrlich (1854–1915) of Frankfurt. Ehrlich was, so to speak, the greatest one-man laboratory, experimental, clinical, and theoretical, in the annals of medicine. The range of his expertise, which straddled fields as diverse as chemotherapy, chemistry, bacteriology, pathology, and immunology, is only partly reflected in the number and diversity of now familiar scientific descriptions which bear his name. These include Ehrlich's (aplastic) anemai, Ehrlich's hemoglobinemic (eosinophilic) bodies, Ehrlich's megaloblasts, Ehrlich's side-chain theory (of antigen-antibody reactions), Ehrlich's reagent (an acidified alcoholic solution of 4-dimethylaminobenzaldehyde used in the eosindole reaction), Ehrlich's diazo reagent or reaction (involving diazotization and coupling of arylamines with sulfanilic acid), Ehrlich's triacid (acid fuchsin, orange G, and methyl green) stain (for dried-blood films), Armanni-Ehrlich degeneration (of Henle's loops in the diabetic kidney), Heinz-Ehrlich bodies (round refractile eosinophilic particles in mature erythrocytes in hemolytic anemia), and Ehrlich-Hata treatment (of syphilis with arsphenamine).

Ehrlich's near-encyclopedic achievements were not due to sheer genius alone, but also to the type of unremitting application which, very often is the 'mother' of genius. This is exemplified in his search for a germicide-impregnated arylaminodye that would specifically kill the syphilis spirochete, *Spirochaeta pallida*, discovered by Shaudinn in 1905. As a 'Gallic' or 'Neapolitan' disease, syphilis had been plaguing Europe at least since the end of the fifteenth century after the return of Columbus' expeditions to the New World. In this search, Ehrlich synthesized, tested, and then discarded the first 605 of such dyes, all ineffective, and found success with preparation No. 606, the arsenic-based Salvarsan. The science of specific targeting of drugs, now so critical to cancer chemotherapy with its bugbear of non specific cytotoxicity, was thus born. Even a tribe (*Ehrlichieae*) of the family *Rickettsiaceae* is named after him. In 1908, he shared with Elie Metchnikoff the Nobel Prize for medicine and physiology.

Before the present century, however, cancer chemotherapy was no more than an offshoot of other efforts. Some examples are the already-discussed Fowler's solution, Ehrlich's anti-syphilitic preparations, and Beatson's oophorectomy that foreshadowed hormonal therapy in some types of cancer. Indeed, the development of cancer chemotherapy into a science in its own right began during the Second World War, with recognition of the extreme vesicant and cytotoxic (particularly lymphocytotoxic) activities of certain war gases, notably the *bis* and *tris* β-chloroethylamines and the corresponding *bis* sulfide. The pioneers in this field were Americans, notably Alfred Gilman, Louis S. Goodman and Frederick S. Philips. Following the lifting of secrecy restrictions at the end of the war, Goodman *et al.* (1946) published their findings which showed that N-methyl-bis(2-chloroethyl)amine (nitrogen mustard, mechloramine, or HN2) was effective clinically against an X-ray-resistant lymphosarcoma. In consequence, literally hundreds of 'biological alkylating agents' have since been synthesized in the United States, Europe, and elsewhere. Many of these have been tested for antineoplastic activity in various experimental (initially transplanted tumour) systems, and some clinically; and many have been used as models in investigations of possible biochemical modes of action against target tissues. The responsible investigators included stalwarts such as C.P. Rhoads, J.H. Burchenal, D.A. Karnovsky, F.S. Philips, C.C. Stock, and K. Sugiura in the United States, G.M. Timmis, F. Bergel, and W.C.J. Ross in England, and G. Domagk in Germany. From this concerted effort came some of the alkylating drugs which are commonly used in cancer therapy, including phenylalanine mustard (*melphalan*), cyclophosphamide (*cytoxan*), chlorambucil (*Leukeran*), 1,4-dimethanesulfonoxybutane (*Myleran* or *busulphan*), triethylene melamine (*TEM*), triethylene thiophosphoramide (*thiotepa*), and the prototype HN2 and its N-oxide (*Nitromin*). Recollections of the early history of the mustards as neoplastic agents have been charmingly presented by Sugiura (1971).

The alkylating agents, however, were developed empirically. Their cytotoxicity is markedly nonspecific, being directed mainly at dividing cells such as those of the bone marrow and intestinal crypt, in addition to cancer cells. A less empiric approach was initiated in the United States in 1948, when Sidney Farber (1903–1973) and his associates showed that certain folic acid antagonists, synthesized and supplied by Yellapragada SubbaRow (1896–1948) and his group at Lederle Laboratories, produced temporary remissions in children's acute leukemia. The most impressive results were obtained with methotrexate (4-amino-N^{10}-methyl-pteroylglutamic acid), an agent which induces significant regressions of even metastatic trophoblastic cancers. Later effective use of actinomycin D with methotrexate in cases of methotrexate-resistant trophoblastic cancer has made this neoplasm one of the few impressive success stories in cancer chemotherapy.

Farber thus introduced a novel and, at the time heady principle into cancer chemotherapy. Attack was now directed at small building blocks of essential cellular macromolecules (proteins and nucleic acids) rather than, as for the alkylating agents, at functional groups in the macromolecules themselves. Folic acid (pteroylglutamic acid) is an essential growth factor which, through the action of folate reductase, produces first dihydrofolate and then tetrahydrofolate, from which are eventually derived compounds involved in the metabolic transfer of one-carbon units. The antagonists such as methotrexate, because of their fraudulent mimicry of the folate structure, can competitively inhibit the reductase action, the one-carbon transfer, and/or the synthesis of thymidylic and inosinic acids. They thus ultimately block biosynthesis of purines, pyrimidines, nucleic acids, and coenzymes. As expected, analogous types of antimetabolites (e.g. purine, pyrimidine, and glutamine antagonists) were soon introduced, such as 6-mercaptopurine, 5-fluoro uracil, and azaserine, with varying degrees of success. Unfortunately, the crucial problem with the efficacy of the antimetabolites in cancer chemotherapy, as it is with other agents in this discipline, is that of non-specificity. Both the normal and the neoplastic cells of the patient depend, qualitatively, upon the same basic mechanisms of macromolecular biosynthesis, and the quantitative differences which may arise are neither predictable nor great. In most cases, the inhibition which is introduced is largely irreversible, and this places stringent restrictions upon dosage regimens in order to minimize harmful side-effects resulting from normal-cell cytotoxicity. In one instance, at least, that of folate reductase inhibition, folinic acid or 'citrovorum factor' has been found to ameliorate the inhibitory effects so that, with proper precautions, the antifolate can be used in unusually small doses.

3.5.5 Summary and New Approaches: Retinoids, 'Norgamems', and other Inducers of Cancer-cell Maturation

Clinically or experimentally, how to kill cancer cells is no problem. Any cancer cell can be destroyed by any one of countless ways, e.g. by heat, hypothermia, osmotic shock, starvation, metabolic blockage, or cytotoxic drugs or radiation. The problem is how to deal with the cells effectively and selectively, i.e. without similarly affecting any of the normal cell populations in the patient. By definition, an effective drug is biologially active, so that selective activity must depend upon exploitation of some specific difference between the target cancer cells and the normal cells. In the absence of such a difference, unwanted side-effects become unavoidable. No such difference is known for human cancer cells (Chapter Nine, Section 9.2.5). Consequently, cytotoxic therapy devoid of dangerous side-effects is unknown in clinical oncology.

There are strong indications that a common feature of cancer cells is blockage of normal pathways towards terminal differentiation (Chapter Nine, Section 9.10.4). Accordingly, an alternative to cytotoxic therapy is induction of terminal differentiation e.g. by retinoids and other agents (Chapter Nine, Section 9.10.3). It has been claimed by Brugarolas and Gonsalvez (1980) that thiazolidine-4-carboxylic acid (thioproline) is a 'completely nontoxic' agent capable of inducing clinical remissions, sometimes 'completely', in patients with epidermoid carcinomas of the head, neck, or other sites, or with other solid cancers, e.g. of the breast, kidney, ovary, thyroid, and parotid gland. The remissions occurred without any signs (e.g. cytotoxicity, inflammatory infiltration, and/or tumour necrosis) of direct cell damage or increased host reactivity. The agent appeared to act by restoring the *nor*mal *orga*nization of the tumour cells' *mem*branes, giving rise to the name 'norgamem'. These are heady claims requiring confirmation and further exploration; but they do stress the importance, in normoneoplastic processes, of cellular interrelationships mediated by interactions at cellular surfaces (Chapter Nine, Section 9.6.4).

On current information, directed cellular maturation as a specific therapy of clinical cancer has a sound theoretical basis (Chapter Nine), but its practical efficacy remains to be established. In the meantime, common sense requires a continuing search for an exploitation of more effective cytotoxic remedies of both new and conventional types. This represents an active area, as variously reviewed in Pinedo (1979), e.g. by Connors for the alkylating agents; by Chabner for the antimetabolites; by Myers and by Crooke for the antibiotics; by Bender for the vinca alkaloids and epipodophyllotoxins; by Rozencweig and Heuson for the steroids; and by von Hoff *et al.* for the new and miscellaneous anticancer drugs.

3.6 Experimental Oncology

3.6.1 Introduction

The birth of experimental oncology was due to a combination of three major factors. The first of these was the attempts of some dedicated early-nineteenth-century clinicians to find out whether or not, in the words of the English surgeon, James Nooth, 'those persons who give their attendance to cancerous subjects' are 'liable to get this cruel disease by absorption, as has been too generally supposed'. The second was the attempts of some oncologists to establish whether or not cancer was transferable within or between species. Together, these undertakings gave rise to tumour transplantation, from which later developed *in vitro* propagation of cells and tissues from tumorous as well as normal sources. The transplantation and propagation have become two of the major subdisciplines of modern experimental oncology.

The third factor was a logical offshoot of the findings of human cancer epidemiology, particularly those of the earlier astute clinicians from Paracelsus to Rehn. This was the need to test the epidemiologically detected cancer-risk factors (such as coal tar and 'aniline' dyestuffs) for their carcinogenicity under controlled conditions, preferably in man but, for obvious practicality, in experimental organisms. This gave rise to a third major subdiscipline of experimental oncology, experimental carcinogenesis. Nowadays, experimental carcinogenesis utilizes intact organisms (animals, plants, and microorganisms) as well as various *in vitro* cultures of plant or animal (including human) origin.

Athough use of animals as models in biological studies dates back at least to the days of Aristotle, its use in oncology is of more recent origin. In 1908, Clunet in France initiated experimental radiation carcinogenesis by exposing rats to X-rays and noting the development of local sarcomas, a finding which was confirmed two years later by Marie *et al.*, also in France. In 1909 Ellerman and Bang in Denmark initiated experimental viral carcinogenesis by inducing viral tumours in chickens, a finding which was both confirmed and extended (by use of a different avian cell-free filtrate) by Peyton Rous (1910) in the United States. Initiation of experimental chemical carcinogenesis, however, proved more difficult. It was marked by many unsuccessful attempts until the scene of action moved out of Europe and into Japan.

Except for radiation oncology, the early history of which has already been discussed (Section 3.4.3), the salient features of the historical development of these various branches of experimental oncology are outlined below.

3.6.2 Transference and Transplantability

3.6.2.1 Interhuman Transference: Nooth and Others.

There is a growing disillusionment that stems from the failure of oncologists to devise a quick solution to the cancer problem, despite the unprecedented commitment of specialists and the public alike to the enterprise. This has sometimes resulted in the voicing of opinions to the effects that dedication is dwindling or dead, and that cancer research is rapidly becoming no more than a means of a comfortable livelihood for an ever-growing band of oncologists and others, i.e. that more people live off than die from cancer. However, the absolute dedication of oncologists to their most frustrating of callings is historic, as exemplified by the two following incidents. First, as recorded in the second edition of his *Observations on the Treatment of Scirrhous Tumours of the Breast* of 1806, James Nooth, the eminent British surgeon, wished to establish, as mentioned above, whether or not 'persons who give their attendance to cancerous subjects' are at risk of contracting the patient's disease by 'absorption'. He thus described his attempt to find out:

> The structure of scirrhous tumours, and the morbid state they are in when under examination, precludes a very nice or satisfactory investigation. Being anxious to know what effects this matter would produce, if inserted by inoculation into the arm of a healthy person (but not being entitled to make that experiment on any human being except myself), I conveyed a minute portion of it into a small incision on my arm; two hours afterwards I felt the part uneasy, with a strong pulsation. On the following day, it was more uneasy, and much more inflammation appeared than generally attends so small a wound inflicted by a sharp instrument; on the third, it remained nearly in the same state; on the fourth day the wound became easier, and the inflammation and pulsation began to subside. A few days afterwards a large dry scab was formed, which I removed, and found the sore perfectly healed. Not choosing to rely on a single experiment as a sufficient proof that a cancerous disposition could not be conveyed into the habit, I repeatedly in-

oculated myself from the year 1777, without ever producing any effects dissimilar to those in the first experiment. I am convinced, that those persons who give their attendance to cancerous subjects, are not so liable to get this cruel disease by absorption, as has been too generally supposed.

An experiment similar to that of Nooth was performed by Jean Louis Alibert (1728–1793), as described by Woglom (1913):

On October 17, 1808, at the Hospital de St. Louis, and in the presence of several physicians and students, Alibert allowed himself to be injected with ichorous material from a cancer of the breast. The experiment was performed at the same time upon M. Fayet, a medical student, and the next morning upon MM. Lonoble and Durand. Except for an inflammatory reaction the experiment was without sequelae. A week later, Alibert inoculated himself a second time, and his colleague, M. Biett. He himself escaped with a result similar to that which followed the first trial, but M. Biett developed a somewhat more severe infection, which involved the axillary and cervical lymph nodes.

3.6.2.2 Animal Recipients: Novinsky, Peyrilhe, and Others

The first of the recorded attempts to transfer cancer between species was that by the French chemist Bernard Peyrilhe. In 1775, he injected human cancerous material into a dog which soon suffered much pain in consequence and had to be destroyed. Other analogous attempts have uniformly failed, e.g. those by Guillaume Dupuytren in 1807, Conrad Lagenbeck in 1840 (Woglom, 1913), and Joseph Leidy in 1851; although Leidy found that the human breast cancer fragments which he had introduced under the skin of a frog had some five months later become vascularized and fibrotic.

The details of tumour transplantability have become generally recognized only within the past three decades. For example, it is subject to the limitations of classical graft-versus-host rejectability. It is likely to be successful when donor and recipient are syngeneic or otherwise histocompatible (e.g. animals of the same inbred strain); or when the recipient organism (e.g. an athymic mouse) or recipient body site (e.g. the hamster cheek pouch) is immunoincompetent. The historical origins of these details, however, are over a hundred years old. During 1875–76, the Russian veterinarian Mistislav Aleksandrovich Novinsky successfully transplanted pieces of two canine tumours, an invasive nasal carcinoma and a tumour of the uterus and vaginal vault, into puppies. In the puppies, the transplant grew and sometimes metastasized, giving rise to tumours which themselves were transplantable into other similar puppies. The trail blazed by Novinsky, who had been described as the 'Forefather of Experimental Oncology' by Shabad (1950), became increasingly well-trodden. In 1889, Arthur Nathan Hanau, a colleague of Conheim at Bonn, reported successful transplantations of metastatic vulvar epidermoid carcinomas between rats; and, in 1894, Henry Morau of Paris, reported analogously for mammary tumours between mice. In the United States, Leo Loeb (1869–1959), a German by birth, worked with rats and transplanted a thyroid carcinosarcoma through seven generations and a spindle cell sarcoma through 40 generations. With A.E.C. Lathrop, he also showed that, in mice, the occurrence of mammary cancer was familial in distribution, was increased by pregnancies, and was reduced by ovariectomy. In Denmark, Carl Oluf Jensen (1864–1934) propagated a mouse alveolar (probably breast) carcinoma through 19 generations, reported an inoculable rat sarcoma, and developed a variety of transplantable rodent-tumour lines which are still being used as standards throughout the world. Other transplantable tumours have since been described, e.g. by Paul Ehrlich in Germany and by E.F. Bashford in England. In 1959, Stewart *et al.* compiled a long list of the then available transplantable tumours. Today, transplantable tumours from man and animals are legion.

3.6.2.3 Propagation in Vitro: Murphy, Harrison, Earle, Gey, and Others. These examples of the great interest in tumour transplantability pay no more than just tribute to its obvious practical and theoretical implications which, as in Shabad's description of Novinsky, indeed mark its discovery as the inception of experimental oncology. The transplantability implies a considerable degree of autonomy of tumours which, therefore, may also grow under suitable *in vitro* conditions. The principle of tumour propagation *in vitro* was first demonstrated by the American James B. Murphy (1884–1950). In 1912, he reported the capacity of malignant rat tumours to grow in embryonated bird eggs. Other pioneers in this field, notably Alexis Carrel (1873–1944) and

Montrose T. Burrows (1884–1947) working at New York's Rockefeller Institute, began to grow tumour cells and tissues in long-term *in vitro* culture, with Burrows himself coining the now familiar term 'tissue culture'.

From such beginnings have grown the increasingly sophisticated techniques of today's *in vitro* culturing and continuous sub-culturing of predominanatly neoplastic cells and tissues from various species of organism including human. The prototype most extensively investigated of the many human neoplastic cell lines which are now available is the HeLa cell line. This line was first propagated by the American George Otto Gey (1899–1970) (cf. his Harvey Lectures of 1954–55), through culturing on roller tubes of a specimen from an agressive cervical cancer, now known to have been adenocarcinomatous. The name HeLa refers to the mysterious donor of the specimen, a Henrietta Lacks (or, perhaps Helen Lane or Helen Larson). The inestimable value of the culture techniques is that they allow detailed study, outside of the complexity of intact organisms, of selected cellular and other features of neoplasia, e.g. its morphology, immunology, virology, growth characteristics and requirements, and biochemistry including biosynthetic features and responsiveness or resistance to therapy. Another is that they permit sparing of the lives and averting of the sufferings of countless experimental animals. However, they also suffer from many disadvantages, due mainly to the artificiality introduced, to clonal selectivity, and to the loss of the complex controls which exist in the intact donor organisms. In consequence, the relevance to these organisms, whether man or mouse, of the *in vitro* results is highly variable and always debatable (Chapter Nine, Section 9.7).

Extension of the techniques, e.g. to comparative studies of neoplastic transformation by oncogens, required development of techniques for the analogous culturing of cells and tissues from normal sources. This latter activity was pioneered in 1907 by the American, Ross G. Harrison, who showed that developing nerve fibres survived for 'nearly four weeks' in simple cover-slip preparations. Later extensions of this discovery, notably by the Americans Gey (mentioned above) and Wilton Robert Earle (1902–1964), demonstrated two important principles of neoplasia. First, most normal cells and tissues, rather like their counterparts from epithelial cancers (carcinomas) do not grow well in culture. Those that do tend either to be embryonic *ab initio* or, having survived a 'crisis point' marked by extensive cell death, to acquire embryonic features during growth. This suggests that the capacity for host-independent growth, like so many features of neoplasia, is intrinsic to normal cells, is suppressed by the latter's maturation, and is re-expressible when there is breakdown of some appropriate component of the complex controls of the intact host. This principle, which suggests a close parallelism between embryogenesis and oncogenesis, is related to the second, i.e. that the induction of neoplastic transformation is not a prerogative of definable 'oncogens'. Thus, Earle's experiments showed that neoplastic transformation of cultured normal fibroblasts (from mice) could be due to the culturing alone, as well as to exposure to an added carcinogen (3-methyl-cholanthrene). This principle of the spontaneous neoplastic transformability of normal cells, including those which survive in artificial culture, is now well established and was observed from the very dawn of the era of tissue culture, i.e. not only by Earle but also by Gey working with rat fibroblasts.

3.5.2.4 Summary. The process of discovery, extension, and exploitation of the principles of tumour transference, transplantability, and *in vitro* culturing and subculturing was initiated at great personal risk to some of its more intrepid and dedicated initiators. The risk, however, was not in vain. Despite their limitations, the techniques which have been evolved in consequence are of inestimable value in the study of many types of tumour properties, individually, and in isolation from the complexity of intact organisms. Although the results which are thus obtained are not always extrapolatable to these organisms, they none the less provide many insights which are not obtainable by any other known means. Indeed, the discovery of tumour transplantability marked the beginning of the era of experimental oncology.

3.6.3 Chemicals and Cancer

3.6.3.1 Chemical Carcinogenesis: Yamagiwa and Ichikawa. Current epidemiological data leave little doubt that chemicals predominate among the known or suspected cancer-risk factors present in the human environment. This fact provides a measure of the import and impact, within the entire history of oncology, of the feat that initiated the era of experimental chemical carcinogenesis.

Through an Ehrlichian-type of patience and single-mindedness (cf. Section 3.5.4), this feat was performed in 1915, by two Japanese workers at Tokyo Imperial University: Katsusaburo Yamagiwa (1863–1930) and his veterinarian associate, Koichi Ichikawa (1888–1948). Every two or three days for over a hundred days, they painted a benzene solution of coal tar on the ears of 137 rabbits; and they continued to examine the animals regularly for any signs of tumour development. Eventually, they observed development of many local skin 'folliculoepitheliomas' and some invasive and metastatic carcinomas.

Jubilation followed, but with true Japanese-style humility and courteousness, Yamagiwa celebrated the triumph with the Japanese *haiku*: 'Cancer was produced. Proudly I walk a few steps.' The results were first published in a Japanese journal, but in German and as a dedication to Rudolph Virchow, who was Yamagiwa's mentor from 1891 to 1894. A more extended version appeared in English, in 1918.

Yamagiwa, the founder of Japanese cancer research, was the third son of a Samurai. From 1895 to his retirement in 1923, he was Professor of Oncology at the University. He was also founder of the Japanese Pathological Society, the Japanese Association for Cancer Research, and, in the tradition of his erstwhile mentor's *Virchow's Archiv*, the venerable Japanese Journal of Cancer Research, *Gann*. He received many honours; but, as sympathetically recounted by Henschen in 1968, he missed the 1925 Nobel Prize which was awarded, instead, to Fibiger for his controversial work on cockroaches and rat cancer.

This pioneer finding of coal-tar-induced cancer in rabbits was later widely confirmed and greatly extended to become one of today's major subdisciplines of experimental oncology. The spate of extensions was heralded by analogous findings in mice, made during 1918–19 by one of Yamagiwa's students, H. Tsutsui. Chemically-induced experimental neoplasms began to multiply all over the world of cancer research, and to become the experimental objects of choice. Test organisms and test agents also multiplied, as did attempts and successes in the field of isolation, purification, identification, and testing of the active principles of the complex mixtures which had been, and still kept on being, identified by epidemiology.

3.6.3.2 Coal Tar and Polycyclic Aromatic Hydrocarbons: Kennaway and Others. The pioneers in this the second stage in experimental chemical carcinogenesis were Ernest Laurence Kennaway (1881–1958), director of the Chester Beatty Research Institute in London, and his celebrated team of researchers at the Institute, notably J.W. Cook and I. Hieger. Using mainly fluorescence spectroscopy for purposes of identification, these workers isolated small amounts of certain polycyclic aromatic hydrocarbons (PAHs) from vast quantities (sometimes tons at a time) of gas-works pitch. One of these isolated compounds was benzo(a)pyrene, which has already become both the most widely-investigated and the supreme archetype of all known PAH-type experimental carcinogens. Kennaway and his team also established the chemical structure of benzo(a)pyrene, through chemical synthesis and other means, and its pronounced capacity to induce skin tumours in mice. Another was 1,2,5,6-di-benz-anthracene, which was shown to be a weak skin carcinogen in mice (Cook *et al.*, 1932).

3.6.3.3 Polycyclic Aromatic Hydrocarbons and Structure-activity Relationships: Cook, Fieser, the Pullmans, and Buu-Hoi. The third major stage in the growth of experimental chemical carcinogenesis was the synthesis of a large number of structural analogues of the coal-tar-derived carcinogenic PAHs, with the object of investigating structure-activity relationships. The notable pioneers at this stage were Kennaway and his team, with Cook leading the way this time (Cook and Kennaway, 1940); Louis Frederick Fieser, the celebrated organic chemist, and his team in the United States (Fieser, 1938); and, in particular, the Pullmans and Nguyen Phuc Buu-Hoi (1915–1972) in France. Over 1,000 scientific publications are credited to Buu-Hoi (Arcos, 1972), a celebrated master by profession and a prince by birth.

Sadly, this then well-conceived enterprise later proved quite fruitless relative to its original intent. It has now become clear that correlation between chemical structure and biological activity, a reality in some cases in pharmacology, is well-nigh impossible in oncology in which the true extent of the already-known multiplicity of dominant variables is yet to be determined. Thus, for perhaps any given 'carcinogen', the 'carcinogenic potency' can vary from zero to very high on the basis of host-related variables alone, e.g. of differences in species, strain, age, sex, or immunological, disease, or nutritional state.

The fourth stage in the growth of the discipline was also doomed to failure. This stage was based upon the notion that carcinogenesis is due to errors (inborn, acquired, or induced) in metabolism of the commonest natural body substance that bears a structural resemblance to the carcinogenic PAHs, i.e. cholesterol. It began with the discovery, by Wieland and Dane in 1933, that the experimental carcinogen 20-methyl-cholanthrene can be produced by chemical means from natural bile acids. This finding was later confirmed by others, e.g. by the above-mentioned Cook's and Fieser's groups of workers. Also, as recently as 1972, Black and Douglas showed that the ubiquitous cholesterol can be oxidized into cholesterol α-oxide in the system represented by the ultraviolet-irradiated human skin. The oxide is an experimental carcinogen; and the system participates in two related phenomena. These are: the natural biosynthesis of vitamin D_3 (the mediator of gut calcium absorption, bone calcium metabolism, and probably, muscle activity) from its precursor 7-dehydrocholesterol, a biosynthesis which can also be effected by the irradiation alone; and the development of skin cancers in association with the inherited genetic disorder xeroderma pigmentosum. Despite all this, appreciation of the carcinogenic propensities of the great variety of cholesterol-unrelated agents has dealt a death blow to the notion. Indeed, recent epidemiological studies have associated hypercholesterolemia with decreased risk of noncardiovascular mortality, inclusive of mortality from cancers of the colon and other sites in men.

3.6.3.4 Dyestuffs and Arylamines: Yoshida and Others. In contrast with the fate of the third and fourth stages, that of the fifth stage was a continuing prosperity, albeit one diluted with the imponderables of extrapolation from the experimental to the clinical. This fifth stage was the extension of the type-structure of experimental carcinogens beyond that of the PAHs. Just as Pott's discovery of chimney-soot scrotal cancer in 1775 stimulated experimental carcinogenesis by PAHs, Rehn's discovery of 'aniline' bladder cancer over a century later stimulated experimental carcinogenesis by arylamino dyestuffs and their synthetic intermediates and related arylamines. The latter endeavour, which benefited from the then extant experiences with the former, was initiated in Japan during 1933–35 by Tomizu Yoshida (1903–1974), of the 'Yoshida sarcoma' fame. With T. Sasaki and others, Yoshida showed that several arylaminoazo-type dyestuffs, but *o*-aminoazotoluene in particular, produced hepatocarcinomas in rats fed diets containing the agents. In rapid succession, R. Kinoshita confirmed the marked hepatocarcinogenicity of *o*-aminoazotoluene in rats; and C.J. Kensler showed the capacity of dietary factors, notably riboflavin, to influence, apparently through detoxification, the hepatocarcinogenic responses.

Two earlier results with the related dye, Scarlet Red, are noteworthy. This fat stain is synthesized from diazotized *o*-aminoazotoluene coupled with alkaline 2-naphthol, and is a stimulator of wound healing in man and animals. Despite its healing capacity, it was shown, in Germany, to produce local atypical 'conditional' (regressing, after cessation of treatment) and other lesions, through injection, in rabbit's ears; and also benign hepatomas, through feeding, in mice. These results have sometimes (e.g. Shimkin, 1977) been interpreted to have foreshadowed the aminoazodye carcinogenesis performed by Yoshida.

Later extensions of experimental arylamine carcinogenesis have delineated with few exceptions, certain basic requirements for this process to become evident. The amino group must be present, be at least mono-unsubstituted or be capable of becoming so *in vivo* (e.g. by metabolic *N*-demethylation of agents such as 4-dimethylaminoazobenzene), be para-substituted, and be activated *in vivo* apparently almost exclusively by metabolic *N*-hydroxy-esterification. Further, the test animal must be susceptible to the carcinogenesis.

Most of these requirements can be illustrated by certain post-Yoshida developments stemming from Rehn's original discovery of 'aniline' cancers (reviewed by Manson, 1976). Aniline is neither para-substituted nor known to be a human or an experimental carcinogen. This contrasts with the aromatic amines such as 2-naphthylamine, benzidine, magenta (fuchsin), auramine, and 4-aminobiphenyl (xenylamine), all of which are para-substituted and cancer risk factors. The aniline suspected by Rehn to have been a human carcinogen was probably an impure mixture with varying amounts of xylidines, toluidines, naphthylamines, and xenylamine and its monomethyl derivatives. The requirement for host susceptibility is illustrated by Rehn's observation of bladder cancer in man and Yoshida's observation of liver cancer in rats. Also, epidemiological studies by Case and others carried out among workers in the British rubber, chemical and dyestuff, pigment and paint, and allied industries, identified 2-naphthylamine as the major culprit (cf. Case, 1956). However, extensive species related studies of experimental carcinogenesis by this agent in dogs and a wide range of other animal species have yielded evidence for significant bladder carcinogenicity only in dogs, rarely in hamsters and monkeys, and not at all in rats or mice. In mice, hepatomas or sarcomas are produced instead.

3.6.3.5 Acetylaminofluorene: Wilson, the Weisburgers, and the Millers. Another chemical carcinogen of much historical and current interest is 2-acetylaminofluorene (AAF). AAF was intended for use as an insecticide in the United States, and was patented in 1940, but never used, for this purpose. This was because, in 1941, Robert H. Wilson and his associates in the United States showed that continuous AAF feeding to rats produced multiple neoplasms, mainly of the liver, lung, kidney, bladder, and pelvis. Particularly in the hands of the Weisburgers (John Hans and Elizabeth K.) and the Millers (James Alexander and Elizabeth) in the United States, AAF became one of the most important of model compounds for the study of metabolism and other aspects of biochemical mechanisms in experimental chemical carcinogenesis (Chapter Nine, Section 9.5).

3.6.3.6 Aflatoxins, Turkeys, and Trout: Jenkins, Wogan, and Others. Other well-investigated and important experimental carcinogens include the aflatoxins, i.e. mycotoxins produced by *Aspergillus flavus*. This fungus commonly contaminates animal feeds stored under warm and humid conditions. It achieved great notoriety in 1961, when it was held responsible for two epizootic outbreaks. One of these resulted in the death of thousands of British turkeys and other poultry from hepatic necrosis, and the other in the loss of even more thousands of American trout from various causes including hepatomas. That the responsible agents were the aflatoxins, mainly aflatoxin B_1 (AFB_1), was soon shown experimentally by various groups in England, the United States and elsewhere. Later studies have shown that some of the biosynthetic precursors of AFB_1, i.e. versicolorin A and sterigmatocystin, are also carcinogenic in trout and other susceptible species (Terao, 1978;Hendricks *et al.*, 1980).

Even more significantly than the above, aflatoxin B_1 has become causally associated with human hepatoma. In this outcome, particularly in West Africa, the agent acts in combination with hepatitis B, the latter probably as a cocarcinogen (Larouze *et al.*, 1977). Among humans, even West Africans, the occurrence of hepatoma is rare in comparison with exposure to aflatoxins and hepatitis B. This suggests that the disease occurs in those exposed individuals who are more hepatoma-susceptible, perhaps genetically, than is the general population. Analogous situations are numerous, e.g. those provided by the risk of lung cancer posed by tobacco smoke (Section 3.4.2.6), the risk of esophageal cancer posed by tobacco smoke and alcohol (Section 3.4.2.7), and the risks of mesothelioma and bronchogenic carcinoma posed by tobacco smoke and asbestos (Section 3.4.2.8). Among other species of organism, these risks may be quite different, as exemplified by cycasin.

3.6.3.7 Cycasin: Laqueur and Others. Another important naturally-occurring carcinogen is cycasin. As reported by Gert L. Laqueur and his colleagues during the 1960s (Laqueur *et al.*, 1963, 1967), cycasin is an inactive glycoside of the active agent methylazomethanol (MAM), the aglycone MAM being released by the action of a bacterial β-glycosidase. Cycasin occurs in the cycad (*C. circinalis*) nut meal eaten by the natives of Guam among whom certain neurologic disorders are unusually frequent. However, cycasin fed to non-germfree rats, or MAM or its synthetic accetate fed to germfree rats, produced no neurological symptoms but, instead, cancers of the liver, kidney, and intestinal tract.

3.6.3.8 Bracken Fern: Pamukcu and Others. Bracken fern, another important carcinogen of natural occurrence, was shown by A.M. Pamukcu of Turkey and his associates (Pamukcu, 1963; Pamukcu *et al.*, 1972) to be responsible for the type of enzootic hematuria which is a symptom of urinary bladder cancer occurring in cattle along the Black Sea area of Turkey. Bracken feeding produces intestinal and urinary tract cancers in rats, but leukemias and pulmonary tumours in mice.

3.7 Summary and Outlook

As outlined in Chapters Two and Three the history of cancer depicts a heroic international attempt to understand the intrinsic nature and to pinpoint the extrinsic causes of human cancer, with the specific purposes to treat and prevent the disease. In both of these enterprises, the direct observations on humans (e.g. by epidemiology) have been supplemented by the indirect studies in various experimental systems. In both also, some progress has been made, but this has remained dwarfed by the problems which remain unresolved. Neither the intrinsic nature nor the true cause of cancer is properly known, and the modest therapeutic successes of the 1940s and 1950s have not been significantly improved upon.

The attempts to pinpoint the extrinsic causes of human cancer have depicted the human environment as a rampant sea of carcinogens. Around the mid-1950s, the focus of carcinogenesis testing was diverted from random 'off-the-shelf' chemicals to certain broad structural types, mainly aromatic amines, nitrosamines, nitrosamides, diazo-compounds, and polycyclic aromatic hydrocarbons. Up to this time, i.e. the period of random testing, some 24 per cent of all the tested compounds were found to be carcinogenic in one or another of the few species or strains of experimental animals in common use. Thus, in the first volume of the *Survey of Compounds Which Have Been Tested for Carcinogenic Activity* (United States Public Health Service Publications No. 49), published in 1941, some 169 of the approximately 696 compounds tested (24 per cent) were active. The second volume, published in 1951, also gave the same percentage (322 compounds found active of 1,329 tested). Even when the period of non-random testing (i.e. after the mid-1950s) is also taken into account, the corresponding value is about 13 per cent. Thus, the combined data from the first seven volumes of the above-mentioned *Survey* and from other published sources up to 1979 show carcinogenic activity for some 1,000 compounds from approximately 7,500 tested. It is a fair estimate that over five million synthetic chemicals have been introduced over the past hundred years (Chapter Nine, Section 9.3.1), not to mention those due to factors such as industrial and vehicular partial combustion processes. Thus, by random testing, over one million new carcinogens, and over 600,000 by the combined random and nonrandom testing, would have been added to the environment during the past hundred years. Moreover, it is impossible to define any substance as a *noncarcinogen* by the criterion of testing in animals, since there can be no certainty that such a substance will not be active in a so-far untried test system. Finally, the combined data from the experimental and the human epidemiological studies have also implicated, among others, sunlight and other radiation, dietary factors, sexual and reproductive factors, and viruses and other microorganisms. This depiction of the human environment as a carcinogenic sea existing even from before the origin of the human species must be as difficult to accept as it raises the question as to how the species managed to survive and prosper as it has.

In the face of such a dilemma, the first line of defence must be common sense precautions. This approach is best illustrated by the combined wisdom from three sources, two in ancient history, and the third source in the American Cancer Society. The first source must be the Buddha, with his doctrine of common sense moderation in panderings to the crass desires of the physical body, and of due obedience to the universal laws of natural interrelationships.

The second source must be John Hill (Section 3.4.2.6.2). In 1761, in his paper entitled *Cautions Against the Immoderate Use of Snuff*, Hill wrote these rare words of wisdom:

Whether or not polypusses [cancers], which attend snuff-takers, are absolutely caused by that custom: or whether the principles of the disorder were there before, and Snuff only irritated the parts, and hastened the mischief, I shall not pretend to determine: but even supposing the latter to be the case, the damage is certainly more than the indulgence is worth; for who is to say that the Snuff is not the absolute cause, or that he has not the seeds of such disorder which Snuff will bring into action . . . no man should venture upon Snuff who is not sure that he is not so far liable to cancer: and no man can be sure of that.

The common sense in these two examples from history has been itemized in recent times in more specific, albeit more restricted, terms by the American Cancer Society, the third source. The Society's 'CAUTION' advises a constant individual look-out for one or more of seven readily-detectable signals of possible cancer. Such signal(s), if discovered, should be immediately followed by appropriate medical consultation. The signals are: *C*hange in bowel or bladder habits; *A* sore throat that does not heal; *U*nusual discharge or bleeding; *T*hickening or lump in breast or elsewhere; *I*ndigestion or difficulty in swallowing; *O*bvious change in wart or mole; and *N*agging cough or hoarseness. This advice is not meant to create alarm, since none of the signals necessarily means the presence of cancer. Precisely this feature, the fact that nothing short of the actual diagnosis of manifest cancer positively identifies the disease, is the prime cause of the problem having remained, from times immemorial, almost as intractable as it ever was. Increasingly, cancer is being seen as a problem of inherited genes and their control, whether or not under the influence of exogenous agent(s), i.e. as the identical problem of normal biological transmission and development. In both of these problems, the body hormones, the subject of the next chapter, play a controlling role.

4 HORMONES AND CANCER

4.1 Introduction: The Growth and Significance of Oncologic Endocrinology

For several reasons, an appropriate discussion of endocrinology represents the ideal transition from the yesterday to the today of oncology. First, modern endocrinology can be seen as a gradual development from the various humoralistic doctrines of ancient times (Chapter Two). It is true that the presumed cause of cancer in these doctrines, most notably the *atrabilis* of Greece, cannot be equated with any particular hormone or any other humoral factor known to modern biology. However, the attempted disproofs of the persistent doctrine of atrabilism led to the alternative humoralistic doctrines (e.g. those based upon iatrochemicals, solidistic and fluid lymph, and blastema) that culminatd in the 'oestrin', 'progynon', and other crude hormonal preparations of the early twentieth century and, eventually, in the complex endocrinology of today. Currently, there is increasing recognition of the exquisite interdependence, based upon feedback controls, that operate within the body's endocrine systems, e.g. the system comprising the hypothalamus, pituitary, adrenal cortex, and germinal glands (ovary and testis) in the control of sexual and reproductive development and function. With this recognition, it does not seem too far-fetched that some of the neurohypophyseal, adrenomedullary catecholamino, and steroidal hormones may play roles in the development of the type of melancholy which, from the days of Galen, through those of Theodoric of the thirteenth century with his 'melancholy' cancers, to even later times, was generally believed to predispose to cancer, mainly of the female breast (Chapter Two, Section 2.4.5). This belief is not too far removed from the modern notion that psychosomatic stress, which is mediated biochemically (though not necessarily caused) by noradrenaline and other hormones, can predispose to some forms of cancer as well as to cardiovascular disease, gastric ulcers, and other maladies (Chapter One, Section 1.1).

Second, endogenous hormones are increasingly being recognized to play a major role in normal development. The estrogens, for instance, are responsible for features as diverse as the control of development and maintenance of the female sex organs, and the regulation of the menstrual cycle in primates and of the estrus cycle in other mammals. (For recent reviews, see Lingeman, 1979; IARC Monographs No. 21, 1979; Brooks, 1983). They markedly influence the functioning of the hypothalamus, that part of the brain stem which regulates the release of luteinizing hormone releasing hormone (LHRH) that controls the episodic secretion of follicle stimulating hormone (FSH) and luteinizing hormone (LH). They also influence the secretion, binding, and/or functioning of other vital agents. Among the latter are premenopausal pituitary adrenocorticotropic hormone (ACTH), resulting in influences upon synthesis of steroid hormone precursors by the zona reticularis; plasma transcortin, resulting in influences upon protein-bound plasma cortisol and, hence, upon corticotrophin secretion, plasma cortisol level, and immune status; plasma prolactin, resulting in influences upon breast development and lactation; and plasma sex hormone binding globulin, resulting in influences upon binding and transport of estradiol and testosterone. Even the effects of androgens within the central nervous system, a major site of action of these hormones, appear to be mediated by estrogens formed from the androgens through the action of aromatase. The androgens not only control development of, and maintain, the typically male features (e.g. testis, seminal vesicle, prostate, and male peculiarities of body shape and texture, hair distribution, and voice) but also are anabolic. In females, they stimulate hypertrophy of the clitoris. Estrogens and androgens are thus essential components of the normal hormonal environment, in which they occur in low levels in males and females respectively. The principal ovarian androgen in young women is androstenedione, with testosterone itself being a less major component. Postmenopausally, the ovary normally involutes and ceases estrogen production, but it continues to produce androgens, accounting for the hirsutism and certain other male features developed by some postmenopausal women, and for the use of postmenopausal hormonal replacement therapy.

The progestins, however, appear to be basically female. Among other effects, they prepare the uterus for implantation, and maintain pregnancy. The major progestin, progesterone, reaches its highest concentration in ovarian blood during the luteal phase, when substantial amounts of estrogens and other steroids are also secreted. Progesterone is a potent anti-estrogen, capable of inhibiting estrogenic effects such as secretion of the fertile type of mucus at mid-cycle, release of prolactin by the pituitary (thus inhibiting lactation), release of LH at mid-cycle, and, at high progestin levels, release of FSH. The body's hormones thus appear to be the prime controllers of gene expression during practically all stages of development from gametogenesis to death. As such, they are particularly evident in what may well be the major if not the sole drive or purpose (depending upon viewpoint) in mammalian evolution, i.e. survival and diversification of inherited genes through sexual reproduction. Fathoming of the nature, extent, and mechanisms of this control is only at its beginning. For instance, it is only now being appreciated that, contrary to textbook dogma, direct interaction between a specific hormone-receptor complex (e.g. that formed between a steroid hormone and its 8S cytosolic receptor which then dissociates into the 4S-5S form) and the cell's nucleus is not confined to the case of the non-polypeptide (e.g. steroidal) hormones. Neither are the cell-surface hormone receptors confined to those for the polypeptide hormones. Prolactin, for instance, has been found in the cell's nucleus, and steroid receptors on its surface; signifying that the cell's use of its activated second messenger system in response to hormonal stimulation may not be exclusive to any one type of hormone. Further, even a single hormone acting on a single cell may have a quite different temporal effect upon the different proteins whose expressions the hormone controls. (For a review, see Campbell and Craig, 1979.)

In view of such important natural roles for hormones, the third reason can hardly come as a surprise. This is that hormones have long been recognized to influence both the development and the regression of neoplasia (Table 4.1). Of course, this dual role is shared by nonhormones such as radiation, cyclophosphamide, and certain agents used in cancer chemotherapy. However, the hormones possess a unique combination of additional features related to the fact that they are natural body components specifically evolved to act upon susceptible cells and tissues in highly specific ways, e.g. in the control of menstruation, pregnancy, lactation, muscular activity, nervous activity, and differentiation. The first clear indications of this dual role of hormones in neoplasia were provided by Ramazzini in 1700

(Chapter Three, Section 3.4.2.2) and by Beatson in 1896 (Chapter Three, Section 3.5.2). Ramazzini's observation of a high incidence of breast cancer among Italian nuns was confirmed in 1842, by his fellow Italian, Rigoni-Stern (Chapter Three, Section 3.4.6), who also extended the observation to other unwed (presumably childless) women. The implied principle, that deprivation of pregnancy hormones can precipitate the development of breast cancer, contrasts with that in Beatson's demonstration of the capacity of ovarian hormone deprivation (by oophorectomy) to aid regression of breast cancer. Analogously, deprivation of testicular hormones (by orchidectomy) was found by White in 1904 to aid regression of prostatic hypertrophy in dogs, and by Huggins and Hodges in 1941 to aid regression of prostatic neoplasia in men (Table 4.1). Ramazzini's discovery might have been the result of chance observation; but Beatson was investigating Schinzinger's suggestion, made in 1889, that oophorectomy might help women with breast cancer. Even earlier, in 1836, Cooper had reported fluctuations in the proliferation of breast cancer during different phases of the menstrual cycle.

In recent years, this dual role of hormones in neoplasia has been debated, confirmed, and extended. Overall, there is little doubt that skilful manipulations of the body's endocrinology hold out a beacon of hope in the management of certain forms of neoplastic and other conditions. However, in oncology, as its history well documents, no real gain ever comes cheaply. With the widespread and increasing endocrine manipulations, the accumulating reports of direct or indirect hormonal involvements in the development of neoplastic and other complications are pinpointing a major cause for concern. These manipulations are aimed, among others, at contraception, induction of ovulation in anovulatory or oligoovulatory women (e.g. by use of clomiphene citrate, which is also used in oligospermic men), muscle-building (cf. anabolic steroids), cancer therapy, enhanced food production, and relief of undesired pregnancy and menopausal symptoms. Oral contraceptives, which are now among the most widely-used of hormonal devices, increase mortality, particularly among women aged over 35 years, from complications such as embolism, and pulmonary, coronary, and cerebral thrombosis (Inman and Vessey, 1968). In such women, particularly those who cannot tolerate oral contraceptives, intra-abdominal implantation of estradiol has been used and recommended as an alternative con-

Table 4.1: Some Landmarks in the History of Hormones and Cancer

1700, 1713	Ramazzini found high frequency of breast cancer in nuns
1842	Ramazzini's finding confirmed, and extended to other unmarried women, by Rigoni-Stern
1896	Beatson reported improvement in clinical breast cancer following oophorectomy
1904	White found castration to improve prostatic hypertrophy in dogs
1905	First recognition of ovarian hormones, by Marshall and Jolly, through observation of estrus induced by ovarian extracts in spayed dogs
1916	Lathrop and Loeb reported early castration to prevent spontaneous mammary cancer development in mice
1923	Isolation, purification, and structural elucidation of steroidal ovarian hormones initiated by Allen; later greatly extended by Gardner and others
1929	Doisy et al. obtained 'folliculin' (estrone) from urine of pregnant women
1932	Folliculin shown by Lacassagne to induce mammary cancer in male mice
1938	Dodds et al. introduced diethylstilbestrol (DES) and reported estrogenic activity of several synthetic nonsteroidal compounds, notably DES
1938, 1939	Suntzeff et al. (1938) and Gardner and Allen (1939) reported malignant and nonmalignant lesions in vagina and cervix of mice treated with estrogens including DES, or with estrogens and androgens together
1939	Lewis prescribed DES for estrogen replacement in ovariectomized women
1940 onwards	Li and his associates isolated, purified, chemically characterized, and investigated the growth regulatory functions of most of the known polypeptide hormones of the anterior pituitary
1941	The International Agency for Cancer Research reported commercial production of DES, and Huggins and Hodges reported beneficial effects of DES and castration in treatment of clinical prostatic cancer
1944	Biskind and Biskind reported carcinogenesis in rats due to induced hormonal imbalance
1946	Smith et al. advocated DES for treatment of 'high-risk' pregnancies in women
1946 onwards	Cantarow and his colleagues demonstrated the capacity of endocrine factors to influence experimental carcinogenesis by chemicals such as acetylaminofluorene
1947	The United States permitted DES implants in poultry for 'caponization'
1948	The United States prohibited DES residues in edible tissues

1950s	Muhlbock and his associates showed capacity of pituitary isografts in mice to produce mammary tumours in absence of the murine mammary tumour virus
1954	The United States permitted DES in beef-cattle feeds, at level of 10 mg DES/head/day
1955	The United States permitted DES implants in ears of beef cattle
1958	The United States' 'Delaney Clause' prohibited food additives with carcinogenic activity
1959	The United States prohibited DES implants in poultry
1962	The United States amended the Delaney Clause to allow use of potential carcinogens in animal feed providing their residues are undetectable in meat from the animals
1968	Symmers reported mammary cancer in transsexuals after hormonal and surgical attempts to correct their primary and secondary sexual anomalies
1970, 1971	Herbst and Scully (1970) and Herbst *et al.* (1971) reported vaginal carcinoma in daughters of women treated with DES during pregnancy
1972	British Committee on Safety of Medicines reported liver tumours in rats treated with oral contraceptive steroidal components
1973	Baum *et al.* reported hepatocellular neoplasms in women using oral contraceptives
1973-1976	In succession, the United States banned use of DES in food animals, overruled the ban in the Court of Appeals, requested its restoration in the Senate, and proposed withdrawal of the New Animal Drug Applications for DES published in the Federal Register
1975	Lyon, Smith *et al.*, and Ziel and Finkle independently reported increased risk of endometrial cancer among women using sequential oral contraceptives and other exogenous estrogens

Note: For detailed references, see Lingeman, 1979; Iacobelli *et al.*, 1980.

traceptive (Emperaire and Greenblatt, 1969; Nezhat *et al.*, 1980).

In general, an appropriate discussion of endocrinology would span the major developments in oncologic thought and practice from the mists of recorded human history to the present. Oncologic endocrinology would be seen as a painful growth from the ancient humoralistic doctrines to the modern concepts of the cell as biology's basic unit, and of the human cell, with its endowment of chromatin and DNA structured into nucleosomes and expressed, perhaps mainly under the direction of hormones, by means of splicing and other mechanisms. Hormonal inadequacies or disturbances would be seen as direct or indirect means of development if not causation not only of cancer as a biological growth but also of the worst (paraneoplastic) effects of the disease, e.g. cachexia, its wasting syndrome. They would also be seen as outcomes of some intrinsic error, e.g. in gene structure or control, or of some error induced by exogenous 'carcinogenic' agents which may be related to dietary, smoking, industrial, or other human practices. Above all, neoplasia would be seen as a question of gene control, the fundamental biochemical process in all development biology. (Some recent books on hormones and cancer: Menon and Reel, 1976; Iacobelli *et al.*, 1980; Leavitt, 1982; Lupulescu, 1983).

4.2 Hormones in Tumour Development, and Some Related Features

4.2.1 The Role of Practices Related to Sex and Reproduction

It is becoming increasingly clear that many of the body's hormones are associated with the etiology and growth of a variety of neoplasms. Among these hormones are estrogens, androgens, progestins, glucocorticoids, insulin, prolactin, and peptide growth factors. Among the neoplasms are leukemia, lymphoma, breast cancer, prostatic cancer, endometrial cancer, and apparently also malignant melanoma, osteogenic sarcoma, and renal cell carcinoma. (For reviews, see various articles in Iacobelli *et al.*, 1980).

In neoplastic development, the natural hormones of the body have long been suspected to be capable of producing a dual effect, increasing the neoplastic susceptibility of one tissue while decreasing that of another. Thus, in early nineteenth-century Germany, Elias von Siebold (1775–1826) reported a high

frequency of uterine cancer among women with multiple pregnancies, difficult labour, and leukorrhea. In a more recent and
carefully-conducted epidemiological study in the United States,
Isadore David Rotkin showed in 1962 that early coitus and
multiple sex partners are associated with increased risk of cervical
cancer. However, in a similar American study, Brian MacMahon
et al. showed in 1973 that early full-term pregnancy and multiple
births are associated with decreased risk of breast cancer, a finding
which is comparable with that of Ramazzini's, made in 1700 (cf.
above; see also Chapter Three, Section 3.4.2.2).

The clear implication of these findings, i.e. that similar practices
associated with procreation can increase the risk of one type of
gynecological cancer but decrease that of another, has been widely
confirmed. However, why this should be so is less clear. If
adherence to the naturally evolved laws of procreation reduces the
cancer risk of the breast epithelium, perhaps by somehow
'priming' the latter for its intended mammalian function, why
should this same practice increase the cancer risk of the cervical
epithelium? Perhaps the latter outcome is a penalty for promis-
cuity, but it remains problematical whether or not factors such as
infective herpesvirus(es) and carcinogens in promiscuous (i.e.
multiple) smegma contribute to the cancer-predisposing disturbances of the cervical epithelium.

4.2.2 Hormonal Influences upon Dietary and Other Cancer-risk Factors

The situation depicted by the hormonally related human cancer-
risk factors is quite complex. Such factors include not only those
practices related to sex and reproduction which can cause serious
hormonal disturbance, but also a variety of other agents. Among
the latter are dietary fat, other exogenous chemicals, radiation,
and, controversially, lactation, obesity, and nutritional status.
Variously, the development of cancers of hormone-sensitive
organs, mainly of the breast, ovary, endometrium, and prostate,
may be affected by such factors. The subject has been extensively
reviewed (e.g. Hirayama, 1978; Miller, 1978; Lipsett, 1979;
Graham, 1980; McMichael, 1980).

Dietary fat as an important determinant of breast cancer risk in
humans, particularly animal-derived fat, has been substantiated by
various types of epidemiological studies. These have included
geographical comparisons (Armstrong and Doll, 1975), migrant

studies (Buell, 1973), and retrospective case-control studies (Nomura *et al.*, 1978; Welsch, 1978). A favourite comparison in these studies has been that between the relative risks of breast cancer in Japan (low risk), and the United States (high risk, high-fat intake). Broadly, this has shown the difference in the risks to be most prominent among postmenopausal women, with the Japanese women showing both the lower risk and the better post-treatment prospects than their American counterparts. Other than any genetic or ethnic differences, this result would implicate the endocrine-related characteristics of the postmenopausal period, e.g. reduced plasma estrogen levels and absence of repro-ductive cycles (Cooke, 1976). It would also encourage veganism (abstention from all foods of animal origin) or, at the least, vegetarianism (as veganism, but without abstention from dairy products). However, although these practices may reduce the risk of breast cancer, they may mimic pernicious anemia in producing a deficiency of vitamin B_{12} (Murphy, 1981).

Studies in laboratory animals, mainly strains of rats and mice which are peculiarly susceptible to spontaneous and induced mammary neoplasia (cf. Chapter Five), have consistently shown that high intake of dietary fat markedly promotes development of the disease, e.g. in Fischer, Long-Evans, and Sprague-Dawley rats (Chan and Dao, 1981; also for other examples and references). In this, polyunsaturated fats or fatty acids are more effective than their saturated counterparts. The mechanism involved is unclear, but it seems that the high-fat diet stimulates pituitary secretion of prolactin, a promoter of experimental breast neoplasia, but not ovarian secretion of estrogen. This effect is seen particularly during the characteristic afternoon of proestrus peak, resulting in chronic, periodic increases in the prolactin-to-estrogen ratio (Chan *et al.*, 1975). The high-fat diet may also stimulate extragonadal estrogen production, as has been clearly demonstrated in ovariectomized Sprague-Dawley rats (Cohen *et al.*, 1981). How-ever, in women, although high dietary fat-induced increase in serum prolactin has been demonstrated (Hill and Wynder, 1976), the precise role of this hormone in the development of mammary neoplasia remains unclear (Nagasawa, 1979). The different physiological activities of the hormone may be associated with the prolactin molecule and its specific parts; and they may thus be dependent upon its synthetic and subsequent metabolic (e.g. hydrolytic) fates within the complex of the hormonal biochemistry in individual organisms. Thus, its mitogenic and lactation-stimulating activities are due, respectively, to a specific peptide portion and the entire structure of pituitary prolactin (Mittra, 1980).

The complex operation of the hormonally related cancer-risk factors is further illustrated by the experimental observation that factors other than prolactin (Ip *et al.*, 1980) enhance mammary tumorigenesis, e.g. by dimethylbenz[a]anthracene, in rats on high-fat diets. One of these factors is selenium (Ip and Sinha, 1981). Selenium, particularly in association with vitamin E, is a potent inhibitor of endogenous lipid peroxidation (Hoekstra, 1975; Griffin, 1979). Hence, when present in sufficient amounts in such experiments, it may act partly by also inhibiting the metabolic oxidative activation of the administered exogenous chemical carcinogens (cf. Chapter Nine). In current thinking, the role of the endogenous hormones in such experiments is at the level of tumour promotion rather than at tumour initiation (but see below).

Among other factors involving the body's hormones in cancer development in humans are male circumcision and female lactation. These, respectively, are associated with reduced risk of cancer of the cervix (among women with circumcised male sexual partners) and breast, but not without controversy. According to MacMahon *et al.* (1970), for instance, 'it is unlikely that lactation has any protective effect against breast cancer in women'. However, female breast cancer is rare among Canadian Eskimos who, despite their high consumption of animal-derived diets, commonly lactate continuously between ages 17 and 50 years (Schaefer, 1969). Further, the incidence of breast cancer has been rising among modern young women showing a tendency to fewer pregnancies and hence to reduced lactation; and it has been observed to decrease in numerous studies of lactating animals. Such considerations have led Cohen and Dix (1981) to conclude that lactation, representing a dramatic, natural, harmless, and convenient change in breast physiology, 'should be carefully evaluated for a protective role against . . . breast cancer before ignored as irrelevant'.

Indeed, hormones and related factors which have variously been associated with risk of cancer of the breast and other hormone-sensitive tissues are numerous (for reviews, see Kelsey, 1979; Kodama and Kodama, 1983). However, as described above for lactation, or elsewhere for other factors including dietary fat (Chapter Nine, Section 9.4), the associations are rarely clear-cut. Other examples include oral contraceptives, which have been associated with increased risk of breast cancer but with reduced risk of fibrocystic breast disease (Kelsey, 1979; Hsieh *et al.*, 1984). Even this increased risk is controversial, particularly in younger women (Hennekens *et al.*, 1984). Analogously, de Waard (1975) in Holland and Hirayama (1978) in Japan reported that breast cancer risk was positively associated with height and weight. However, Adami *et al.* (1977) in Sweden and Wynder *et al.* (1978) in the United States found no significant association between this risk and obesity. Hormonal roles in neoplasia are hence clearly complex. Even neoplastic transformation *in vitro* has sometimes been shown to be dependent upon hormones, e.g. the transformation of cultured mouse fibroblasts by X-rays, in which thyroid hormone is an essential requirement (Guernsey *et al.*, 1980).

As a final demonstration of the complexity of hormonal involvement in neoplastic development, there is the widespread belief that hormones act as promoters rather than initiators of the process. This is particularly applicable to the role of estrogens unopposed by progesterone or androgens (the 'estrogen window' hypothesis) (cf. Korenman, 1981). However, the problem with this belief is that the presumed initiators in humans are yet to be identified with certainty. In the two-stage hypothesis of Berenblum and others, initiation is thought to require structural mutation(s) of target cell DNA (Chapter Nine, Section 9.5). The body's hormones are not known to be mutagenic. Yet, they can induce neoplasia without the assistance of any known mutagen, e.g. simply by their manipulations.

4.2.3 Hormonal Manipulations

It has long been known that manipulated disturbances of the body's hormonal balances can, in presumably susceptible subjects, induce the appearance of neoplasia. This was first shown in 1932, when Lacassagne in France reported the capacity of administered 'folliculin' (estrone) to produce breast cancer in male mice. This finding then attracted much investigative effort, particularly in the United States by William Ullman Gardner during the 1940s (Gardner, 1947, 1948) and by Morton S. Biskind and Gerson R. Biskind and their associates during the 1940s and 1950s (Biskind and Biskind, 1944; Biskind *et al.*, 1953). In a particularly interesting experiment, Biskind and Biskind induced hormonal imbalance in castrated female rats bearing ovaries transplanted to the spleen, causing the rats to remain anestrous due to hepatic inactivation of the estrogen secreted into the portal circulation. The resulting low levels of circulating estrogens caused anterior pituitary hypersecretion of gonadotropins and consequent unopposed stimulation of the transplanted ovaries. During one year's observation, the ovaries had progressively formed masses of corpora lutea, luteomas, and granulosa cell tumours. A contributory factor might have been anterior pituitary hypersecretion of prolactin. Although, in mammals, this polypeptide hormone is best known for promotion of mammary growth and lactation, it is also necessary for maintenance of the corpus luteum in species of rodents and in sheep and rabbit. In ewes, it has an inhibitory effect on ovulation; and, in women, its hypersecretion appears to be associated with ovulatory failure (cf. Hamada *et al.*, 1980). Analogously, Biskind and Biskind found testicular interstitial cell tumours in castrated male rats bearing splenic transplants of testes.

In related studies, Otto Mühlbock and his colleagues in Holland (e.g. Mühlbock and Boot, 1959) showed during the 1950s that mammary tumours can be produced in certain inbred strains of mice bearing pituitary isografts, independently of the murine mammary tumour virus (MTV). They also showed that resistance to MTV tumorigenesis is genetic, related to the H-2 locus, and associated with suppression of viral replication.

Such experimental findings also suggested a possible cancer risk to man from one or more of the various hormonal manipulations which are becoming increasingly common. The use of natural or synthetic hormones or hormonomimetics developed gradually with understanding of the chemistry and biochemistry of natural hormones. As shown in Table 4.1, ovarian hormones were first recognized in 1905 when Marshall and Jolly reported the capacity of ovarian extracts to induce estrus in spayed dogs. They led to various attempts to isolate, purify, and chemically characterize these hormones, giving rise to early preparations such as the 'oestrin' (the terminological source of today's 'oestrogen' or 'estrogen') of Guy Fredrick Marrian, the 'progynon' of Adolph Butenandt, and the 'folliculin' of Edward A. Doisy *et al.* which was distinguished by its source, the urine of pregnant women. After Edgar Allen, in 1923, isolated, purified, and chemically characterized one of the ovarian follicular hormones, the field was opened for detailed studies of their steroidal structure, their estrogenic functions, their biosynthesis from acetate through cholesterol, synthesis and testing of their structural or functional analogues such as diethylstilbestrol (DES), and related studies of hormones of other (e.g. polypeptide and biogenic amine) types. In recent years, new polypeptides with hormone activity have been increasingly discovered, e.g. two polypeptides from porcine intestine, one related to secretin and the other to pancreatic polypeptide and neurotensin (Tatemoto and Mut, 1980). Others have included, from both porcine (Hakanson *et al.*, 1979) and human (Benjannet *et al.*, 1980) sources, a pituitary polypeptide related to the common evolutionary precursor of the melanocyte stimulating hormones α, β, and γ), as well as β-lipotropin, ACTH, and β-endorphin.

The notable later pioneers in the new field thus opened were the above-mentioned Gardner, his fellow-Americans Herbert M. Evans and Choh Hao Li, the Englishman E.C. Dodds, and the New Zealander F.D. Bielschowsky, and their associates. Among other features, Gardner investigated the role of steroid hormones in neoplasia in relation to their imbalances and to heredity factors. Evans (cf. his Harvey Lectures of 1923–24), and Li and others (e.g. Li and Graf, 1974), investigated the role of the polypeptide hormones of the anterior pituitary in the regulation of normal and pathological growth. The investigations of Li and his associates, carried out since the 1940s, also included the isolation, purification, and structural characterization of seven (interstitial cell-stimulating hormone, lactogenic hormone, adrenocorticotropic hormone, β-melanotropin, follicle stimulating hormone, β-lipotropin, and growth hormone) of the currently known adenohypophyseal hormones. Dodds *et al.*, in 1938, reported estrogenic activity for several synthetic agents, but most notably DES, which they introduced for the first time. Bielschowsky, working with parabiotic and endocrine-modified animal systems, introduced and developed, during the 1950s, the now classic concept of pituitary-thyroidal and pituitary-adrenal-gonadal relationships.

That hormonal manipulations can carry a human cancer risk was first forcefully underlined by Herbst and his associates during the early 1970s (Herbst and Scully, 1970; Herbst *et al.*, 1971). They reported what must surely be one of the most disturbing of recent findings in environmental oncology (somewhat paralleling that of excess lung cancers among smokers), i.e. a significantly increased frequency of clear-cell vaginal adenocarcinoma in young women (between the ages of 15 and 22 years) whose mothers had been treated with DES during pregnancy. This type of therapy was advocated initially in 1946, by Smith *et al.*, for 'high-risk' pregnancies, i.e. those with threatened abortion or with prior pregnancy loss. Up to around 1979, some 350 cases of vaginal adenocarcinoma in young women have been studied, most of which are associated with DES or the related substances dienestrol and hexestrol (Herbst and Cole, 1978; IARC Monographs No. 21, 1979). Numerous other authors have reported widespread histopathological changes or cancers in individuals exposed prenatally or postnatally to DES. These changes have included, in females, vaginal adenosis, cervical ectropion and transverse ridges, microglandular hyperplasia (the 'pill lesion'), small endometrial cavities, 'T'-shaped uteri and dilated cornual areas, and congenital renal and ureteral abnormalities. On males also, they have included a variety of genital tract abnormalities such as epididymal cysts, hypotropic testes, capsular induration of the testes, and cryptorchidism. (For references, see IARC Monographs No. 21, 1979). Replacement therapy with DES, first initiated by Lewis in 1939, has been associated with the development of adenocarcinoma of the endometrium in young women with gonadal dysgenesis (Culter *et al.*, 1972), or of the ovary in mainly older women (Hoover *et al.*, 1977). DES-associated endometrial adenocarcinomas have been observed by others (e.g. Wilkinson *et al.*, 1973; Louka *et al.*, 1978) in various women, including a 42-year-old patient with Sheehan's syndrome (Reid and Shirley, 1974) and several patients with metastatic breast cancer (Hoover *et al.*, 1977; Khandekar *et al.*, 1978). Cancers of the breast (O'Grady and McDivitt, 1969; Bulow *et al.*, 1973), liver (Galanaud *et al.*, 1976; Hoch-Ligeti, 1978), and skin (Sadoff *et al.*, 1973) have been reported to have developed in men treated with DES, mainly for prostatic cancer.

DES is clearly a dangerous invention, even more so than thalidomide. In one form or another (e.g. as the underivatized compound, or as its dipropionate or diphosphate), it is or has been produced in many European and American countries but not in Japan, in vast quantities; and it is or has been widely used for many purposes (cf. IARC Monographs No. 21, 1979). In human medicine, these purposes have included: alleviation of symptoms arising during the climacteric and following ovariectomy; treatment of senile vaginitis and vulvar dystrophy; post-coital emergency contraception; maintenance of pregnancy; prevention of post-partum breast engorgement; and chemotherapy of female hypogonadism, advanced breast cancer, and prostatic cancer. In veterinary medicine, it has found use in replacement therapy for underdeveloped females; in incontinence and vaginitis of spayed bitches; in the checking of milk secretion in pseudo-pregnancy; in the induction of heat in anestrus; and in the treatment of prostatic hypertrophy in dogs, and of uterine inertia and pyometria. As a growth promoter, it has been in use in beef cattle since 1976, and in poultry since 1978.

Despite these great human benefits of DES, its attendant dangers demand the search for suitable, less harmful substitutes wherever feasible. A notable step in this direction has recently been taken in the United States. Here, in a randomized comparative trial, another non-steroidal anti-estrogen, tamoxifen, was found to be as effective as, but significantly less toxic than, DES in the clinical management of advanced postmenopausal breast cancer (Ingle *et al.*, 1981). It cannot be beyond today's ingenuity to extend such findings to the other persisting uses of DES.

Increased risk of human cancer in association with administered hormones or hormonoids is not restricted to DES. In 1968, Symmers reported mammary cancer development in transsexuals treated hormonally and surgically in attempts to correct their anomalies. Use of oral contraceptives was first reported to be associated with hepatocellular adenoma in 1973 by Baum *et al.*, and with endometrial adenocarcinoma in 1975 by Lyon, and by Silverberg and Makowski. By 1979, Ishak was able to review well over 100 independent reports of the hepatopathological association alone, involving hepatocellular carcinomas as well as focal nodular hyplasia (also variously described as focal cirrhosis, hepatic pseudotumour, solitary hyperplastic nodule, hamartomatous cholangiohepatoma, hepatic hamartoma, mixed adenoma, and benign hepatoma). The 'sequential' regimen (estrogen for the first 14–16 days, followed by 4–6 days of estrogen-plus-progestin) produced endometrial hyperplasia more readily than the combined regimen (estrogen-plus-progestin) in every pill, probably because of the 14–16 days of unopposed estrogenic stimulation in the former.

Other than the liver and endometrium, several body sites have been reported to develop one type of abnormality or another in association with contraceptive pill usage (cf. reviews in Iacobelli *et al.*, 1980). Among these sites are the vasculature, vagina, cervix, ovary, and breast. Some epidemiological studies have shown that, among users of the pill, the risk of mortality from vascular diseases, mainly ischemic heart disease, is some fourfold that among non-users (Mead *et al.*, 1980; Layde and Beral, 1981; Vessey *et al.*, 1981). The report of Layde and Beral, representing a continuation of the Royal College of General Practitioners' Oral Contraception Study, agreed with previous reports of the relative risk increasing with age (particularly 35 years and over) and cigarette smoking but not with duration of pill use. This report also positively implicated subarachnoid hemorrhage and parity as risk factors, which have not been previously implicated. Such findings, inclusive of those of new associated risk factors, are particularly ominous, in view of the widespread and increasing use of the pill. For instance, some 54 million women were using the pill in 1978.

The question of the pathological effects of the pill on the breast is still controversial. Estrogens are associated with the production of neoplasms of the breast and other organs in many species of animal (cf. Casey *et al.*, 1979); and it has been claimed (Hertz, 1969) that most animal carcinogens are probably also human carcinogens. In humans, however, the breast lesions associated with usage of the pill have been described as epithelial and/or other types of atypical hyperplasia occurring within fibroadenomas, or, results of a survey by the Boston Collaborative Drug Surveillance Program (1973) have suggested that pill usage may, in fact, protect against the development of breast neoplasms. Several other studies have shown pill usage to be associated with no increased risk of breast cancer development (Vessey *et al.*, 1971, 1979; Paffenbarger *et al.*, 1977; Matthews *et al.*, 1981). Further, Spencer *et al.* (1978) and Matthews *et al.* (1981) have reported that pill usage is associated with improved prognosis in the disease, except possibly in patients with a close family history of breast cancer. The reason for this possible exception is unknown. Perhaps it is associated with the unusual features (e.g. bilaterality and early age of onset) (cf. Chapter Six) of familial breast cancer, or with different biological effects of contraceptive steroids on the growth and spread of familial and non-familial breast cancer.

At present, the role of contraceptive steroids on the development of malignancies of the female reproductive organs remains unclear (see various discussions in Knab, 1977, and Iacobelli *et al.*, 1980; also WHO Technical Report Series No. 619, 1978; Swan and Brown, 1981). However, their harmful role in the development of vascular and related disorders is already obvious, calling for much caution in their indiscriminate use. Indeed, the possible dangers of incautious hormonal manipulations were indicated long ago by results other than those already described from the days of Ramazzini and Rigoni-Stern. For instance, vaginal and cervical neoplasms have been described in DES-treated mice (e.g. Gardner and Allen in 1939). Gardner and Allen also reported neoplasms in mice treated with equilin compounds. The sulfates of such compounds (mainly of equilin itself and 17 α-dihydroequilin, but also of equilenin) occur together with the sulfates of estrone and other estrogens in the 'Premarin' (Ayerst) and those related estrogenic representations of pregnant mares' urine that are so widely used in estrogen replacement therapy. The increasing awareness of the neoplastic and other health hazards posed to man by DES, anovulatory contraceptives, and other hormonal preparations brought home the painful lesson that presumptions of reliability of animal-to-man extrapolations and of the absolute safety of physiological agents can be worthless drug-manufacturers' assurances when such agents happen to be as biologically potent as are the body's hormones. Estradiol-17β, for instance, is one of the most 'physiological' of agents because of its great importance in mammalian reproduction. However, in susceptible mice, it has been reported to produce neoplasms of the breast, uterus, vagina, testis, pituitary, and lymphoid organs (reviewed by Casey *et al.*, 1979). Indeed, ovarian hormones have been found to influence tumour growth and spread in some unexpected instances, e.g. the B_{16} mouse melanoma (Proctor *et al.*, 1981). This situation may have an analogy in human melanoma which, like human breast cancer (cf. Sledge and McGuire, 1983), has been found to possess estrogen receptors (Fisher *et al.*, 1976).

4.2.4 Attempts at Legislative Control of Exogenous Hormones and Other Environmental Agents Posing a Risk of Human Cancer

More than ever before, man is now playing with some of the most intimate secrets of nature. However, the potential dangers (and benefits), and hence the need for caution, are far greater in his dealings with the universe within than without himself. Sensible control of his synthetic hormones, for instance, is no less important than that of his nuclear weapons. Recognition of this fact has led to a series of near panic legislations and counter-legislations about use and abuse of DES and other potential human carcinogens, e.g. in the United States, as shown in Table 4.1.

The legislative task is as difficult as it is vital. Just part of the difficulty is reflected in the contrasting interests of profit-making concerns against those of human health, and in the already-discussed (Chapter Three; Section 3.7) 'earthful of carcinogens' which is being depicted by various experimental tests. This difficulty is also reflected in the increasing manipulations of the hormonal systems which are such vital controllers of the developmental processes by which all metazoans, including man, are formed. Neither of the two fundamentals of biology, the genetic inheritance and its control during development, is properly understood. Yet, both have become the subjects of intense manipulations, the former in DNA recombinations and the latter in various ways being the more serious because of its use of human subjects as opposed to the use of mainly bacteria in the former. Thus, natural or synthetic estrogens, androgens, progestins, and/or hormonoids are being prescribed for purposes as diverse as are endocrine replacement, induction of ovulation, contraception, prevention or induction (rarely successful) of abortion, induction or suppression of lactation, correction of primary or secondary sexual anomalies, anabolism, and treatment of postmenopausal distress, anemia, and cancer. For therapy of cancer and certain other conditions also, the practice of endocrine surgery or radioablation has grown steadily since Beatson's original discovery in 1896.

4.2.5 *The Proliferation of Synthetic Hormones*

Already, synthetic hormones and hormonoids are legion (Table 4.2) (for reviews, see Lingeman, 1979; Schally *et al.*, 1984). They include, among the steroidal classes alone, ethynylestradiol, the progestagenic 17α-hydroxyprogesterones medroxyprogesterone and megestrol acetates, the androgenic 19-nortestosterones dimethisterone and norgestrel, and the anabolic oxymetholone and 17-methyltestosterone. In addition, there is a long list of typically plant or microbial (phyto)estrogens such as coumestrol, genistein, and zearalenone, and typically animal hormones such as the equilin and equilenin which appear to be restricted to equine species. All of these agents possess steroidal hormonogenic activities. So do many others, among them certain therapeutic agents such as reserpine, the *Rauwolfia* alkaloids, and the synthetic chlorpromazine and iproniazid, as well as, according to some reports (cf. Bitman and Cecil, 1970) various polychlorinated biphenyls and the related pesticide DDT (reviewed by Lingeman, 1979).

Table 4.2: Some Hormone Preparations in Common Use

Compound	Chemical structure
Estrogens	
Chlorotrianisene	1,1',1''–(1–Chloro–1–ethenyl–2–ylidene)tris (4–methoxy–benzene)
Conjugated estrogens	A mixture of compounds, mainly sodium estrone sulphate
Dienestrol	4,4'–(1,2–Diethylidene–1,2–ethanediyl) bisphenol
Diethylstilbestrol	4,4'–(1,2–Diethyl–1,2–ethenediyl)bisphenol
Diethylstilbestrol dipropionate	4,4'–(1,2–Diethyl–1,2–ethenediyl) bisphenol dipropionate
Ethinylestradiol[a]	(17α)–19–Norpregna–1,3,5(10)–trien–20–yn–3,17–diol
Mestranol[a]	(17α)–3–Methoxy–10–norpregna–1,3,5(10)–trien–20–yn–17–ol
Methallenestril	β–Ethyl–6–methoxy–α,α–dimethyl–2–naphthalene propanoic acid
Estradiol–17β	(17β)–Estra–1,3,5(10)–triene–3,17–diol
Estradiol 3–benzoate	Estra–1,3,5(10)–triene–3,17–diol(17β)–3–benzoate
Estradiol dipropionate	Estra–1,3,5(10)–triene–3,17–diol(17β)–dipropionate
Estradiol–17β–valerate	(17β)–Estra–1,3,5(10)–triene–3,17–diol 17–pentanoate
Polyestradiol phosphate	(17β)–Estra–1,3,5(10)–triene–3,17–diol polymer with phosphoric acid
Estriol	(16α,17β)–Estra–1,3,5(10)–triene–3,16,17–triol
Estrone	3–Hydroxyestra–1,3,5(10)–trien–17–one
Estrone benzoate	3–(Benzoyloxy)estra–1,3,5(10)–trien–17–one
Quinestradiol	(16α,17β)–3–(Cyclopentyloxy)–estra–1,3,5(10)–triene–16,17–diol
Quinestrol	(17α)–3–(Cyclopentyloxy)–19–norpregna–1,3,5(10)–trien–20–yn–17–ol

Progestins

Chlormadinone acetate[a]	17–(Acetyloxy)–6–chloro–pregna–4,6–diene–3,20–dione
Dimethisterone[a]	(6α,17β)–17–Hydroxy–6–methyl–17–(1–propynyl)–androst–4–en–3–one
Ethynodiol diacetate[a]	(3β,17α)–19–Norpregn–4–en–20–yn–3,17–diol diacetate
17–Hydroxyprogesterone caproate	17–[(1–Oxohexyl)oxy]pregn–4–ene–3, 20–dione
Lynoestrenol[a]	(17α)–19–Norpregn–4–en–20–yn–17–ol
Medroxyprogesterone acetate[a]	(6α)–17(Acetyloxy)–6–methylpregna–4, 6–diene–3,20–dione
Norethisterone acetate[a]	(17α)–17–(Acetyloxy)–19–norpregn–4–en–20–yn–3–one acetone
Norethynodrel[a]	(17α)–17–Hydroxy–19–norpregn–5(10)–en–20–yn–3–one
Norgestrel[a]	(17α)–13–Ethyl–17–hydroxy–18,19–dinorpregn–4–en–20–yn–3–one
Progesterone	Pregn–4–ene–3,20–dione

Androgens

Testosterone	(17β)–17–Hydroxyandrost–4–en–3–one
Testosterone enanthate	(17β)–17–[(1–Oxoheptyl)oxy]androst–4–en–3–one
Testosterone propionate	(17β)–17–(1–Oxopropoxy)androst–4–en–3–one

Others

Clomiphene[b]	2–[4–(2–Chloro–1,2–diphenylethenyl)phenoxy]–N,N,diethylethanamine
Clomiphene citrate[b]	2–[4–(2–Chloro–1,2–diphenylethenyl)phenoxy]–N,N diethylethanamine 2–hydroxy–1,2,3–propanetricarboxylate(1:1)

Notes: a. Used in estrogen–progestin oral contraceptive preparations.
        b. Used for induction of ovulation.
Source: Adapted from IARC Monographs No. 21, 1979.

It may, hence, not be surprising if certain other polychlorinated aromatics also belong to this category. For example, 2,4,5-trichlorophenol (2,4,5-T) and its product dioxin, the culprits of the Seveso disaster of 1976, and of the United States' defoliation blasts in Vietnam, are increasingly being reported to have abortifacient, teratogenic, carcinogenic, and other harmful effects.

To all of these, humans are exposed in one way or another.

Women in particular are also exposed to synthetic antagonists of natural hormones, such as the anti-estrogenic tamoxifen, the anti-androgenic cryproterone, and the ovulation inducer clomiphene.

4.2.6 Structural and Other Analogies Between Natural Hormones, Cancer-inducing Polycyclic Aromatic Hydrocarbons, and Agents Such As Interferon and Phorbol Esters

It is a curious fact that certain exogenous and endogenous agents which have been associated with neoplasia in man and animals bear a close structural analogy with the reduced phenanthrenoid nucleus of all natural steroidal hormones. The exogenous agents include all known cancer-associated polycyclic aromatic hydrocarbons (PAHs), some of which, like benzo[a]pyrene and the dibenzanthracenes, are present in tobacco smoke, alcoholic brews, and burnt foods. They are also present in vehicular and industrial exhausts, and hence also in the general atmosphere. Through the latter, they can pollute other public utilities such as water, fish, and, through soil, food crops. It may thus not be mere coincidence that the neoplasms and other pathologies produced experimentally by the PAHs in susceptible species, usually mice, involve mainly hormone-sensitive organs, e.g. breast, prostate, ovary, adrenal, and skin. The endogenous agents include some of the cholesterol metabolites, notably bile acids (cf. Chapter Three, Section 3.6.3.3). Some of the latter, whether through discharge into the intestinal lumen via the hepatobiliary system or through local formation by the action of gut flora, have sometimes been associated with intestinal neoplasms in man.

Not all of the hormone-related cancer-risk factors to which man is becoming increasingly exposed, however, bear a structural resemblance to natural hormones. This is illustrated by several synthetic non-steroidal agents, such as DDT, certain polychlorinated biphenyls, hexestrol, dienestrol, chlortrianizene, and DES, all of which possess estrogenic activity. The notorious DES, for instance, has been shown by its founders Dodds *et al.* in 1938 to be estrogenic even after peroral administration, suggesting its utilization of normal absorptive mechanisms. They also found it to be more potently estrogenic than ovarian estrogens, and to be capable of cheaper commercial production than natural estrogens. Subsequent investigations have shown DES to bind to estradiol receptors; like the endogenous steroidal hormones and cholesterol, to be metabolized and conjugated in the liver and to be excreted largely in the feces, via the bile and intestines; and to pose a cancer risk both clinically and experimentally (cf. Lingeman, 1979; IARC Monographs No. 21, 1979).

It thus seems likely that the body's hormones are intimately involved, in one way or another, in the cancer-associated effects of many types of exogenous agent. These agents may share the normal (e.g. differentiational) pathways of hormone action, producing synergistic, competitive, or inhibitory effects. Even some non-hormonal natural body substances such as interferon, the most recent of the white hopes in cancer therapy, has been shown to share such pathways of both polypeptide and steroidal hormones (Blacklock and Stanton, 1980). In a related instance, the neurohypophyseal hormone vasopressin and the experimental tumour promoters, the phorbol esters, have been shown to stimulate DNA synthesis by a common mechanism involving ornithine decarboxylase and 2-deoxyglucose uptake (Dicker and Rozengurt, 1980).

4.2.7 Section Summary

In one way or another, most of the major categories in the spectrum of known human cancer-risk factors (Chapter Three, Section 3.4; Chapter Nine, Section 9.3) appear to be associated with the body's natural hormones and/or hormonal systems. There are endocrine manipulations by surgery, radiation, and chemotherapy; utilizations of natural or synthetic agents with hormonogenic or anti-hormonogenic activities; and public or personal exposures to such agents which do or do not resemble the body's hormones structurally, but may resemble them functionally. Whether or not all cancer-risk factors may indeed have such an association remains to be discovered. However, it is significant that the commonest human cancers known from remote antiquity have been those involving hormone-sensitive tissues, particularly those of the female breast and of the male and female urogenital system. Even bronchogenic carcinoma, one of the commonest of modern cancers because of its increasing prevalence in relation to recent smoking habits and industrial and other pollutions, is associated mainly with the oncogenic polycyclic aromatic hydrocarbons, i.e. agents showing some structural analogy with the steroid hormones and some preferential organotropism in hormone-sensitive tissues.

Through means such as contraception, food, and therapy, hormone disturbances are now induced in millions of people worldwide. Such disturbances influence the oncologic role of other, particularly dietary and therapeutic, factors, e.g. in cancers of the breast and possibly also the endometrium, ovary, and prostate (Miller, 1978; Lipsett, 1979). Drugs and nutrition can stimulate or inhibit the secretion of hormones, alter their rates and routes of metabolism, and, among other features, disrupt their mechanisms of action through receptors, second messengers, and binding to DNA. Estrogen replacement alone is being practised in about 24 per cent of women over age 70 years in the United States, mainly for the prevention of osteoporosis and resulting bone fracture. However, for this purpose, the effectiveness of the treatment is greatest when the replacement is started soon after the menopause, and is continued over the remaining life of the patient. Interrupted treatment is accompanied by accelerated bone loss, so that the treated patient may eventually be no better off than her untreated counterpart (Lindsay *et al.*, 1978); while the use of low-dose estrogens combined with progestogens may increase the risk of stroke and vascular disease. Clearly, much caution is needed in the manipulations of these powerful tools of Mother Nature.

4.3 Hormones in Tumour Regression

The Schinzinger-Beatson principle of hormonal therapy in clinical cancer (Section 4.1) received some early experimental verification. Thus, castration was found by White in 1904 to improve prostatic hypertrophy in dogs, and by Laythrop and Loeb in 1916 to reduce the incidence of spontaneous mammary neoplasia in mice.

However, the operation of this principle, as of that relative to hormonal roles in cancer development (Section 4.2.2), has been shown to be quite complex. In 1905, for example, Lett *et al.* collected and analyzed data involving 99 cases of inoperable breast cancer in women treated by ovariectomy. They found evidence for significant regression only in women with the premenopausal disease, and, even so, in only about one-third of these. The result of this finding was a disillusionment with the efficacy of hormonal therapy in clinical breast cancer, particularly since the disease predominates among postmenopausal women, in whom the ovaries produce insignificant amounts of steroid hormones. It is now known that, in such women, estrone continues to be produced elsewhere in the body, through aromatization of androstenedione secreted by the adrenal cortex (Grodin *et al.*, 1973).

Significant interest in Beatson's observation was not revived until 1941. In this year, Charles Brenton Huggins and his associates in the United States showed that orchidectomy sometimes improved prognosis in disseminated prostatic cancer in men (cf. Huggins and Hodges, 1941). With the later introduction of cortisol and other adrenocortical hormones into clinical practice, it became possible to maintain adrenalectomized patients by glucocorticoid replacement. Then, in 1952, Huggins and Bergenstal showed that adrenalectomy sometimes aided regression of breast cancer in postmenopausal women as well as in men. As a logical extension of this therapeutic approach, because of the known dependence of steroidogenesis upon pituitary function, surgical removal of the pituitary gland was soon shown by Luft and Olivercrona (1953) and by Pearson *et al.* (1956) to produce similar effects in breast cancer. Finally, the irreversibility of the endocrine ablations involved stimulated alternative (additive) procedures, such as the use of estrogen antagonists including androgens (Nathanson, 1952) and tamoxifen (Cole *et al.*, 1971; Ward, 1973). For this same purpose, Haddow *et al.*, as early as 1944, had introduced the use of large doses of estrogens.

These notable advances in the therapy of clinical cancers of hormone-dependent tissues increasingly pinpointed a major problem. Even among cancers of the same histogenesis, grade, and stage, only some showed a dependence upon hormones for their continued growth and survival. Although endocrine therapy has remained the most effective of currently available treatments for advanced breast cancer in particular, in terms of both quality and duration of the induced remission, the problem of selection of responding patients has also remained unsolved. Based empirically upon clinical experience, a favourable response appeared likely in patients who showed a long disease-free interval between mastectomy and the appearance of distant metastases; who developed metastases in skin and lymph node rather than in bone, brain, or viscera; or who had responded earlier to another type of endocrine therapy. In very young women, breast cancer usually progressed rapidly and failed to respond favourably to hormonal therapy.

Some heroic attempts have since been made to make the selection process more accurate than through empiricism. Notably, during the 1960s, Bulbrook and his associates (cf. Atkins *et al.*, 1968) investigated a number of 'discriminant functions', based upon measurements of the relative amounts of steroid hormone metabolites excreted in the urine of patients with breast cancer, particularly etiocholanolone and 17-hydroxycorticosteroids. Although these functions showed some correlation with the clinical response to hormonal therapy, the correlation was too weak to influence therapy decisions significantly, and it has not been duplicated in later studies (cf. Segaloff *et al.*, 1980). The effort, however paved the way to another attempt, the search for specific hormone-binding cellular components or hormone receptors that may aid in the selection process,

It had been known for over two decades that agents such as tritiated hexestrol (Glascock and Hoekstra, 1959) and tritiated estradiol (Jenson and Jacobson, 1960) will bind preferentially to estrogen-responsive organs (e.g. uterus, vagina, and anterior pituitary) in laboratory animals. Analogously, some breast tumours in women later shown to respond to adrenalectomy (Folca *et al.*, 1961), and also some in rats (King *et al.*, 1965; Mobbs, 1966), were found to bind labelled estrogens (hexestrol and estradiol, respectively) more avidly than did other tissues. From 1970 onwards, Elwood V. Jensen and his associates in particular, but also many workers in several countries, began to show that even some highly advanced clinical breast cancers retain a dependence upon endogenous hormones through possession of the specific receptors for the hormones, notably estrogens. It has now become well-established that objective remission following endocrine therapy in patients with breast cancer is better when the cancer tissues contain significant amounts of estrogen receptor activity (termed 'estrophilin' by Jensen) than when they do not. However, this correlation is far from absolute (cf. reviews by McGuire *et al.*, 1975; De Sombre and Jensen, 1980; Sledge and McGuire, 1983).

The selection of patients with cancer of the breast or another hormone-responsive tissue for endocrine therapy is thus still uncertain. For instance, McGuire *et al.* (1975) concluded that although absence of significant levels of estrophilin in clinical breast cancer correlated with a general refractoriness to endocrine therapy, their presence predicted a favourable response in only about 55 per cent of the cases. It may well be that the tumours' dependence is upon multiple endogenous factors, which may or may not be exclusively hormonal. Breast tumours which contain significant levels of receptors for both estrogen and progesterone, whether premenopausal or postmenopausal, sometimes but not always respond better to endocrine therapy than do those tumours with significant levels of only the estrogen receptor (Osborne *et al.*, 1980; Skinner *et al.*, 1980). The problem of prediction of response to therapy on the basis of hormone receptor content is thus complex, and it is not confined to hormonal therapy in cases of estrogen receptor-positive patients with advanced breast cancer. In such cases, cytotoxic therapy is also problematical (Jonat *et al.*, 1980; Lippman and Allegra, 1980; Sears and Olson, 1980; Paone *et al.*, 1981). The question as to why some of these cases do not respond to hormonal or other therapy has been considered by Maas *et al.* (1980) who advanced reasons based upon factors such as technical inadequacies, unknown effects of non-steroidal hormones such as prolactin and immunological factors, and the differential responses of multiclonal tumours, each of which may contain both estrogen receptor-positive and receptor-negative clones of tumour cells.

Overall, endocrine manipulations in clinical cancer management have been becoming increasingly involved. Gonads, adrenals, pituitary, and/or other endocrine organs are being surgically removed or radiologically inactivated in different cases; their functions are being suppressed, stimulated, or replaced by various means; and the making, testing, and use of hormones and hormonoids are on the increase. Yet, many unanswered questions remain, e.g. questions related to the biochemical basis of the hormone dependence of tumours, to whether tumours progress from an initially high dependence to an eventual independence, and to the significance of aberrant hormone synthesis by tumours. One certain outcome, however, is that hormonal effects upon cancer development and regression are complex but are closely related to the normal effects of these ancient and ubiquitous gene regulators during normal development.

4.4 Hormones in Gene Regulation

The growing recognition that cancer has many of the hallmarks of a complex of developmental diseases sharing the common feature of differentiational aberrations in variable combination and character has underlined the importance to oncology not only of gene regulation but also of gene regulators. Among these regulators, hormones appear to be the most ancient, ubiquitous, and important (some reviews: Young *et al.*, 1980; Bell *et al.*, 1980; Brooks, 1983).

Several observations support the notion of the great ancestry and ubiquity of hormones and their regulatory functions. Among these are the now classical observations by Neville-Wilmer that amoeboid-flagellate interconversions in *Naegleria* are dependent upon soluble factors in the culture medium. Also, land plants, whose photosynthesis together with that of the more ancient Thallophytes (algae, fungi, lichens) were responsible for the intitial reducing-to-oxygenated (and ozonated) atmospheric conversion that enabled evolution of modern animals, depend for their development upon hormones such as auxins, gibberelins, cytokinins, ethylene, and abscisic acid. So do insects (e.g. upon ecdysone for metamorphosis) which characteristically co-evolved with plants to produce the plant–insect symbiosis that has remained one of the essential features of the biosphere.

Further, a given type of hormonal activity can be of widespread natural distribution. Peptidergic neurons, for example, which synthesize and secrete peptides possessing either endocrine or local 'paracrine' or synaptic actions, are of widespread occurrence among innervated organisms. The neurosecretory counterparts, since their first discovery by Ernst Scharrer in 1928, have been found in nervous systems ranging from those of coelenterates to man and have indeed been postulated to represent the evolutionary antecedent of 'conventional' neurons that use small molecules such as acetylcholine and biogenic amines as neurotransmitters. Two of the peptide hormones secreted by peptidergic neurons, particularly by those of the posterior pituitary but also by some extra-hypothalamoneurohypophyseal axons, are the nonapeptides vasopressin and oxytocin. Vasopressin or antidiuretic hormone stimulates renal resorption of water, and oxytocin stimulates milk ejection and uterine contraction, and may be involved in parturition. Arginine vasopressin (AVP) has been found in most mammals, except in some members of the pig family in which lysine vasopressin is predominant, but it sometimes occurs together with AVP, e.g. in the wart-hog and peccary. Arginine vasotocin seems to be ubiquitous among lower vertebrates, and oxytocin among fish, reptiles, birds, amphibians, and mammals.

It would seem that, like other biologically active polypeptides, the polypeptide hormones belong to specific families showing structural and functional relatedness, e.g. the four families represented in the pancreas by insulin, glucagon, somatostatin, and pancreatic polypeptide (Blundell and Humbel, 1980).

The importance of hormones as gene regulators is indicated by their multiple roles during many (perhaps all) stages and phases of sexual reproduction, the key process in evolution and its diversification, and of normal and abnormal development. Thus, among the pituitary hormones alone, follicle stimulating hormone (FSH) stimulates follicular development in the ovary and spermatogenesis in the testes; while luteinizing hormone (LH, or ICSH, i.e. interstitial cell stimulating hormone) promotes ovarian luteinization and testicular leydig cell function. Among others, growth hormone (GH) controls growth-related protein anabolism, lipolysis, and other aspects of metabolism; while prolactin (Pr) controls lactation and mammary gland development. The effects of the pituitary polypeptide hormones are usually trophic, e.g. those of adrenocorticotropic hormone (ACTH) upon adrenocortical functions, involved in steroidogenesis.

Individually, these functions are thus controlled by more than one hormone. The above-mentioned GH and Pr functions, for instance, also involve the steroid hormones, particularly estrogens and progesterone. Also, in *Xenopus laevis*, meiotic maturation of oocytes is initiated by progesterone and other steroids, but also by insulin (cf. review by El Etr *et al.*, 1980). In this effect, the agents seem to act through influences upon calcium movements and/or translocation from membrane stores. The effect is hindered by cyclic adenosine monophosphate (cAMP), or by agents such as cholera toxin which increase oocyte cAMP, possibly through interference with the formation/activity of a maturation promoting factor (MPF). MPF is produced in the progesterone-stimulated oocytes, in which it stimulates maturation phenomena such as germinal vesicle breakdown.

The complexity of the endocrinology of just one gland, the pituitary, is only just beginning to be appreciated. This gland has somatotropic, lactotropic, thyrotropic, adrenocorticotropic, gonadotropic, non-secretory (or 'chromophobe'), and other distinct cell types. Each of these cell types is associated with distinct control functions.

Yet, the pituitary represents just one part of the total complexity of the body's endocrine system. For instance, the adrenal gland almost matches the structural and functional complexity of the pituitary, e.g. in the neural crest derivation of the phaeochromocytes of the catecholamine-synthesizing adrenal medulla, and in the three separate anatomical zones (zona glomerulosa, zona fasciculata, and zona reticularis) of the ACTH-responsive, steroidogenic adrenal cortex. Further, the pituitary is only one component of the hypothalamus-pituitary-adrenal-gonadal axis. This axis, in turn, is closely interrelated with other endocrine and neurosecretory axes, e.g. the adrenocortical-gonadal-fetoplacental-steroidogenic axis. Further, there are strictly controlled functional interrelationships, e.g. between the steroid hormone (or steroid hormone precursor such as de-hydroepiandrosterone), catecholamine (or catecholamine precursor such as dihydroxyphenylalanine, or DOPA), sex hormone, or pregnancy gonadotropin synthetic functions of, respectively, the adrenal cortex, the adrenal medulla, the gonads, and the placenta.

The total complexity is stressed further by other facts which have recently come to light. Among these is the fact that glucocorticoids control T-cell proliferation and, with it, immune status (reviewed by Smith *et al.*, 1980; Tubiana *et al.*, 1984). In lymphoid cells, the glucocorticoids also have pronounced metabolic and lethal effects (reviewed by Young *et al.*, 1980), and they regulate transcription (reviewed by Bell *et al.*, 1980). Also, in their biosynthesis and metabolism alone, hormones call upon practically all of the biosynthetic and metabolic categories of the organism. Thus, biosynthesis of the steroidal hormones including cortisol, corticosterone, aldosterone, and the estrogens and androgens can start from just cholesterol or even further back from just acetate. Analogously, the catecholamines are produced from L-tyrosine or even 3-hydroxyphenylalanine, and the related neurotransmitter serotonin (5-hydroxytryptamine) from L-tryptophan. Serotonin is the enterochromaffin cell secretagogue which is also formed in patients with carcinoid tumours and which, like agents such as bradykinin and prostaglandin E_1, produces flush and other effects in such patients. Also, biosynthesis of the polypeptide hormones utilizes the body's protein synthesizing machinery. Finally, hormone metabolism depends upon the same systems responsible for the metabolic activation and inactivation, conjugation, degradation, and selective excretion and reabsorption of other normal tissue components, or of drugs, poisons, and carcinogens.

The body's hormones exhibit other expected features of natural gene regulators. Thus, hormones are powerful agents, effective in low physiological concentrations; they are thermolabile; and their synthesis is under fine (negative and positive) feedback control. Their activity is both geared to the demands of developmental stage-specific and various cyclical (e.g. menstrual, circadian, and seasonal) and stress variations, and dependent upon complex factors such as specific receptors, second messengers in selected instances, enzymes, and other mediators (e.g. components of the protein-synthesizing machinery) of hormonal effects upon gene expression. Thus, biosynthesis of just the 'salt and water' mineralocorticosteroid aldosterone by the rat adrenal zona glomerulosa is regulated primarily by ACTH and angiotensin II and secondarily by a variety of other factors including potassium, sodium, and serotonin (Müller, 1971).

In developmental processes, the complexity of hormonal control appears to reflect the complexity of the processes themselves, as just the sex hormones illustrate (cf. reviews in Lingeman, 1979). First, a single hormone may dominate in control of a particular aspect of development. Examples are 5α-dihydrotestosterone (DHT), which dominates in differentiation of the urogenital sinus (the anlage of the prostate) and the urogenital tubercle (the anlage of the external genitalia); and testosterone, in differentiation of the wolffian duct system (the anlage of the epididymis, vas deferens, and seminal vesicles).

Second, a single hormone and/or one or more of its analogues may be involved in a broad spectrum of control functions. For example, estrogens (mainly estrone, estradiol, and estriol), usually in combination with other hormones such as prolactin and progesterone in mammary gland development and lactation, or with growth hormone in protein metabolism and lipid and carbohydrate metabolism, are thus involved in multiple aspects of development. These aspects include development of primary and secondary sexual characteristics; infant nourishment; body lipidization; skin texturing and ageing; and, within the bony skeletal system, ossification, modelling, growth and the postpubertal hypophyseal joining that delimits stature. They appear also to include the bone shortening and porosity that accompany old age, and the osteoporosis that is associated with many cancers, particularly of the breast, thyroid, and lung. The capacity of estrogens to simulate uterine growth has been exploited for their bioassay.

Third, a single class of hormones may exert opposite effects under different conditions. The 'double threshold theory' of Folley, for instance, is based upon the capacity of estrogens in low or high circulating levels respectively to activate or inhibit lactotropic activity of the anterior pituitary.

Fourth, a single hormone, either the whole or a specific part of its structure, may exert different control functions upon target cells. For instance, the whole of the prolactin molecule appears necessary for stimulation of lactation, but a specific part for that of mitosis. Synthesis, but not translation, of casein mRNA occurs in virgin breast tissue under the influence of prolactin, with translation occurring in lactating breast and requiring stimulation by a peptide fragment of prolactin (Mittra, 1980). Analogous differential effects of the whole and parts have been described for growth hormone, and they may well apply to other hormones. Future studies may well show that hormones are directly involved in gene regulation at different levels of protein synthesis, e.g. to the transcriptional, RNA-splicing, translational, and post-translational levels.

Fifth, two or more hormones may act upon distinct subcomponents of a single organ. For instance, breast tissues, including those from male breast cancer, can have multiple hormone receptors, including receptors for estrogens, progesterone, androgens, and glucocorticoids (reviewed by Everson *et al.*, 1980). Also, during breast development in man, estrogens and progesterone stimulate, respectively, ductular and lobular-alveolar tissue development. In the disease-free human ovary as well as in its benign and malignant neoplasms cytoplasmic receptors have been found to include those for 17β-estradiol (ER), progesterone (PR), 5α-dihydrotestosterone, and cortisol (Galli *et al.*, 1981). The distribution of these receptors was non-uniform in the malignant neoplasms: ER and PR occurred in 50 per cent but all four receptors in only 44 per cent of the 18 malignant neoplasms investigated by Galli *et al.* In another report, PR was found in the benign lesions but not in the disease-free ovary (Holt *et al.*, 1979).

Sixth, two hormones may have mutually antagonistic effects. Progesterone, for example, antagonizes estrogen-induced endometrial growth, cervical ferning and sperm-penetrability, protein-associated anabolism particularly in the secondary sexual organs, and lipolysis. Analogously, androgen-induced prepubertal growth in the extremities is antagonized by estrogens, so that women with delayed puberty tend to have longer extremities than those with earlier puberty.

Finally, in developmental processes, hormonal action appears to be closely coupled to, and directed by, species-specific genetic inheritances. Thus, in breast, estrogens, stimulate both ductular and lobular-alveolar development in the guinea pig, cow, and goat, little or no ductular development in the dog, and, as indicated above, mainly ductular development in man.

The already-known regulatory roles of hormones are thus legion. In addition to those already mentioned, dominant roles in glucoregulation, thermoregulation, and in regulation of blood pressure, sympathetic outflow, muscular activity of the gut, gastric secretion, and stress that can induce hemorrhagic lesions are played by a variety of brain oligopeptides, among them thyrotropin-releasing hormone (Tache *et al.*, 1980). The adrenal-corticoids regulate sensitivity of noradrenaline receptor-coupled adenylate cyclase in the brain, suggesting that the pituitary-adrenal axis may be involved in mood and stress-related psychosomatic disorders (Mobley and Sulser, 1980). The brain neurones show differential sensitivity to hormones, e.g. the testosterone-sensitive neurones respond to estradiol but not to dihydrotestosterone on the one hand and testosterone and estradiol on the other may act on different brain sites (Kendrick and Drewett, 1980). In the case of progesterone, a prominent pregnancy active hormone (Section 4.1), neither its role nor mechanism of action in the brain is properly understood. However, there are marked differences between progesterone receptors in brain and uterus, and corticosteroid binding globulin enters uterine but not brain cells (Al-Khouri and Greenstein, 1980).

Mechanistically, hormonal action is poorly understood, but some valuable insights are already available. Broadly, but not exclusively (cf. Section 4.1), the polypeptide hormones first bind to specific receptors on the surfaces of appropriate target cells. The binding then activates a second messenger system (usually a cyclic nucleotide or soluble calcium), which may be the same for different targets. Consequently, the specificities involved from complexation to response must be due to factors in addition to phosphorylase activation. For example, cyclic adenosine monophosphate (cAMP) is activated intracellularly after binding of glucagon to liver, vasopressin to kidney, and ACTH to adrenal cortex. However, the respective responses are all different: glucose release, change in water permeability, and steroid hormone synthesis and release. This indicates the operation of cell-specific allosteric and other (unknown) processes.

In the case of the steroid and amine-type hormones, the response may be elicited by more direct mechanisms. These agents appear to enter cells non-specifically, but then to bind to their specific receptors found usually in the cytosol of appropriate cells. In a given tumour, the receptors may be of multiple specificities; for example, receptors for estradiol and progesterone have been found in human breast tumours. The hormone-receptor complexes, after undergoing certain changes relative to the receptors, then enter the nucleus and interact with chromatin to activate and/or repress specific genes, and thus to modulate specific mRNA species in both normal and neoplastic processes (cf. review Sledge and McGuire, 1983). Little is known about the fine molecular details of the intranuclear mechanisms involved in hormone-mediated gene control. However, enough is known to depict a bewildering complexity. Participating factors may include the polyamines (putrescine, spermine, and spermidine) generated from the L-ornithine decarboxylase-adenosyl methionine system, other intranuclear cations, the histone acetylases and phosphorylases, some of the nonhistone chromatin proteins, and RNA splicing mechanisms. Such factors, particularly the modifications of the nuclear proteins including not only the histones but also others such as some of the high-mobility group (HMG) proteins, may then, by as yet unknown mechanisms, influence specific gene regulation. Various such modifications are known to occur post-translationally, e.g. phosphorylation, acetylation, and possibly ADP-ribosylation of HMG-1, and poly(ADP-ribosylation) of the structurally related HMG's 14 and 17. Some of the smaller HMG proteins, particularly HMGs 14 and 17, like the rapidly turning-over acetylated histones, are more prominent in chromatin that is transcriptionally active, than inactive. Other intranuclear factors may be involved in the hormonally mediated gene-regulatory effects. These include factors such as 'protein A24'. This nucleolar protein has a Y-shaped structure, represented by histone H2A forming the stem and one arm of the structure and the polypeptide ubiquitin (found in all organisms inclusive of microorganisms, plants, and mammals) linked through a Gly-Gly peptide forming the other arm. In isolated nucleosomes, A24 occurs at less than one molecule per nucleosome, so that it may be associated with a specialized nucleosomal subset. Ubiquitin, in free form, predominates in active chromatin, contrasting with the predominance of the conjugated form in inactive chromatin. The factors also include a highly phosphorylated nucleolar protein (C23) of 114,000 daltons; an N-terminal blocked protein (BA) of about 31,000 daltons, which is more prominent in quiescent than rapidly growing tissues such as Novikoff and Morris hepatomas, Walker 256 carcinosarcoma, regenerating rat liver, and PHA-stimulated human lymphocytes; and a protein (C14) of about 70,000 daltons. Protein C14 stimulates RNA synthesis and decreases with progression of thioacetamide-induced liver hypertrophy in rats. Yet others include contractile proteins, such as actin, myosin, tubulin, and light and heavy tropomyosin; DNA and RNA polymerases; and a 'nucleosome assembly factor'. This factor, an acidic and apparently multimeric protein of about 100,000 daltons in its native state, induces nucleosome formation from DNA and histones under physiological conditions. (For detailed discussions of the structural and other features of the HMG proteins see reviews by Walker and other authors in Johns, 1982.)

Clearly, eukaryotic gene regulation, whether by hormones or other agents, is a highly complex affair that has been selectively evolved and has, in turn, influenced the course of evolution. Except in some simple biological systems, the source and pace of adaptation and speciation have been greatly dependent upon sexual partners involving sexual dimorphism in phenotype, function, recognition, and behaviour. In turn, sexual dimorphism shows marked dependence upon hormones. Thus, during the first phase of gestation, male and female human embryos develop identically, but this is followed by gonadal differentiation into ovaries and testes whose characteristic hormones then direct development of, respectively, female and male phenotypes. The fact that the female phenotype can develop in the absence of gonadal differentiation suggests that gonadal hormones are not necessary for female embryonic development; but male embryonic development requires, at least, Müllerian regression hormone and testosterone (Wilson *et al.*, 1981). Although few genes, notably the gene encoding the H-Y antigen, seem to govern sexual dimorphism, their control is complex, involving interactions between regulatory sites on the sex chromosomes and possibly also the autosomes (Haseltine and Ohno, 1981). Among the hormones involved, testosterone rather than 5α-dihydrotestosterone controls extragenital sexual dimorphism in organs other than skin and reproductive tract, but other steroid metabolites and their receptors are also required to produce the diverse physical and other differences seen in males and females. Among the others are differences in disease susceptibility, in response to drugs and toxins, and in the metabolism and assimilation of dietary constituents (Bardin and Catterall, 1981). Gonadal hormones also influence permanent and largely irreversible sexual differentiation in the central nervous system and, thus, sexual differences in behaviour patterns (McLusky and Naftolin, 1981; McEwen, 1981). Postnatally, certain sexually dimorphic behaviour patterns are influenced by gonadal hormones interacting in complex ways with psychological, sociocultural, and other factors (Rubin *et al.*, 1981).

The great importance of the body's hormones in gene regulation is only beginnning to be fully appreciated. Even more important for present purposes is the likelihood that they may play important roles in the *control* of neoplastic development, at least in the preclinical stages. Thus, epidermal tissues, whether normal as in the case of human keratinocytes or malignant as in the case of human colon carcinoma cells, grow well in artificial serum-free culture media supplemented with suitable hormones (Maciag *et al.*, 1981). Analogously, mammary, endometrial, thyroid, prostatic, and other cancers of endocrine-responsive epithelial tissues show variable dependence for their growth upon the same hormones that control the growth and differentiation (or maintenance of function) of the corresponding normal tissues themselves. However, it remains a moot point whether such hormonal functions can be adequately represented in model systems that lack the complex hormonal interdependencies that exist in whole organisms. For instance, it is a well known paradox that estrogens can produce hyperplasia and hypertrophy of the uterus, vagina, and other responsive organs in castrated animals, but by themselves have no effect on the growth rates of cultured cells from such tissues (Sonnenschein and Soto, 1980).

4.5 Outlook: Some Fundamental Implications of Neoplasia, with Special Reference to Maldifferentiation and Ectopic Hormone Synthesis

The fact that species-specific differences in genetic inheritances can vary the gene control activity of the same hormone is no more surprising than is the incapacity of a petunia seed in an onion patch or of a mouse zygote in a rat uterus to develop into an onion plant or a rat. Analogously, the same abnormality in the hormonal or other type of environment may produce different pathological effects upon different species or genetically distinct individuals of a given species. For example, exposure to DES, tobacco smoke, or any other carcinogen neither produces cancer in all exposed species or individuals, nor the same type of cancer in those developing the disease. Thus, the first level of gene control is at the genetic inheritance itself.

Gene control in neoplastic processes thus appears to be at least as complex as it is in the normal counterparts. If hormones are as important in the former processes as they are in the latter, it seems unlikely that the role of hormones in neoplasia can be restricted to any simple category such as that of 'promotion', as envisaged in the two-stage carcinogenesis concept developed during the 1940s mainly by Isaac Berenblum of Israel and Philippe Shubik of the United States (Berenblum, 1941; Berenblum and Shubik, 1947). Upon suitable target cells, which may fall within the range of normalcy dictated by the astounding genetic heterogeneity of natural species of organisms, a natural hormone may be sufficient to 'initiate' as well as 'promote' carcinogenesis. In the mouse, for example, Huseby (1980) recently showed that estradiol, possibly with a cocarcinogenic influence of pituitary hormones, produced a direct neoplastic effect on Leydig cells. The testicular tumours were not due to the action of some systemic metabolite, or of any conventional exogenously-derived carcinogenic 'initiator'. This two-stage concept stemmed largely from the observation that the noncarcinogenic croton oil, whose active component is now known to be a phorbol ester, can enhance mouse skin tumorigenesis by a tumour 'initiator' such as 3-methylcholanthrene. It was foreshadowed by some earlier findings, particularly by Murray Jacob Shear's observation, in the United States in 1938, of the capacity of a basic fraction of creosote oil, which he considered to be a 'cocarcinogen', to enhance mouse skin tumorigenesis by benzo(a)pyrene. Later studies have shown that certain goitrogens, hormones, and other endocrine factors can influence experimental carcinogenesis by agents such as 2-acetylaminofluorene (cf. Chapter Three, Section 3.6.3.6).

When the complexity of gene-environment interactions in normal life processes is considered, it is always possible to postulate the involvement of one or more 'initiating' carcinogens at some stage during these processes. However, as discussed above, a variety of hormonal manipulations appear sometimes to be sufficient in themselves either to produce cancer (Section 4.2) or to cause its regression (Section 4.3), and in a manner which can differ according to species, strain, or individual. As reviewed by Thelma B. Dunn (1979), for example, adminstered estrogen produces granular cell myoblastomas and cancers of the cervix, vagina, and breast in some strains of female mice, but pituitary tumours in others. In male mice, it produces testicular tumours, but kidney tumours in male hamsters. In rats, it produces mammary tumours, but mammary and uterine tumours in female rabbits, and human fibromyoma-like conditional (hormone-dependent) uterine and abdominal tumours in female guinea pigs. Indeed, some of the effects may also be specific to sex and developmental stage. Thus, testosterone given to pregnant rats causes genital maldevelopment in the female but not male fetuses. The prominent pathological effects of the same transplacentally active agent such as DES can be embryotoxic during cleavage, implantation, and placental stages, but teratogenic during organogenesis, and carcinogenic during histogenesis.

An associated phenomon which is becoming so familiar that it may well be a general feature of neoplasia is that of deranged (ectopic or eutopic) synthesis of hormones by tumours. Discovery of this phenomenon of 'paraendocrine neoplasia' stemmed from W.H. Brown's report, in 1928, of a case of hyperadrenocorticism, or of the 'Periglandular Syndrome: "Diabetes of Bearded Women"'. By 1961, over 40 analogous cases had become well-documented, all showing various combinations of the features (e.g. weakness, hypokalemia, hyperglycemia, glycosuria, edema, obesity of trunk, purple striae atrophica on abdomen and flanks, polycythemia, excessive bruising and amenorrhea in women, and osteoporosis) associated with the classical syndrome described around the turn of this century by the Boston neurosurgeon, Harvey William Cushing. Liddle *et al.* investigated 37 cases of this 'ectopic ACTH syndrome' (cf. Liddle *et al.*, 1969). These involved, among others, cancers of the lung, pancreas, thymus, prostate, mediastinum, parotid, ovary, breast, and liver, and pheochromocytoma and ganglioma. Their basic findings were that the syndrome is due to uncontrolled (uncontrollable by administered dexamethasone) production of apparently normal (as judged by various biological, physical, chemical, and immunological criteria) ACTH usually in association with other ectopic products (e.g. melanocyte stimulating hormone, gastrin, parathyroid hormone, antidiuretic hormone), all capable of performing their normal functions but independently of normal host controls. The ACTH overproduction, for instance, resulted in adrenal hyperstimulation, overproduction of corticosteroids including plasma and urinary 17-hydroxycorticosteroids, and the clinical manifestations of the classical 'Cushing syndrome'. Liddle *et al.* speculated that 'many of the now obscure manifestations of malignancy might some day be understood in terms of the noxious effects of tumour products which are carried like hormones to other parts of the body where they exert unwanted effects'.

All of these findings have since become sufficiently well-documented and extended to other tumours and other ectopic and eutopic tumour products to make the basic principles involved some of the cornerstones of modern oncology (some reviews: Hall, 1974; Odell *et al.*, 1974; Waldenstrom, 1978). The basic principles are that tumour development is a reordering of cellular genes to yield phenotypes selected, almost evolution-like, for survival advantage and towards an increasing degree of relative autonomy that abrogates the ordered intercellular and intertissular sociology of the host organism. The genes which are reordered are normal host genes, so that structurally aberrant products that may lead to tumour cell destruction by the host's homeostatic (e.g. immunological) systems either are not produced, or may be produced but remain ineffectual as stimulators of specific tumour rejection. In many later detailed studies of the phenomenon, products interpreted initially to represent those of novel genes have turned out to be normal gene products such as biosynthetic precursors. Gastrin, for example, usually contains 17 amino-acid residues, but it sometimes also contains 13 (in 'mini' gastrin, or G-13), 34 (in 'big'gastrin, or G-34), or some larger number (in 'big big' gastrin) of such residues. Apparently all of these modifications can exist in the normal stomach as sulfated or nonsulfated forms, with the normal circulating form being nonsulfated G-17, or 'little' gastrin. Presumably 'big big' gastrin is the biosynthetic precursor of the other gastrins formed through its graded proteolysis. Thus, one of these modifications, rare but actually normal, can sometimes be erroneously described to represent a product of a novel gene acquired by the tumour during its progression, or by the normal progenitor cell of the tumour as a prelude to or cause of malignant transformation of that cell.   ·

The above-mentioned speculation of Liddle *et al.* has also been documented only too well. It is now well known (Hall, 1974) that uncontrolled synthesis or lack of synthesis (through abnormal differentiation) of hormones, enzymes, antigens, and other potently active normal cellular products by tumours is the biochemical basis of the 'paraneoplastic' effects. These effects include the cachexia (general wasting away) and the enhanced susceptibility and vulnerability to even normally mild intercurrent infections which are mainly responsible for the dehumanization and fatality of malignancy.

It is not known whether the abnormal synthesis is itself the cause or a mere consequence of neoplasia. However, it is becoming increasingly clear that the reordering of normal genes which occurs during neoplastic development is in the same mould as that occurring in normal development. In either case, it is an expression of the innate capacities of the inherited cellular genome; although, in the former case, there are degrees of disordered expression or, in the words of Azzopardi and Evans (1971), of 'divergent differentiation'. The synthesis of ectopic hormones in neoplastic development, for instance, is effected not only by APUD, neural crest, or other normal endocrine progenitor cells but also by cells of multiple embryologic origin (Baylin and Mendelsohn, 1980; Vuitch and Mendelsohn, 1981). Conversely, the same type of neoplasm may produce a variety of ectopic products. Among such products of breast cancer, for instance, are ACTH, calcitonin, parathyroid hormone, chorionic gonadotropin, and norepinephrine (Cohle *et al.*, 1979).

Biochemical endocrinology may indeed hold as many of the secrets of neoplastic development as it undoutedly does in the normal counterpart. More broadly, these secrets appear to be held by the same phenomena which are at the root of all biology: the genetic inheritance, its evolution and diversification, and its developmental control. The role of the genetic inheritance itself in neoplasia is the subject of the next chapter.

5 HEREDITY AND CANCER: COMPARATIVE ASPECTS

5.1 Introduction: Unity, Diversity, and the Genetic and Medical Paradigms of Health and Disease

Inherited genomes cannot function independently of either their own innate capabilities or their environment. Physiologically, it is unlikely that a mouse genome, in any environment, could develop into a man. Pathologically, a peculiarly human disorder such as the skin-cancer-predisposing xeroderma pigmentosum or the smoking-associated oat-cell lung carcinoma is not known either to occur naturally or to be inducible in experimental animals. Analogously, even an 'environmental' human disease such as malaria or *Schistosoma haematobium*-associated bladder cancer is not known to occur in the insect or snail vector harbouring the implicated pathogen. Oncogenic viruses such as the feline leukemia virus or the chicken sarcoma virus of domestic animals with which humans are in constant contact are not known to produce cancer in man. Conversely, human viruses such as some of the adenoviruses are non-oncogenic in humans, their natural hosts, but they can produce fatal cancers when artificially introduced into some animals (Chapter Three, Section 3.4.4.2.3). Consequently, the essential basis of perhaps all aspects of normal and pathological developments is ecogenetic. The terms 'genetic disease' and 'environmental disease' are hence relative and operational within this generalized framework.

Currently, there are two major but quite different concepts of human health and disease. The first of these, the medical or environmental paradigm, has traditionally regarded all populations and all individuals as being essentially uniform in their homeostasis and in their inherent risk of disease, both of which are variable in a specific environment-dependent manner. This concept stresses the importance of specific environments in health maintenance and disease causation. Its prominent feature is specific environmental effects in a common genotype.

It is this concept which has engendered the widely encountered

177

notion, popularized during the 1960s, that up to 90 per cent of all human cancers are directly caused by the environment and, hence, are only marginally, if at all genetic (Haddow, 1967; Higginson, 1968; Higginson and Muir, 1973; Boyland, 1969; Doll, 1977; see also Chapter Nine, Section 9.4). This statement was based upon human cancer statistics showing that, for these cancers, incidence rates vary significantly between populations, and upon calculations assuming the lowest observed incidence rates for specific cancer types to represent the inherently uniform and specific environment-independent risks.

The second concept, the less traditional and less popular but growing genetic or genetic-environmental paradigm, recognizes significant inborn differences between populations or individuals, both in homeostasis and in susceptibility or resistance to disease. It stresses the importance of intrinsic (genetic) factors interacting with extrinsic (environmental) factors to produce states of equilibrium in health and of disequilibrium in disease. Its prominent feature is specific genotypic effects in a common (e.g. public) or a more restricted (e.g. private) environment.

The genetic paradigm is thus all-inclusive. It accommodates, at the two extremes of the disease spectrum which it describes, disorders in which the role of one or more specific components, genetic or environmental, is overwhelming; and, at different points between these extremes, those disorders, which may include most of the common human cancers, for which both types of component play important roles. These components, because of their complexity, are particularly difficult to identify and control.

The extreme cases, the operationally defined genetic or environmental diseases, have different implications and consequences, e.g. relative to prevention, diagnosis, and treatment. For instance, environmental diseases of the nutritional-deficiency or infectious type are being diagnosed specifically by biochemical or other means, and are being controlled more-or-less specifically., e.g. by appropriate dietary corrections, chemoprophylaxis (specific, or nonspecific), or immunoprophylaxis (active or passive). Infectious diseases such as cholera, influenza, gonorrhea, syphilis, leprosy, malaria, tuberculosis, and rheumatic fever are controllable by specific chemoprophylaxis, i.e. by treatment with a drug before, during, or shortly after the infective exposure, usually to a specific agent. When the drug treatment is directed simultaneously against several agents, and particularly when at least one of these agents is endogenous to the patient, the pro-phylactic effect tends to be nonspecific. Most of these diseases, as well as others, including tetanus, diphtheria, mumps, rubella, and typhoid are controllable by active or passive immunoprophylaxis, i.e. by direct vaccination of the individual with an appropriate antigen or toxoid, or by treatment of the individual with an appropriate antiserum from another individual or from an immunized animal. (For reviews, see Mortimer, 1978; Jackson, 1979). The clinical approach to the genetic diseases, in contrast, is genetically oriented. It is also, perhaps always, nonspecific, mainly because of current technological inadequacies (e.g. regarding the requisite genetic rectification), but also because no genetic lesion is yet known which simultaneously is exclusive to, and occurs in all cases of, the disease with which the lesion is associated. These features of the approach apply equally whether in relation to screening for high-risk individuals, e.g. by amniocentesis or other modes of prenatal diagnosis for high risk pregnancies (for a review, see Omenn, 1978) or by pedigree analysis or other modes of detection of persons at high risk of cancer, or to patient retrieval, genetic counselling, treatment, follow-up, or after-care.

The principle of basic differences between the two approaches is well illustrated by the nutrition-related disorders, e.g. a non-hereditary dietary protein-deficiency disorder such as kwashiorkor on the one hand and, on the other, one of the related hereditary disorders, the 'inborn errors of metabolism' first described by Garrod around the turn of the century. Kwashiorkor, an African word signifying 'the disease the child gets when the next baby is born' (*Butterworths Medical Dictionary*, 1978), describes a pellagra-like condition characterized by anemia, edema, stunted growth, skin lesions including depigmentation, bulky soft stools, and reversal of albumin/globulin ratio. Occurring most commonly among chronically malnourished children, mainly in Africa, South Africa, and the East and West Indies, it shows no significant ethnic, familial, or other indications of a genetic disorder, such as are shown by the large number of known hereditary metabolic disorders (McKusick, 1975; Milne, 1974). Among the latter are disorders related to inherited defects in absorption and transport of essential body requirements. The latter include amino acids (e.g. the 'blue diaper' or tryptophan malabsorption syndrome, phenylketonuria, and Hartnup disease), carbohydrates (e.g. the amylase deficiency, fructose intolerance, and lactase deficiency syndromes), fats (e.g. abetalipoproteinemia, intestinal.amyloidosis, and mucoviscidosis or cystic fibrosis of the pancreas), electrolytes (e.g. familial chloride diarrhea, hepatolenticular degeneration or Wilson's disease, and vitamin D resistant rickets), and vitamin B_{12} (e.g. pernicious anemia, congenital deficiency of intrinsic factor, and hereditary folate malabsorption). Appropriate dietary correction often cures the environmental disorder; but, at best, it may only alleviate the symptoms of the genetic disorder.

In either event, one outcome of modern advances in hygiene (particularly of the use of soap and hot water), and in medicine, nutrition and related disciplines, is the propagation, within the human gene pool, of potentially disease-producing genetic elements which, in the absence of these advances, might have been selectively eliminated, i.e. by infertility or pre-reproductive death of the affected individual. Thus, according to most estimates (for a review, see Scriver *et al.*, 1978), chromosomal anomalies are now known to be present in, and presumably to be responsible for, about 50 per cent of all spontaneously aborted fetuses and about 5 per cent of all perinatal mortality; and to persist in about 0.5 per cent of all live births. Diverse genetic variants capable of producing handicap during a lifetime occur in about 10 per cent of live-born infants; and about 15 per cent of diagnoses among hospital admissions with severe mental retardation reflect a Mendelian and about 45 per cent some other genetic component.

For various reasons, it is difficult to quantify the role of man's activity in modulating the course of human evolution by propagation of artificially induced, potentially disease-producing genetic elements. Thus, diverse chromosomal and/or genetic anomalies are associated with exposure to man-made chemicals and radiation. However, they also occur with normal ageing; and, whether spontaneous or induced, their occurrence is almost confined to somatic cells (Chapter Seven, Section 7.3.5) which, like specific chromosomes themselves, are not involved in vertical transmission. Whether or not they carry anomalies, specific chromosomes are notoriously transient structures that manifest themselves only during certain cell-cycle stages, and they finally disappear forever with the demise of their host organisms. None the less, some of the anomalies, such as those affecting sperm mobility, can rarely be induced in the otherwise naturally highly-protected germ cells (Chapter Two, Section 2.6.16), in contrast with their much greater frequency in the less protected and highly dispensable somatic cells. Also, some chromosome anomalies or, preferably, the propensity to develop these anomalies, which may be associated with man's activities, are heritable. An example is the balanced (Robertsonian) translocations in Down's syndrome, which are accentuated by procreation in mothers aged 35 years or more (Chapter Seven, Section 7.5). Finally, the use of modern cytogenetic techniques such as amniocentesis can have opposing consequences. For instance, it may eliminate a potentially disease-producing genetic element, by voluntary abortion of a conceptus found to harbour the element; or it may itself induce such an element. The role of medical care in propagation of the Mendelian, multigenic, or chromosomal diseases which are harboured by some 12 per cent of pediatric hospital admissions (Scriver *et al.*, 1978) is also difficult to quantify, because of factors such as the patients' advanced years restricting procreativity, and the natural protection of the germ line from the ravages of ageing seen in the somatic line.

It thus seems unlikely that man's intervention in the natural course of evolution is responsible for most of his potentially disease-producing genetic burden. As is known for many non-human species, e.g. for populations showing marked interregional differences in disease transmission efficiency among insects (Powell *et al.*, 1980) or in physiological tolerance among Amargosa pupfish (Hirschfield *et al.*, 1980), the bulk of the genetic burden among humans appears to be due to natural evolution. For instance, factors such as genetic drift, selection, and founder effects are believed to be mainly responsible for the many known Mendelian conditions displayed at unusually high frequency by various ethnic subgroups (McKusick, 1975). Some well-known examples are porphyria variegata among Afrikaaners; hereditary tyrosinemia among French Canadians; sickle cell anemia and α and β thalassemias among African Negroes; α-thalassemia among the Chinese and certain other Asiatics; β-thalassemia among Italians, Greeks, Sephardic Jews, and certain other Mediterranean peoples; congenital nephrosis among Finns; the Ellis-van Creveld syndrome among the Amish; homozygous familial hyper-cholesterolemia among the Lebanese; acatalasemia among the Japanese; and Tay-Sachs disease among the Ashkenazi Jews. Indeed, it seems likely that most if not all distinct human populations may each possess a peculiar predisposition to at least one genetic disorder. This may be because such populations have evolved in comparative isolation until very recently in evolutionary terms, at least until the time of the Phoenicians or even of the great explorations of the late fifteenth century onwards. This, together with the subsequent phenomenal rise of industrialization and transportation, has been leading towards establishment of an essentially single, uniform human society marked by progressive lifting of the ages-old religious, social, economic, and related barriers to free interminglings and intermarriages. Continuation of this process may well result in eventual elimination of the more extreme examples of marked ethnic predisposition to a variety of neoplastic and other diseases. Ashkenazi Jews, for instance, are peculiarly prone not only to the already-mentioned Tay Sachs disease but also to others including Kaposi sarcoma, lymphoma, Bloom's syndrome (a cancer-predisposing condition), abetalipoproteinemia, recessive dystonia musculorum deformans, factor XI (PTA) deficiency, familial dysantonomia (Riley-Day syndrome), Gaucher's disease (adult form), Niemann-Pick disease, and pentosuria (Goodman and Motulsky, 1979).

Although the isolated evolution has not been sufficiently prolonged to establish either distinct non-interbreeding human species or, apparently, exclusive ethnic segregation of specific disease-associated genes, it seems to have been long enough to establish ethnic peculiarities to at least some of the diseases which segregate in two or more ethnic populations. For instance, among Negroes, some of the usual clinical features of α-thalassemia are very rare, notably hemoglobin H and Bart's hydrops fetalis which, respectively, are usually associated with doubly heterozygous α-thalassemias 1 and 2 and with homozygous α-thalassemia 1. Recent studies have indicated that Negro α-thalassemia 1 resembles Oriental α-thalassemia 2 in its single α-globin gene anomaly (Higgs *et al.*, 1979), and that its phenotype may represent homozygosity for α-thalassemia 2 (Serjeant *et al.*, 1980).

The apparent lack of exclusive ethnic segregation of disease-associated genes is exemplified by the hemoglobin E trait. This β-globin anomaly is found mainly among certain South-East Asian populations, notably the Burmese, Malays, Indonesians, Siamese, and Cambodians, and it has been reported to be absent from the African Negroes, the American Indians, and the Japanese (Shibata, 1961). However, sporadic cases of the trait are increasingly being reported among Negro and many other populations including Indians, Persians, Turks, Egyptians, Qatarians,

Greeks, and Germans (El-Shirbiny *et al.*, 1980). This would suggest the presence of the trait in perhaps all human populations.

Continuing genetic analysis of many types of neoplastic and non-neoplastic disorders of man, by old methods such as those of population genetics including pedigree analysis and by new methods such as those of restriction enzyme analysis and cloning of cellular DNA, are providing valuable insights into the complex pathogenetic mechanisms which operate even for the simply inherited disorders. For instance, one of the two major categories of the extensively reviewed (e.g. Furbetta *et al.*, 1979; Bellevue *et al.*, 1979; Gallo *et al.*, 1979; Bank *et al.*, 1980) heritable disorders of the simply inherited globin genes is the hemoglobinopathies represented by sickle cell anemia in which both β genes are of the mutant (β^s) type. This category involves qualitative changes in globin, usually single base substitutions in DNA that generate corresponding single amino acid substitutions in globin. However, no fewer than 100 such changes are known to generate the at least as many normal variants of just one (HbA, or $\alpha_2\beta_2$) of the two adult forms of the major human hemoglobin tetramers. The second adult form is HbA_2, or $\alpha_2\delta_2$; and the other major tetramers are the embryonic hemoglobins Gower I ($\zeta_2\epsilon_2$), Gower II ($\alpha_2\epsilon_2$), and Portland ($\zeta_2\gamma_2$) together with the fetal hemoglobin HbF ($\alpha_2\gamma_2$). The γ globin genes are of at least two major types, Gγ and Aγ, respectively encoding a glycine or an alanine residue at the triplet codon for position 136 on the γ globins.

The second major category, represented by the thalassemias, involves qualitative changes, usually reductions but also imbalances, in synthesis of structurally normal globin genes. This can be due, in different instances, to some defect in a control element, either at the level of control genes in the linked Gγ-Aγ-δ-β gene locus on chromosome 11 or in the α-α gene locus on chromosome 16, or at the level of transcription, processing of the primary transcripts, or translation of the mRNAs. Further, the thalassemias themselves represent a heterogeneous group of disorders with variable clinical features. For example, anemia is usually mild in the HbG and heterozygous forms but severe in the homozygous forms of β-thalassemia (Bank *et al.*, 1980), and it is usually milder in the α-thalassemia of Negroes than of South-East Asian and other populations (Bellevue *et al.*, 1979). In addition to these heterogeneous patterns, there are others comprising the 'thalassemia intermedia syndromes', i.e. the $\beta/\delta\beta$, $\alpha_2\beta/\beta$, and the β/β-heterocellular HPFH (hereditary persistence of fetal hemoglobin) patterns (Gallo *et al.*, 1979). In two (δβ and HPFH) forms of thalassemia, the only globin detectable is the fetal form (Bank *et al.*, 1980), but nothing is known about why HbF persists in these cases, about how the switchings from the embryonic to the fetal to the adult forms occur, or even about the chromosomal location of the embryonic globin genes.

Despite the paucity of current knowledge about the molecular genetics of the interindividual variations, the many already known differences would leave no chance whatsoever that any two human individuals, except identical twins, are genetically identical. There are, for instance, the well-known differences in features such as voice; fingerprints; skin and hair textures; the ABO blood groups and their scores of subgroups; the Rh factors; the HLA haplotypes, which alone occur in at least 300 million different combinations (Bodmer and Bodmer, 1978); and the variations in platelets and isoenzyme patterns. The inheritance of such marked and varied differences in blood has aided identification of the ancient origins of ethnic populations such as the American Indians (to North-East Asia) and the Basques (to the remnants of neolithic tribes fleeing the Indo-European invasions before 1000 BC). Hereditary deficiency of erythrocyte glucose-6-phosphate dehydrogenase has accounted for the serious anemia sometimes experienced by Sardinians, Jews, and other Mediterranean people treated with the antimalarial drug primaquine.

In recent years the known list of recognized 'genetic' cancers has been steadily growing, already sufficiently to attract many reviews of the subject (e.g. Schimke, 1978; Feingold, 1978; Strong, 1978; Harris *et al.*, 1980; Lynch, 1976; Harnden *et al.*, 1984; see also Chapter Six). These and related reports are documenting a prominent trend — that of an increasing realization of the existence, among humans and other species, of considerable inborn genetic variability in susceptibility or resistance even to those types of cancer which are most strongly associated with environmental factors. Examples are lung cancer associated with smoking and upper digestive tract cancers with alcoholism, in which even the habits themselves may have a genetic basis (Tokuhata and Lilienfeld, 1963; Cohen *et al.*, 1977; Goodwin, 1976, 1979; Mendelson and Mello, 1979). For these associations, the concept of a hereditary role, even a decade ago, not only was unsuspected but also would have been 'laughed out of class' if then proposed.

Certainly the most searching but, hopefully, never-to-be-repeated test of the concept has been the most extreme of all cancer-associated exposures known to history, the atomic blasts of Hiroshima and Nagasaki. These, with their searing clouds of gamma and neutron rays, have already claimed around 200,000 human lives and might be expected to have completely over-whelmed the interindividual differences. Yet, even from the midst of this Dantean inferno of death and destruction, some have survived. Among the survivors, some have developed various malignancies while few, including Dr and Mrs Akizuki, have re-mained free of cancer, 35 years later, i.e. long after the known latency period of radiation-induced cancers. Dr Akizuki, believing that he was spared in order to tell the gruesome details of the immediate aftermath of those blasts, reported as follows (Honey-combe, 1980):

> The sky was as dark as pitch, covered with dense clouds of smoke; under that blackness all the buildings on earth were [appeared to be] on fire . . . as if the earth itself sent forth flames . . . the ground was scarlet. Three kinds of colour (black, yellow, and scarlet) loomed over the people, who ran about like so many worms seeking to escape. But that ocean of fire, that sky of smoke! . . . They walked with strange, slow steps, groaning from deep within them, as if they came from the depths of hell. Their faces had the appearance of masks. It was like a scene from the Buddhist scriptures, their laments echoing everywhere, as if the earth itself was in pain . . . the crowd of ghosts that had looked whitish in the morning were now turning black.

In less dramatic ways, the existence of markedly variable spontaneous and induced neoplasia between and within species is becoming increasingly obvious.

5.2 Interspecific Comparisons

5.2.1 Spontaneous Cancer

5.2.1.1 Overview. With the pioneering studies of Maud Slye and others particularly since the First World War, it has been becom-ing increasingly evident that the natural incidence of cancer both between and within animal species is significantly nonrandom. As reviewed by Willis (1967), for instance, the earlier evidence indicated that spontaneous neoplasms are rarer in sheep and pigs than in most other domestic animals, in rabbits and guinea pigs than in rats and mice, and in cats than in dogs. In dogs, the neoplasms predominate during and after middle age, involving mainly the breast, skin, testis, bone, tonsil, and lymphatic system, but rarely the stomach and intestines which, in contrast, are two of the commonest cancer sites in man. In turn, some types of spontaneous neoplasms which are rare in man are common in animals. These include leukemias and lymphomas in mice, cats, and chickens, papillary tumours of the conjuctiva which are among the commonest of tumours in horses and cattle, testicular tumours in dogs and horses, and embryonic renal tumours in pigs, rabbits, and rats.

For practically all types of spontaneously-occurring animal neoplasms, significant interspecific differences are known. For instance, spontaneous renal neoplasms are rare in mice (Terracini and Campobasso, 1979). So are spontaneous tumours of all types, including hematologic tumours, in non-human primates (Lingeman *et al.*, 1979). This contrasts sharply with the situation in man, who appears to be the most cancer-afflicted of all known metazoan species (Chapter One, Section 1.2.3); but he is also the most well-investigated to the old ages at which cancer most clearly manifests itself. None the less, non-human primates, in common with all metazoan species, are not immune to spontaneous neoplasia. For example, spontaneous tumours found in Rhesus macaques and other non-human primates include oral tumours (Shalev *et al.*, 1980) as well as lymphomas showing some clinical features of other naturally-occurring animal lymphomas and of non-Hodgkin human lymphomas (Terrell *et al.*, 1980). As in man, the lymphomas in macaques may not have a viral etiology which, in turn, is not always evident even in the case of species showing a high susceptibility to hematologic tumours. In the chicken, for instance, the several types of lymphoid neoplasm which are known include one type which is apparently caused by the leukosis virus, another by the reticuloendotheliosis virus, a third (an acute type) by the Marek's disease herpesvirus, and yet other types for which a viral or any other etiological association is unknown, including that with a virus such as RAV-O, which is an endogenous avian leukosis virus of subgroup E (Crittenden *et al.*, 1979).

Hematologic neoplasms are also common in mice, occurring mainly in association with certain oncornaviruses such as the murine leukemia virus; but mice rarely develop the many types of epithelial neoplasm, such as bladder carcinoma, which are common in man. Indeed, spontaneous bladder neoplasms are rare or unknown in most animal species, they having been rarely observed, according to a recent review (Wood and Bonser, 1979) in rats, rabbits, pigs, dogs, horses, mules, cattle, a cat, a fishing cat, and a mongoose.

Like the non-human primates, species with low overall incidence of spontaneous neoplasia are not immune to specific types of the disease. For instance, large white pigs are prone to a form of lymphoma showing an autosomal recessive mode of inheritance (Brownlie *et al.*, 1978), and sheep to a peculiar type of bronchiolar-alveolar carcinoma ('pulmonary adenomatosis') called 'jaagsiekte', a South African term denoting the type of respiratory acceleration which characterizes the disease (Hod and Milchan, 1979).

Proper interspecific comparisons would require observation of feral animals in their natural environments up to the older ages at which cancer predominates, but this has rarely been done. Most of the available data refer to the common laboratory animals, particularly inbred animals introduced largely to facilitate transplantation of experimental tumours. As outlined below for some of the commoner types of neoplasm occurring in humans, even the laboratory animals show marked variations in their natural susceptibilities to both spontaneous and induced neoplasia. (For extensive discussions, see Strong, 1978; and various authors in the *Pathology of Tumours in Laboratory Animals*, published serially since 1973 under the editorship of V.S. Turusov and the joint auspices of the World Health Organization and the International Agency for Research on Cancer).

5.2.1.2 Mammary Cancer. The comparative incidence and other features of mammary neoplasia in the murine and other species have been extensively reviewed (e.g. Nandi and McGrath, 1973; Hamilton, 1974; Stewart, 1976; Casey *et al.*, 1979; Squartini, 1979; Mesa-Tejada and Spiegelman, 1983; Hynes *et al.*, 1984). In general, this disease, which is among the oldest known and commonest of neoplasms in women, is rare among large domesticated animals including the pig, sheep, goat, and horse. It is also rare among cows, despite their large mammary glands, and among non-human primates, despite their menstrual cycle being comparable to that of women (Casey *et al.*, 1979). This suggests that neither breast size, menstrual cycle, nor phylogeny is a necessary correlate of breast cancer susceptibility. In contrast, the disease is three to four times less common in women than in dogs, whose estrus cycle, occurring once every 6–9 months with a 3–6 months' period of anestrus, differs markedly from the menstrual cycle of women and other primates.

According to most reports, breast tumour development in the dog is dependent upon ovarian hormones, with over half of the tumours occurring in the two caudal pairs of the five pairs of mammary glands. Dogs develop a great histologic variety of breast lesions, including benign or apparently benign dysplasias, benign tumours, and malignancies of the sarcomatous, carcinomatous, and mixed sarcomatous-carcinomatous types. Mammary neoplasia is also common in cats and mice. However, among all the species (e.g. cats, dogs, mice, and humans) in which it has been found to be common, only in mice has a viral etiology been established. Moreover, the murine tumours develop mainly from the luminal or secretory cells of acinar origin, and the rat tumours are mainly benign fibromas, adenomas, and fibroadenomas. The murine tumours involve the ductules and alveoli mainly, and the rat tumours are mainly non-malignant, contrasting with the predominant epithelial or ductal origin and the pronounced metastatic propensity of the human tumours.

Thus, neither the disease in the large domestic animals, nor in the non-human primate, the dog, the mouse, or the rat would appear to be a suitable model for the human counterpart. This is despite the fact that B particles resembling the murine mammary tumour virus (MTV), anti-MTV antibodies, reverse transcriptase, and some sequence homology with MTV RNA have occasionally been found to occur in association with human breast cancer (for references, see Squartini, 1979; Mesa-Tejada and Spiegelman, 1983). In contrast, the feline disease displays some analogies with its human counterpart: a predominant epithelial origin, a pronounced tendency to metastasize (especially to the lung), significant hormone dependence, and occurrence mainly at older ages. For these reasons, the feline disease has sometimes been proposed as a suitable model of the human disease, but it remains still insufficiently explored to allow proper evaluation of this proposal.

5.2.1.3 Ovarian Cancer. In terms of evolutionary significance, the ovary can be regarded as the most important of the body's organs. Upon the ovary's prime function, oogenesis, rests species propagation which, actually in some species and at least theoretically in others, can occur through parthenogenesis, i.e. independently of spermatogenesis and fertilization. Also unlike the mammalian breast, which shares many of its structural and functional features with skin tissues reflecting its likely evolution from sweat glands, the ovary displays some unique features analogously to those of the ovarian function-controlling organs such as the pituitary and adrenal. The adrenal, for instance, is unique in that it can hardly be regarded as a single organ in view of its cortex and medulla having distinct hormonal functions and responses and apparently distinct embryologic origins. The uniqueness of the ovary is lifelong, starting with its earliest organogenesis when it is endowed with specialized germ cells (oogonia) which, at or even before birth, develop into the ovary's full, irreplaceable and specific complement of diploid primary oocytes. The latter, at ovulation, undergo meiosis to form haploid secondary oocytes and haploid first polar bodies, followed by modified mitosis to form mature haploid ova and haploid second polar bodies. Thus, and also through prematurative degeneration of some of the ova and of the Graffian follicles ('folliculi ovarici vesiculosi') which rupture to release them, the oocytes are gradually lost to become rare or totally absent in old age. During ovarian activity, cyclical changes occur, marked by the growth of some selected oocytes into mature follicles, within a complex relationship between germ cell and stroma. Granulosa and theca cells form corpora lutea which, like the conditional neoplasms, grow and then disappear in the stroma. This entire, highly complex and selective process is also highly controlled, e.g. by pituitary and ovarian hormones; is accompanied by appropriate changes in vascularization and blood supply; and is strictly modulated during pregnancy, lactation, and ageing. With increasing age, for instance, the delicate balance between hormonal stimulation and ovarian response gradually deteriorates, resulting in marked changes in ovarian structure and function. Superimposed upon this generalized mammalian pattern are interspecific differences. Between humans and mice, for instance, the differences seem to be related to factors such as the smaller size of the murine ovary, the continuous estrus cycles (as opposed to the human menstrual cycle) of the animal's reproductive life, and its shorter post-reproductive life. Also, in mice compared with women, an inactive reserve of fibrous ovarian tissue is less pronounced, stromal cells are more prominently differentiated into thecal and interstitial cells, and the corpora lutea are less persistent and more tracelessly resorbed.

The relationships between these differences and those characterizing the ovarian neoplasms of mice and women remain unclear. In general, the murine tumours are rarer, less metastatic, and histologically less diverse than are their human counterparts; but, despite these differences, the complexity of even the murine tumours is such as to make exact definitions, e.g. of histologic origins or of distinction between benign and malignant lesions, extremely hazardous. The subject has been well discussed recently by Lemon and Gubareva (1979) who, in a review of the literature and a study specifically of some 3,000 ovarian tumours in about 5,000 white non-pedigree mice of the 'Rappolovo' strain, were able to classify the tumours broadly into three groups. The first group comprised potentially hormonally active tumours resembling histologically either the female gonad (granulosa-cell tumours, theca-cell and theca-granulosa-cell tumours, and luteomas) or parts of the male gonad (androblastomas, and Sertoli cell and Leydig cell tumours). In the second group were tumours that are always hormonally inactive (tubular adenomas, cystadenomas, fibromas, and angiomas); and, in the third, miscellaneous rare tumours (teratomas, mucin-producing tumours, endotheliomas, and sarcomas).

Many other examples of species-specific differences in ovarian neoplasia are known. For example, the disease accounts for 1.4 per cent of all neoplasms in dogs, compared with 1.8 per cent in horses, less than 0.7 per cent in pigs, and 4 per cent in ruminants generally. The granulosa-cell neoplasms are predominant in cattle, these and cystadenomas in dogs, and teratomas in horses (Zembrzycka, 1979). In women, ovarian cancer accounts for about 20 per cent of all genital cancers and about 80 per cent of all ovarian malignancies (Hauser, 1979). The incidence of ovarian cancer, in cases per 100,000 population, varies from 2.8 in the Japanese to 15.1 in the Swedes; it is substantially higher among Europeans than among Asians or Africans; and it increases with age but at different rates among all populations investigated (Waterhouse *et al.*, 1976; Roemer *et al.*, 1979).

5.2.1.4 Lung Cancer. Among humans, lung cancer is already the prime cause of male cancer mortality in most highly industrialized Western countries. It is threatening to become so in those developing countries which, particularly since the smoking–lung cancer 'scare' of the 1960s, have been receiving the diverted, irresponsible, specialized and even government-placating-and-hoodwinking attentions of the biggest 'monsters' of the tobacco industry (Taha and Ball, 1980; Smith and Troop, 1983).

The human disease, whether or not it is associable with smoking or another specific environment, differs considerably from the animal counterpart in many ways, including in spontaneous or induced incidence, inducibility, sex-specific distribution, number and type of primary tumours per individual, location within the lung, and clinical course and features (reviewed by Stewart *et al.*, 1979). Thus, spontaneous lung tumours are rare in most species of animal including the rat, mouse, hamster, guinea pig, pig, cow, and chicken. However, they are being observed with increasing frequency in dogs, most likely because dogs are now living longer due to effective immunizations against infections and to better general care by humans, and because of more careful examination by veterinarians and researchers. In animals, the neoplasms that do appear, whether spontaneously or by experimental induction, are mainly multiple, multicentric-in-origin, and peripherally-located alveologenic tumours, with variable contributions from hemangioendotheliomas and, very rarely, squamous cell tumours. In contrast, the human neoplasms are predominantly single and centrally-located oat-cell carcinomas and squamous cell carcinomas, with some adenocarcinomas. Oat-cell carcinomas are as unknown in animals, with a Java sparrow from the Philadelphia Zoo (Stewart, 1966) being perhaps the only known exception, as are the lung hemangioendotheliomas in man. Other notable differences include predominance in males and rapid progression to fatality, which are pronounced features of lung neoplasia in humans but not in animals. In man also, the tumours frequently metastasize in a prominent pattern, preferentially to the brain and adrenal gland; in animals, the metastasis is rare and patterned metastasis rarer, except in some mice. In such mice, the preferential metastatic sites are the pleura, mediastinum, heart, and kidney (Turusov *et al.*, 1974).

5.2.1.5 Other Types of Cancer, and a Major Principle of Oncology. The natural phenomenon of marked interspecific differences superimposed upon a background similarity in innate susceptibility to spontaneous neoplasia, as illustrated above, applies to practically all known types of neoplasm. This has been amply demonstrated in comparative studies, e.g. those between the neoplasms in man and their counterparts in the rat or the mouse as reviewed by various authors in the already mentioned WHO/IARC volumes of *Pathology of Tumours in Laboratory Animals* (cf. Section 5.2.1.1). For example, in man, periosteal osteomas and osteosarcomas are rare, and leukemias originate mainly in the bone marrow; contrasting with the commonness of these bone tumours in mice, particularly after infection with polyoma virus which has no known association with neoplasia in man, and with the mainly thymic origin of murine leukemias (Stanton, 1979). Liver cancers are significantly more metastatic, malignant and fatal, in man than in mice. They are often associated with liver cirrhosis in man but extremely rarely in mice. They develop almost exclusively from morphologically benign hyperplastic nodules or liver-cell adenomas in mice, but this situation is practically unknown in man in whom liver-cell adenoma is extremely rare and is not known to be premalignant. In the mouse, distinction between benign and malignant liver tumours is difficult; in man, hyperplasia, liver-cell adenoma, and liver-cell carcinoma are distinct entities; and certain features such as bone are common in the hepatoblastomas of man but not of mice (Turusov and Takayama, 1979). In mice, the occurrence of spontaneous hepatomas seems to be influenced by three main factors, all host-related: genotype, sex, and body weight (Heston and Vlahakis, 1966).

An appropriate illustration of the composite similarities and differences is probably best provided by a comparison of the teratomas of man with those of mouse (Pierce *et al.*, 1978; Demjanov *et al.*, 1979; Fraley *et al.*, 1979; Raghavan *et al.*, 1980; see also Chapter Nine, Section 9.10.2). In both species, the tumours are composed not only of morphologically similar pluripotent embryonal carcinoma cells which are the tumours' stem cells but also of multiple somatic tissues at various phases and stages of differentiation. However, the many differences which exist include the following features, all of which are relatively common in the human neoplasms but are rare or absent in the murine counterparts: highly organized tissues such as teeth, finger, and eye anlage; thyroid derivatives; carcinoid tumours; mixtures of malignant derivatives of extra-embryonic tissues in the form of trophoblastic or yolk-sac carcinoma; malignant alteration of somatic tissues, e.g. to squamous cell carcinoma, adenocarcinoma, or carcinosarcoma; and metastatic propensities. These similarities and differences may well mimic the similarities and differences which are inherent to the genetically-determined developmental capabilities of the respective species-specific genetic inheritances.

The above-mentioned natural phenomenon may hence well constitute one of the major principles of oncology, a principle which is equally applicable to induced neoplasia.

5.2.2 Induced Cancer

The principle of marked interspecies neoplastic differences is also applicable to induced neoplasia (see also Chapter Nine, Section 9.2.4). For instance, nitrosamines are ubiquitous in the human environment, but their causal relationship with any type of human cancer remains suspected but unproven. In animals, nitrosamines, like other classes of chemical carcinogen, are well known to produce tumours of variable histogenesis in susceptible individuals according to species, age and other factors such as dose, and route of administration. As recently reviewed or shown by Cardy and Lijinksy (1980), for example, nitroso-2,6-di-methylmorpholine induces tumours of the pancreas in Syrian hamsters but of the esophagus in rats; nitrosomethyldodecyl-amine induces bladder tumours in rats and Syrian hamsters; dinitroso-2,6-dimethylpiperazine induces esophageal tumours in rats; nitrosoheptamethyleneimine induces tumours of the lung in European hamsters, but of the lung and esophagus in rats, and of the forestomach and esophagus in Syrian hamsters; and nitrosomethyldiethylurea induces tumours of the central nervous system in rats. In guinea pigs, however, only liver tumours are produced by the first three compounds mentioned and no tumours by the remaining two. This contrasts with the non-hepatotumorigenicity of any of the five compounds in rats and hamsters.

As mentioned above (Section 5.2.1.4), oat-cell carcinoma of the lung is, to all intents and purposes, unknown in animals, but it is one of the commonest of human cancers. Accordingly, from epidemiological evidence, it is highly inducible in man, particu-larly by cigarette smoke; but, despite numerous attempts, it has not been induced in animals by cigarette smoke or any of its fractions (cf. Stewart *et al.*, 1979; see also Chapter Nine, Section 9.2.4). In man, this cancer occurring in non-smokers does not differ in any material particular from its counterpart in smokers (Enstrom, 1979).

In contrast with the practically unknown incidence of oat-cell cancers in animals (Section 5.2.1.4), bladder cancer occurs spontaneously in some animals (e.g. dogs and hamsters), though more rarely than in man. In susceptible animal species, bladder tumours are inducible by various agents, and the induced tumours show striking epithelial and other similarities to their spontaneous counterparts (Wood and Bonser, 1979). One such agent, 2-naphthylamine, used in the manufacture of dyestuffs such as auramine, has, as already mentioned (Chapter Three, Section 3.4.2.4), a long-known association with human bladder cancer. This agent, which also occurs in cigarette smoke and other sources of human exposure such as coal tar and gas retort houses, induces bladder cancer in some dogs, monkeys, and hamsters, but not in several other animal species including the mouse, rat, and rabbit. In the mouse, it induces liver tumours. Auramine itself also induces liver tumours in the mouse; and also in the rat, but in which it also induces local sarcomas and intestinal tumours. In the dog and rabbit, auramine is non-tumorigenic. Analogously, human bladder cancer is also associated with the cancer-chemotherapeutic agent cyclophosphamide; but, in the mouse, the agent induces hematologic, lung, and other tumours not involving the bladder. (For reviews of these topics, see Manson 1976; Tomatis *et al.*, 1978).

Even in organisms of a single genotype, the tumorigenic response to a putative carcinogen can vary with respect to time, type and occurrence or non-occurrence of tumour(s). Prehn (1979) has shown that in the BALB/c ByJ female mouse-methylcholanthrene system, a major part of the phenotypic variability in tumour susceptibility is due to variability among the immunological phenotypes of the animals.

Two other examples, of direct significance to man, may be noted. First, coumarin, a natural product in plants and essential oils, has been widely used in foods, perfumes and alcoholic beverages for about 80 years. It induces histologic liver damage in the rat and dog, but not in baboons even after intake of up to 67.5 mg/kg/day for two years. It is an experimental mouse skin carcinogen, but it has been associated with bile duct tumours in coumarin-fed rats in which the agent is metabolized differently than in man. (For references, see Cohen, 1979.) Is coumarin, then, a 'potential human carcinogen'? Second, chronic, long-term human exposure to ultraviolet (uv) radiation is associated with lentigo maligna-type melanoma, and melanoma also occurs in patients with xeroderma pigmentosum (xp), who are ultrasensitive to uv radiation (cf. Chapter Seven, Section 7.5). However, neither uv-induced melanoma nor xp is known among any nonhuman animal (Kripko, 1979).

The capacity of an exogenous agent to induce a given tumour in man or animals thus seems to be significantly restricted by the intrinsic propensity of the organism to develop that tumour spontaneously. Thus, liver angiosarcoma occurs rarely in humans; and, in presumably susceptible individuals, it can be induced by agents as chemically unrelated as vinyl chloride and thorotrast (Falk *et al.*, 1979; Baxter *et al.*, 1980). The former agent is an organic substance to which man becomes exposed through inhalation and/or skin contact, and the latter an inorganic substance administered intra-arterially since 1928, mainly for cerebral angiography in neurosurgical patients.

On the basis of literature data compiled from three major sources (The National Cancer Institute Bioassay Program, The Monograph Series from 1972 to 1978 of the International Agency for Research on Cancer, and the US Public Health Service Document No 149), Purchase (1980) made a comparison of the reported carcinogenicity of 250 selected chemicals in the mouse and rat. Of these chemicals, 110 were found to induce tumours of one type or another in both species, 21 in mice only and 17 in rats only, with a site-specific non-concordance of about 32 per cent.

5.3 Intraspecific Comparisons

5.3.1 Spontaneous Cancer

5.3.1.1 General Features. The above-described phenomenon of interspecific differences in susceptibility to spontaneous or induced neoplasia can reflect only part of the genetic heterogeneity which confers upon Nature's organisms both interspecific and intraspecific genetic signatures in health and in resistance or susceptibility to disease. Indeed, the intraspecific differences extend beyond the level of races, strains, breeds, and individuals, as they are also displayed phenotypically in a single organism, thus extending to the levels of both genetic structural and genetic expressional differences.

In animals, the phenomenon of significant intraspecific differences in susceptibility to types and incidences of neoplasia has been long recognized, e.g. since 1909 when Bashford observed natural mouse colonies displaying different susceptibility to spontaneous mammary and other tumours, with incidences varying from high to low or even undetectable. Since then, these observations have been greatly extended, and similar observations have included other animal species. In dogs, for instance, spontaneous mammary tumours of several types, whether occurring singly or multiply in one or more of the glands, are far commoner in collies, boxers and chihuahuas than in most other breeds (Casey *et al.*, 1979). Among strains of the Syrian golden hamster, both incidence and multiplicity of spontaneous tumours are higher in the albino hamsters (AH) than in the cream (CH) or white (WH) hamsters, with tumours of the thyroid predominating in AH, of the pancreatic islet cell in CH, and of the adrenal gland in WH. Some of the tumours, e.g. malignant melanomas in AH and CH but not in WH, show exclusive strain specificity; others show pronounced sex preference, e.g. the thyroid or adrenal tumours; but neither in incidence nor in multiplicity do the tumours show a correlation with the strain-specific lifespans.

The introduction of inbred strains of animals, particularly of mice by Little in 1928, greatly facilitated studies of hereditary transmission of many types of tumour in animals. (For reviews, see the already-mentioned continuing series publication: *Pathology of Tumours in Laboratory Animals.*) In one of these studies, the incidence of spontaneous tumours in C3H-A and C3H-A fB mice was shown to be higher in the USA than in Australia (Sabine *et al.*, 1973). This key observation, i.e. of a role for the external environment in spontaneous tumour incidence, requires clarification of the precise nature of that role, i.e. whether it is etiological or merely a differential influence upon the rate of expression of a uniform and pre-existent (inherent) tumour susceptibility.

5.3.1.2 The Inbred Mouse-mammary Tumour System. The continuing studies with inbred strains of animals have amply demonstrated that such strains can be tailored to almost any desired specification regarding innate susceptibility to specific types of cancer. Studies in the inbred mouse-mammary tumour system, which has been particularly well-investigated in this regard, have amply demonstrated what may well be the two essential requirements for tumour genesis and development in general: a host-specific (genetic) susceptibility to the tumour, and extragenetic (intrinsic and/or extrinsic) factors which interact with the susceptibility to enhance, inhibit, or otherwise influence its expression. Thus, in the mouse system, the first requirement is the host genome to which the murine mammary tumour virus (MTV) in one or more of its genetically transmitted forms (MTV^{gt}) may contribute. The second is met by some of the animal's endogenous hormones (mainly estrogen, progesterone, and prolactin, but also growth hormone together with the system of adenohypophyseal and hypothalamic hormones such as ACTH which control steroidogenesis in the adrenal cortex, ovary, and certain adipose and other tissues) (cf. Chapter Four); and also by one or more of the several milk-transmitted forms (MTV^{mt}) of the mammary tumour virus. Historically, MTV^{mt} is the maternal 'extrachromosomal factor' described in 1933 by the staff of the Roscoe B. Jackson Memorial Laboratory, and which was later shown by Bittner to be the milk-transmitted 'milk factor', to be distributed widely among the animal's organs, tissues and body fluids (Dmochowski, 1949), and to be a virus (Lyons and Moore, 1962). MTV^{mt}-carrying mouse strains (e.g. the C3H strain, in which Bittner discovered the milk factor, and the R3, A, DBA, GR, and DD strains) have a high spontaneous incidence of the disease; those lacking MTV^{mt} but carrying MTV^{gt} (e.g. the BALB/c strain) have a moderate incidence made manifest usually at later ages and after the hormonal stimulation of pregnancies and pseudo-pregnancies; and those lacking both MTV^{mt} and MTV^{gt} (e.g. the C57BL and 020 strains) have a low to undetectable incidence. The salient features of these strains and of some of their derived hybrid strains have recently been reviewed by Squartini (1979) and are summarized in Table 5.1.

Some additional points of interest to this discussion are as follows. In susceptible strains, mammary tumours are inducible by a suitable chemical or physical 'carcinogen'; but even in these instances stimulation by hormones appears to be as essential (DeOme *et al.*, 1962) as it is in the case of the virally-associated neoplasms. Even in some resistant strains, breast neoplasms can develop simply as a result of breeding. For instance, in the 020 strain, the spontaneous incidence has been reported to be nil in virgins, 5 per cent in breeders, and 13 per cent in forced breeders (see review by Squartini, 1979). Mühlbock and Boot (1959)

Table 5.1: Differential Susceptibility of Common Laboratory Strains of Inbred Mice and of Their Breast Tissues to Spontaneous Mammary Neoplasia

Strain	Incidence, Morphology, and other Features of Tumours
Carriers of MTV^{nt}	
GR	Also carries MTV^{e}. High incidence of mainly early-onset pregnancy-dependent type-P tumours in breeders, and adenocarcinomas (types A and B) as well as pale-cell carcinomas in virgins
C3H	High incidence of hormone-independent acinar or type-A adenocarcinomas, with some type-B adenocarcinomas and, very rarely, adenoacanthomas
R3	High incidence of pregnancy-dependent plaques progressing through type-B adenocarcinomas with hemorrhagic cysts towards autonomy
DBA	High incidence of adenocarcinomas (types A and B) with an acinar structure together with solid and cystic variants
DD	High incidence of plaques and of adenocarcinomas (types A and B) with some adenoacanthomas
A	High incidence of adenocarcinomas (types A and B), with some adenoacanthomas
Non-carriers of MTV^{nt}	
C57BL	Extremely low tumour incidence; e.g. Squartini et al. (1979) found only a single mammary tumour (an adenoacanthoma) among 1,563 C57BL mice observed through 40 inbred generations
O20	Low incidence of mammary tumours: 0% in virgins, 5% in breeders, and 13% in forced breeders. There is a marked rarity of purely acinar tumours, papillary growth, or squamous metaplasia; but marked features are anaplasia, spindle cell formation, and highly cellular stroma resulting in poor distinction between the epithelial and stromal cells and a carcinosarcomatous appearance
C3HfC57BL	Like the C3HeB strain, this strain is free from MTV^{nt} but carries a type of MTV^{e} termed 'nodule inducing virus'. Both strains have a moderate incidence of mainly late-onset adenocarcinomas (types A and B) and adenoacanthomas in breeders
R3fC57BL	Like two other R3-derived strains (R3fBALB/c and R3eB), this strain has a relatively low incidence of mainly late-onset type-B adenocarcinomas and adenoacanthomas, with some adenoacanthomas of types A and C, carcinosarcomas, and miscellaneous tumours
DBAb	Low incidence of mainly 'deviating' types of tumour, including tumours with keratinization (adenoacanthomas), tubular adenocarcinomas with abundant stroma, carcinosarcomas, and papillary tumours
BALB/c	This strain, though free from MTV^{nt}, is highly susceptible to MTV infection. It has a low to moderate incidence of mainly late-onset adenocarcinomas, with some adenocarcinomas of types A and C and miscellaneous tumours
AfC57BL	As in the C57BL strain, mammary tumours are extremely rare in this strain.

Source: Adapted from Squartini (1979).

showed that hormonal stimulation alone, in the absence of any known exogenous carcinogen, can be a sufficient inducer of the disease. The hormonal effect on tumorigenesis of any type, which it does operate, appears to be direct, i.e. not to be due to the action of some systemic metabolite, nor even perhaps to an alteration of the animal's general endocrine status. This was recently demonstrated by Huseby (1980), for instance, who grafted testes of neonatal BALB/c mice to the spleen of castrated isologous recipients and placed estradiol-containing pellets of cholesterol next to the explants. Leydig cell tumours were found to develop only when the pellets were in close apposition to the explants but not when they were at a distance away or were absent. It may thus well be that the capacity of hormones to influence the genesis, development, and hormone-dependence of neoplasia has the same fundamental basis as their capacity to influence gene expression: i.e. susceptibility of organism, presence of appropriate receptors in susceptible tissue or organ, and specificity of hormone-receptor interaction, of receptor activation, and of nuclear translocation and DNA-binding of the hormone-receptor complex (cf. Chapter Four, Section 4.4).

5.3.1.3 Other Systems. Although in the mouse-spontaneous mammary tumour system, the major components of the second requirement mentioned above (i.e. that pertaining to modifiers of the expression of genetic-susceptibility) appear to be MTV^{mt} and endogenous hormones, their identity is often unclear in other systems. This is evident, for instance, in the (C57BL/6N × C3H/HeN)F_1 (B6C3F$_1$) hybrid mouse system, which is extensively used mainly as control in the Carcinogenesis Testing Program of the US National Cancer Institute. Mice of this inbred strain spontaneously develop a great variety of neoplastic and non-neoplastic disease that increase in frequency and diversity as the animals age. Recently, Ward *et al.* (1979) found the most common neoplasms in 2,543 such mice to include hepatocellular adenomas and carcinomas, lymphomas, leukemias, and pulmonary carcinomas and adenomas. Among the major non-neoplastic diseases were cystic hyperplasia of the uterus, nephritis, ovarian and uterine cysts, lung inflammations, brain mineralization, and focal hyperplasias in several tissues.

5.3.1.4 Multiple Genic Involvement in 'Mendelian' Cancer? In the face of such a diversity of spontaneous pathological expressions, it seems difficult to postulate a pathogenetic basis other than aberrations of specific facets of the largely unknown but clearly bewilderingly complex system of intragenomic extragenomic interactions that govern normal gene expression during development. In these interactions, both the extragenomic component and the intragenomic component, even in those cases conventionally described to show mendelian patterns of inheritance, are rarely, if ever, unifactorial. For example, in the celebrated swordtail-platyfish crosses investigated by Anders and his colleagues (reviewed by Anders, 1978) in which the crosses develop many melanomas, pterinophoromas, neuroblastomas, thyroid carcinomas, kidney tumours, reticulosarcomas, and other spontaneous neoplasms, the involvement of a specific tumour gene (*Tu*) was postulated. However, *Tu* appears to be present in several copies on the sex and other chromosomes; and, in melanoma production, to be linked to perhaps 13 different genes governing some 13 different compartments.

5.3.2 Induced Cancer

5.3.2.1 Inducers of Cancer, Cytochrome P-450, and Inducers of Cytochrome P-450 Mono-oxygenase Activity. The foregoing discussions have alrady implied that, whether between or within species, differences in induced neoplasia may have a common genetic-environmental basis. This is the capacity of the inducing agents to interact with, and thus to stimulate expression of, host-intrinsic differential susceptibilities to the disease. The exact identity of these agents (when they exist), or even whether they are specific and are thus identifiable is not known for many types of neoplasm in man and other species. In man, these neoplasms include breast and ovarian cancers (two of the major cancers in women), colonic and rectal cancers (two of the major cancers in men), and most cancers of childhood. However, for human cancers of certain types, various inducers are known with some certainty, e.g. tobacco smoke ingredients, probably aromatic hydrocarbons (AH) such as benzo(a)pyrene (BP) and 3-methylcholanthrene (MC), for bronchogenic carcinoma, and certain arylamines for transitional cell carcinoma of the urinary bladder.

During the 1960s, an important development in aid of understanding the biochemistry of tumour induction by chemically inert substances such as AH and arylamines was pioneered in the United States by the Millers, the Weisburgers and Gutmann and, in the United Kingdom, by Boyland and by Clayson, initially from experimental studies of tumorigenesis, in rodents, by 2-acetylaminofluorene and 4-aminobiphenyl. This development was that, for many such inducers, their metabolic activation into strong electrophile-yielding intermediates is an obligatory, though *per se* insufficient, prelude to their tumour-inducing activity. (See Chapter Nine, Section 9.5.2.) Extensive concomitant and subsequent reports from practically all of the world's major cancer research centres have shown that the activation is effected mainly by one or more of the at least a dozen distinct forms of 'cytochrome P-450'. The cytochrome represents a multicomponent, membrane-bound, electron-transfer system of both cytoplasmic and nuclear carbon monoxide-binding hemoproteins associated, mainly in the liver but also in many other tissues, with NADPH-dependent arylhydrocarbon hydroxylase (AHH) and other mono-oxygenase activities for diverse chemical substrates of both exogenous and endogenous origins. The reports have also shown that a major feature of the mono-oxygenase activities is their inducibility by many factors, inclusive of their tumorigenic and non-tumorigenic substrates themselves. (For reviews, see Arnott *et al.*, 1979; Nebert *et al.*, 1979.)

5.3.2.2 Mono-oxygenase Inducibility: A Genetically-Controlled Phenomenon. In 1973, following earlier demonstrations of AHH inducibility in human cultured lymphocytes, Kellerman *et al.* reported its trimodal (low, intermediate, and high) distribution among humans, with the higher activities being more prominent in patients with lung cancer than in healthy control subjects including the patients' spouses (Kellermann *et al.*, 1973 a-d). These reports also purported to show simple inheritance of the AHH inducibility, but this has later been questioned on a number of grounds (Mulvihill, 1976). However, the gist of the findings by Kellermann *et al.* has since received experimental support (see the reviews by Arnott *et al.* and Nebert *et al.*). This is that significant genetically-controlled AHH (and perhaps related) inducibility differences exist among humans; that the inducibility is higher among patients with lung, oropharyngeal, and perhaps other types of chemically inducible cancers than among their normal counterparts; and that the inducibility differences may be one of the factors contributing to the associated interindividual cancer-susceptibility differences.

In other studies, it has been shown that the inducibility differences, smoking habits (which also may be under genetic control), familial factors, and obstructive lung disease may act independently and synergistically to enhance the risk of lung cancer (Tokuhata and Lilienfeld, 1963; Cohen *et al.*, 1977).

This phenomenon of genetically-controlled AHH inducibility differences has been more thoroughly investigated in animals, particularly mice, than in humans. For instance, the inducibility is high in some inbred strains of mice such as the B6 and C3 strains and low or undetectable in others such as the D2 and AKR/N strains derived, respectively, from C57BL/6, C3H, DBA/2, and AKR mice. The differences are thus probably due to allelic polymorphism at the gene loci controlling responsiveness to the inducers of AHH activity. The non-responsive strains may then lack, qualitatively or quantitatively, some important product of the arylhydrocarbon (*Ah*) or a related regulatory locus, such as the inducer-binding cytosolic receptor protein of Polan *et al*. A genetic model comprising at least six distinct alleles and two distinct loci is indicated by the observations that AHH inducibility segregates as an autosomal dominant trait in crosses between the B6 and D2 strains, but as an additive trait in crosses between the C3 and D2 strains; and that AHH non-inducibility segregates as an autosomal dominant Mendelian trait in crosses between the B6 and the AKR/N strains (Nebert *et al.*, 1979).

The phenomenon of the natural existence of marked differences in metabolic capacities is well known. Among humans, such differences are increasingly being described on an intergroup or interindividual basis; and, in some instances, familial studies have indicated the mode of inheritance of the metabolizing capacity. For instance, extensive (EM) and poor (PM) metabolizers of the antihypertensive drug debroisoquine have been identified (Mahgoub *et al.*, 1977), and the PM phenotype has been described as an autosomal recessive trait (Evans *et al.*, 1980). Analogous genetic polymorphisms have been described, e.g. in capacity to acetylate sulfonamides, hydrazines, and other amino-derivatives including some of the human bladder cancer-associated arylamines (Lower, 1978); to hydrolyze esters such as paroxon and succinyl choline; and to oxidize at aliphatic, alicyclic, or aromatic carbon or nitrogen centres in drugs or poisons such as guanoxon, debroisoquine, guanethidine, phenacetin, and polycyclic hydrocarbons (Lunde *et al.*, 1977; Idle *et al.*, 1978; Sloan *et al.*, 1978; Irving, 1979; Evans *et al.*, 1980).

It seems that significant ethnic differences along these lines also exist. For example, it was recently shown that Negroid as compared with Caucasoid alcoholics have higher levels of erythrocyte superoxide dismutase (Del Villana *et al.*, 1980), a situation which may be considered in association with the already-mentioned acatalasemia of the Japanese (Section 5.1). Life on this planet is generally believed to have begun and to have initially evolved in a reducing atmosphere until photosynthesis introduced the aerobic conditions that still persist. As the above discussion on the effects of mono-oxygenase activity on inherently inert chemicals exemplifies, adaptation to the aerobic lifestyle is fraught with potential hazards, against which enzymes such as catalase and superoxide dismutase afford some protection. Biological oxidative processes require an electron-acceptor, a role which is fulfilled by, among other agents such as cystine and oxidized glutathione, molecular oxygen, whence the potentially harmful superoxide radical anion ($0_2 .^-$) is formed. The dismutase catalyzes the dismutation of the anion into the vital molecular oxygen and still potentially harmful peroxydi-anion (yielding hydrogen peroxide). The final task of superoxide detoxification depends upon catalase, which converts the hydrogen peroxide (by another dismutation) into water and oxygen. (For a review, see Fridovitch, 1978.) Carried to its logical conclusion, this would lead to the expectation of Negroes, Caucasians, and Japanese, or at least the corresponding alcoholics, exhibiting increasing susceptibilities to chemically induced neoplasms which are dependent, for their induction, upon superoxide or hydrogen peroxide participation. However, except for stomach cancer, this expectation remains unsupported.

Clearly, the inborn differences in metabolic capacity constitute only a part of the genetic basis for the marked cancer-susceptibility differences. This is further substantiated by a variety of experimental observations. For instance, in comparative studies with strains of rodents selected for their widely different responses to colon carcinogenesis by 1,2-dimethylhydrazine (DMH), the same differential responses are elicited by DMH as by its activated metabolite or 'proximate carcinogen' (Deschner *et al.*, 1984; see also Chapter Nine, Section 9.5). Also, complex genetic mechanisms have been described for natural cell-mediated cytotoxicity to inoculated tumour cells in mouse strains such as BALB/c, B6, and their F_1 crosses (Clark and Harmon, 1980).

Further, some inbred strain differences in cancer susceptibility are due to the presence in specific chromosomal loci of oncorna proviral DNA sequences. In the AKR/J mouse strain, for instance, products of the *Akr*-1 locus on chromosome 7, as well as the proviral sequence acting as a dominant gene in an appropriate genetic background, are essentials for leukemogenesis. Other genetic factors may also be operative. The $FV-1^b$ allele in BALB/c and other mouse strains, for instance, acts as a dominant gene to suppress leukemogenesis; and control of tumour outgrowth is dependent upon a complex interaction between the H-2 haplotype and the specific strain of virus (Lilly, 1972). In the SJL/J mouse strain, spontaneous lymphoma development is also suppressed by a specific gene, the *Rcs*-1 gene (Bubbers, 1984). (For a more detailed discussion, see Harnden *et al.*, 1984).

Thus, among the known determinants of the differences in innate cancer susceptibility are genetic elements controlling differences in metabolic handling of carcinogens, and in stimulation or suppression of tumorigenesis. Each of these categories may itself be complex. For example, the co-operation of at least two oncogenes can be required to transform normal mouse embryo fibroblasts (Weinberg, 1983) or to produce lymphoma in chickens (Hayday *et al.*, 1984) (see also Chapter Nine, Section 9.6.3). The phenotypic expression of any of these various genetic elements intimately involved in tumorigenesis will perhaps always be influenced by the genetic and extragenetic environments of that element. In nature, single genes do not function in isolation, so that mendelianism is a relative concept.

5.4 Summary and Outlook

Whether in susceptibility to spontaneous or induced neoplasia in man or animals, the comparative studies clearly indicate the existence of marked interspecific and intraspecific differences, e.g. relative to both type and incidence of the disease. In this, whatever role the extragenomic including extracorporeal environment may play, there can be little doubt that susceptibility or resistance to neoplasia is non-uniform in Nature, that inherited genetics contribute significantly to the non-uniformity, and that the basic principles of oncology are more in keeping with the tenets of the genetic paradigm than with those of the medical paradigm described in the introductory section of this chapter. That this non-uniformity is at least as pronounced within the human species as it has been shown above to be both within and between other species, comprises the subject of the next chapter.

HEREDITY AND CANCER: HUMAN ASPECTS

6.1 Introduction: Aspects of the Traditional and Methodological Underestimation of Inherited Cancer Predisposition in Man

In the etiology of human cancer the millennia of speculations and the recent decades of unprecedented intensification of controlled investigations have not identified the indisputable cause(s) of any type of the disease. Despite the recent accumulations of overwhelming evidence for the close associations between various environmental (mainly smoking, dietary, cosmic, and sexual) factors and some types of cancer, these associations are, at best, demonstrably causative of the increased cancer-incidence rates rather than of the cancers themselves (Chapter Nine, Section 9.4). These implicated factors are such that they have always involved or are involving most or all of mankind, but among whom only a small proportion is known ever to develop the associated cancers. Moreover, the latter can also develop in the absence of the associations. Bronchogenic carcinoma, for instance, not only develops among some non-smokers but, as such, it is indistinguishable in any material particular from the smokers' equivalent (Enstrom, 1979; Enstrom and Godley, 1980). Also, the lifetime expectancy of its development among heavy smokers is under 10 per cent. This same principle of the high selectivity of carcinogenic responses among the genetically heterogeneous human population (Chapter Five, Section 5.1) is equally applicable to other human cancer-environmental associations. A particularly impressive example of the latter is the association between skin cancer and solar radiation. This factor has been impinging upon the Earth for some five thousand million years before the origin of the human species, and has been affecting all humans ever since this origin. Despite this, the incidence of skin cancer worldwide has consistently shown a marked dependence upon constitutive factors such as pigmentary trait, ethnic origin, and family history (Section 6.4.1). Association is not causation.

A likely basis for the selectivity of cancer is corresponding differences in innate cancer predisposition. This implies that, among the heavy smokers described above, the innate predisposition to bronchogenic carcinoma is, on average, some nine times higher among those who do than do not develop the disease in a lifetime. Moreover, such smokers themselves, like any other subgroup undergoing a potentially lethal major biological experience, are likely to be genetically more homogeneous than the general population. This further implies that the range of the innate predisposition may be wider among the general population than among the heavy smokers. The molecular basis of the predispositional differences is unknown, although various studies have implicated genetic factors including those associated with arylhydrocarbon hydroxylase inducibility, sister chromatid exchanges, or chronic obstructive pulmonary disease (for a review, see Murata and Tanaka, 1983). The basis thus appears to be multifactorial and, as such, to be beyond the capability of current genetic analysis (see below).

It may well be that the real causes of all human cancers are ecogenetic, with the relative importance of the genetic and environmental influences being variable in different instances. The epidemiologically based interpretation of human cancer as a predominantly environmental disease (Chapter Five, Section 5.1; Chapter Nine, Section 9.3), in the words of Mulvihill (1980), 'ignores the facts that the cause of cancer in most patients is unknown and that gene frequencies, as well as environment, can differ worldwide'.

It is salutory, however, that recognition of the genetic involvement in the causation and development of human cancer represents a growing recent trend. Among the prominent features of this trend are spontaneous cancer occurrences, i.e. without the mediation of any known or perhaps even any likely extrinsic cause; significant non-random cancer distributions, e.g. among individuals, families, and ethnic groups; and involvement of certain specific, normal, and developmentally vital inherited genes. Of these genes, the recently discovered oncornavirally-related 'oncogenes' (cf. Chapter Nine, Sections 9.2.6 and 9.6.3) may represent only a minor part. Since cancer can, at least theoretically, afflict any individual, it seems unlikely that these genes are necessarily mutated or otherwise structurally abnormal. None the less, some 200 of the over 2,000 mendelian disorders described by McKusick (1975), among them XP and familial polyposis coli, are already known to carry an excess risk of one type of cancer or another. Colon cancer has been known for almost two decades to develop in about half of all carriers of the polyposis trait by age 40 years, and in nearly all by age 70 (Veale, 1965).

There is no evidence that cancer itself is an inherited disease. A widely encountered term such as 'inherited breast cancer' must be seen in this light. What is indicated by the available evidence is that a predisposition to one form of the disease or another is inherited in varying extents and kinds, presumably by all humans and as an intrinsic part of the capabilities of the inherited individual genome. Whether or not this predisposition becomes expressed in the form of a clinical cancer during a lifetime would depend upon its subsequent interaction with appropriate intrinsic (e.g. hormonal) and/or extrinsic (e.g. dietary) factors.

On present understanding, few cancers show a strong genetic component, e.g. some cancers of the colon, skin, ovary, and breast. That the others are thought to show a weak and sometimes even an undiscernible genetic component is almost certainly due, at least partly, to current methodological inadequacies. Thus, although the mode of inheritance is clearly dominant or recessive in some instances, it is more often unclear. For instance, colon cancer is associated with familial polyposis coli (cf. above) but also with the Peutz-Jehger and several other syndromes (Section 6.4.2), and it occurs mostly in people with no such condition. These facts suggest that the genic involvement in this cancer is not the same in all instances. A multifactorial (i.e. unknown) mode of inheritance is inferred when, in those increasingly observed familial examples of usually multiple neoplasms (cf. Meisner *et al.*, 1979; Lynch *et al.*, 1981), a simple mendelian mode is not clearly deducible. Further, in comparable familial cancers with such a simple mode, the inheritance pattern may vary from one family to the next. Also, whether the mode is dominant or recessive is often complicated by the relativity of these concepts. In a given allelic series, for instance, the same allele may be dominant to some of the alleles but recessive to others, and its expression may be conditional upon the presence, absence, or activity of one or more specific extragenetic factors of either endogenous or exogenous origin. Conventionally, such ecogenetic effects are described by *penetrance* (the proportion of heterozygotes in which the allele or predisposition is expressed) and *expressivity* (the range of severity of the phenotype in those heterozygotes in which it is overtly expressed). However, a phenotypic alteration may not be readily evident even in the presence of a structurally or functionally altered allele. For instance, the sister allele may compensate for the functional alterations such as an under-production of the allelic product. Alternatively, as is not uncommon in transformed cells (cf. Chapter Nine, Section 9.8.4), either of the sister alleles may undergo extensive amplification, with the possibility of even over-compensation for the alteration. Another methodological inadequacy is the incapability or, at best, limited capability of current cancer genetics to determine the likely genetic basis for the widespread phenomenon of marked interindividual differences in carcinogenic response to the same cancer-associated environmental factor, e.g. tobacco smoke or radiation (cf. above; and also Chapter Five, Section 5.1).

At present, therefore, the proper study of the genetics of cancer predisposition in man is hampered by many difficulties. In pedigree analysis, upon which this study so largely depends, additional difficulties centre upon generalized human-specific features such as man's long generation time, the uncontrollability of his matings, the fewness of his familial offspring, his still unfathomed genetic heterogeneity (cf. Chapter Five, Section 5.1), and the complexity and rapid changes of his society. Then, also, there is the complexity including genetic and environmental multifactoriality of the real or presumptive causes of his neoplasms, the slow and multi-phased development and heterogeneity of the neoplasms themselves, and the predominance of his most common neoplasms during middle and older ages. This last-mentioned fact alone often renders difficult not only prospective studies, but also satisfactory fulfilment of essentials such as retrospective collection of reliable family data. Such data may be inadequately recorded, based upon faulty diagnosis, or, perhaps more often than not, incorrectly and/or selectively remembered.

Such difficulties are widely recognized. Schimke (1978), for instance, illustrated the problems inherent in interpretation of mode of inheritance and in genetic counselling which can arise when even a presumably simply inherited condition such as one of the subtypes of familial colon cancer is complicated by co-occurrence, within the pedigree, of another simply inherited condition such as Marfan's syndrome. The latter is a well-known autosomal dominant non-cancerous condition.

The difficulties can be further illustrated by recent experiences with the exomphalos-macroglossia-gigantism syndrome first described in 1964, by Wiedemann. Showing a marked tendency to segregate in families, this syndrome is characterized by omphalocele, hemihypertrophy, gigantism, and marked susceptibility to hypoglycemia and neoplasia, probably through an intimate mediation of hypothalamic dysfunction (Matsuura *et al.*, 1975). Through various applications of the available analytic methods to the associated familial and related data, different workers have ascribed practically every conceivable mode of inheritance to the syndrome. Thus, Filippi and McKusick (1970) described the mode to be autosomal recessive; others regarded it as autosomal dominant (Kosseff *et al.*, 1972; Forrester, 1973; Ben-Galim *et al.*, 1977); Sommer *et al.* (1977) postulated 'delayed mutation' involving the Knudson hypothesis-like 'premutation' or 'prezygotic mutation' and a later 'telomutation' or 'postzygotic mutation'; and Lubinsky *et al.* (1974) also mentioned premutation while proposing an autosomal-dominant sex-dependent mode of inheritance. Yet others (Wiedemann, 1973; Gardner, 1973; Berry *et al.*, 1980), from their observation of monozygotic twins discordant for the syndrome, proposed a multifactorial involvement. Among the multiple factors proposed by Berry *et al.* were the genetic background of the affected patient, the latter's paternal and/or maternal environment, and other familial factors predisposing to twinning and to diabetes mellitus with its distorted carbohydrate metabolism.

Another example is provided by thyroid cancer. Inheritance in the medullary carcinoma sometimes shows features of autosomal dominance (Keiser *et al.*, 1973), but of autosomal dominance, recessiveness, or multifactoriality in the papillary carcinoma (Lote *et al.*, 1980). In two affected kindreds, reported by Lote *et al.*, there was a pronounced absence of factors usually associated with the disease, such as previous medical irradiation, Gardner's syndrome, arrhenoblastoma, or Sipple's syndrome or any of the multiple endocrine adenomatosis (MEA) syndromes.

In leukemia also, the possible involvement of predisposing genetic factors, such as the Philadelphia chromosome (Chapter Eight, Section 8.4), has been suggested by various studies. For instance, reports of familial segregation of the disease, which were first made during the 1930s (Petri, 1933; Ardashnikov, 1937), have been steadily accumulating. A recent review of the accumulated evidence has shown that chronic lymphocytic leukemia (CLL) is more likely than the other types of leukemia to be familial (Conley *et al.*, 1980). To Conley *et al.*, a genetically conditioned disorder of immune regulation (possibly one involving a histocompatibility gene or gene complex on chromosome 6) may be the genetic factor predisposing to CLL and other lymphoid neoplasms, but also to autoimmune diseases such as pernicious anemia, hemolytic anemia, Hashimoto's thyroiditis, and systemic lupus erythematosus.

Despite the magnitude and variety of such difficulties in proper genetic analysis of the variable cancer predisposition among humans, their resolution, which is hardly beyond human ingenuity, is vital for both theoretical and practical reasons. Theoretically, this would improve understanding of the molecular biology and related aspects of cancer causation and development. Practically, it would aid in the identification, genetic counselling, and general care of individuals at particularly high risk of cancer. For instance, a patient with xeroderma pigmentosum or an individual identified as being highly predisposed to lung cancer would, in all probability, be more readily persuaded than the general population respectively to avoid strong sunlight or cigarette smoking. Analogously, a female member of a breast-cancer-prone family would be kept under constant surveillance including self-examination for breast lump, and would be given the option of preventive mastectomy when and if signs of incipient breast cancer appear. Similarly, a patient with familial polyposis coli would be given the option of surgical removal of the diseased colon as a precaution against later development of colon cancer, which is one of the most fatal and, in the West, most common of cancers in both sexes (cf. Miller, 1983). However, each of the options in all of these instances (sunlight avoidance, giving up smoking, and surgical removal of breast or of colon with the attendant messy colostomy) may well be regarded by the affected individual as no option at all. This stresses the importance of the theoretical reason mentioned above, i.e. exploitation of the improved understanding in the interest of correction of the high cancer predisposition at its (genetic) source. Clearly, this constitutes a tall order, a matter for the distant future. This fact is underlined by the consideration that, even at present, the genetic basis of an inherited predisposition to any disease is widely regarded as a 'mutation', as if this basis is necessarily foreign to the normal evolutionary and developmental genetics of the human species.

In the remainder of this chapter, the basic features of inherited predisposition to human cancer, as they are currently understood, are briefly outlined. More detailed reviews of this topic are available (e.g. Heston, 1976; Schimke, 1978; Purtilo *et al.*, 1978; Murata and Tanaka, 1983; Harnden *et al.*, 1984).

6.2 Historical Aspects

Recorded observations, mainly anecdotal, of nonrandom occurrences of cancer date back to remote times. In the second century AD, Galen noted a concentration of cancers of the breast and other body sites among melancholy women, although he did not clarify the issue of whether such women belonged to specific families (Chapter Two; Section 2.4.5). However, centuries later, in 1853, Velpeau recorded: 'I have seen families in which three sisters, daughters of one mother, who had died of cancer of the breast, were attacked between the ages of 30 and 40 years with cancerous tumours in the same situation'. Velpeau thus noted two of the main features of familial breast cancer: high penetrance and early age at onset. Among the other main features of this disease is involvement of the breast bilaterally, and of other organs, mainly reproductive, apparently, according to Lynch *et al.* (1978), with an autosomal dominant mode of inheritance.

Several other instances of familial cancer were recorded before the phenomenon, within the past two decades or so, began to attract major attention. Thus, it is well known that Napoleon Bonaparte and several of his family members were afflicted with gastric cancer. In 1972, Kaposi described 'multiple idiopathic pigmented sarcoma'. Now known as 'Kaposi's disease' or 'Kaposi sarcoma', it is a low-grade recrudescent multicentric angiosarcoma or an infective granulomatous disease sometimes presenting with sarcomatous transformation. It is a disease of blood vessels, originating typically in skin of the lower extremities and usually responding to chemotherapy. Other than familial, it is associated with homosexuals; and it also shows some ethnic propensities, chiefly among African Negroes, Ashkenazi Jews, and Italians and Jews in the United States (Lo *et al.*, 1980). In other examples, Osler, in 1907, described hereditary multiple telangiectasia of the skin and mucous membranes; and Warthin described familial cancer of the uterine corpus in 1925. In 1926, Lindau described familial visceral abnormalities coexisting with angiomas of the retina and central nervous system, a condition now known as von Hippel-Lindau disease. In 1938, Goetsch described early onset lymphangiomas and hemangiomas spanning the borderline between neoplasms and malformations. In more recent times, in 1959, McGirr *et al.* described familial thyroid cancer.

Even before its current rise to prominence, the phenomenon of familial and related nonrandom tumour occurrences had already begun to attract sufficient attention to warrant mechanistic conjectures. In 1932, for instance, Adair *et al.* proposed a 'heredofamilial predisposition' to neoplasia. This they based upon contemporary literature reports and upon their observations of a 53-year-old woman with 16 lipomas, and with two sons and a grandson afflicted by multiple lipomas. In 1940, Ewing proposed a 'congenital tissue predisposition' to account for his observations of varied and multiple familial lipomas.

A notable feature of these early observations is the variety of types of neoplasms which they involved.

6.3 General Aspects: Mendelian and Other Factors

At present, there are at least six major classes of clue suggesting the existence and importance of inherited genetics as determinants of variable cancer predisposition among humans. First, cancer occurrences, whether worldwide or within the individual, are highly selective. The disease afflicts only some individuals, or only one or few of an affected individual's tissues, irrespective of the presence, absence, nature, extent, or duration of any cancer-associated environmental factor (Chapter Nine, Section 9.2.4). Second, the biochemical and other manifestations of cancer are physiological mimicries. They reflect abnormal functioning of inherited genes, and they may vary among cancers of the same histological type (Chapter Nine, Section 9.2.5).

Third, the occurrence of clinical cancer itself identifies that subgroup of individuals who are more genetically predisposed to the disease than are comparable but clinical cancer-free subgroups. In the former subgroup, some but not all of the patients bearing first primary cancers develop second primaries; and the latter occur with variable degrees of shortening of their usually long latencies. These facts imply the existence of variable cancer predispositions even among the cancer-bearing patients. Some of the latter appear to have become primed, by virtue of their initially high inherited predispositions possibly accentuated by their first cancers, for rapid development of their second. The development of the second primaries is sometimes independent of therapy, such as in patients with Kaposi sarcoma. Such patients are prone to second primaries, mainly of the lymphoreticular system (Safai *et al.*, 1980). More usually, the development is iatrogenic (cf. Chapter Nine, Section 9.2.2), sometimes involving known hereditary cases. For instance, osteogenic sarcomas develop at various body sites after radiotherapy of some patients with retinoblastoma; and skin cancers develop at sites of radiotherapy or others with medulloblastoma associated with the nevoid basal cell carcinoma syndrome (Strong, 1977). The variability of the latency-shortening mentioned above is illustrated by the case of the two sisters, described by Li *et al.* (1981), who developed second primary cancers of the breast, one sister four years and the other eleven years after diagnosis and radiotherapy of their Hodgkin's disease. Many studies have shown that siblings with Hodgkin's disease have around a sevenfold risk of developing breast cancer (Grufferman *et al.*, 1977). Second primaries associated with the therapy of Hodgkin's disease also include leukemias, squamous cell carcinomas, and adenocarcinomas (Bolvin *et al.*, 1984). Those similarly associated with childhood leukemia include chemo-resistant leukemia, and those with adult teratoma include acute leukemia and bladder carcinoma (Hoekman *et al.*, 1984).

Fourth, practically all types of cancer can occur in families (Schimke, 1978). The relative risk of such familial occurrences does not change significantly even when it is adjusted for nongenetic risk factors (Murata and Tanaka, 1983).

Fifth, certain known genetic marker traits are associated with few cancers, albeit usually weakly. Blood group A is associated with about 20 per cent higher risk of stomach cancer than blood group O, in both high-risk countries such as Japan and low-risk countries such as the United States (King and Petrakis, 1977). Certain haplotypes of the HLA system, notably HLA-A2 and B-sin2 in Chinese nasopharyngeal carcinoma, are clearly associated with certain cancers (cf. Dausset and Svejgaard, 1977; McMichael, 1983). This system plays important roles in immune regulation, ageing, and other vital developmental and some pathological processes, but its role in its namesake GvH reaction is only a sec-

Table 6.1: Some of the Polyposis and Related Syndromes Associated with Heritable Colon Cancer

Syndrome	Inheritance	Other associated features
Cancer family syndrome	?AD[a]	No polyps
Cronkite–Canada syndrome	Not known to be familial	Adenomatous; entire gi tract
Familial combined colon and breast cancer	?AD	No polyps
Familial polyposis coli	AD	Adenomatous; colorectum
Gardner's syndrome	AD	Adenomatous; colorectum, rarely duodenum and stomach
Generalized gastrointestinal adenomatous polyposis	?AD	Adenomatous; small and large intestines, stomach
Generalized gastrointestinal juvenile polyposis	Not known	Polyps throughout small and large bowel intestines, stomach
Juvenile polyposis coli	AD	Cystic hamartomas throughout gi tract, usually benign; simultaneous adenomatous polyps; adenocarcinoma in relatives; connective tissue abnormality
Peutz–Jehger's syndrome	AD	Hamartomas throughout gi tract except esophagus, usually benign but some may show malignant degeneration; hamartomas of muscularis mucosa
Solitary polyps	?AD	Colon
Turcot's syndrome	AR[a]	Adenomatous; colorectum

Note: AD=autosomal dominant; AR=autosomal recessive.
Source: Adapted from Schimke, 1978; Lynch and Lynch, 1979.

Table 6.2 Some Cancer–associated Conditions Showing Autosomal Dominant Inheritance

Condition	Associated neoplasms	Other associated features
Adnexal tumour syndrome	Trichoepithelioma, milia, and cylindroma; multiple cutaneous syringomas	Anlage cell of these tumours is probably the embryonic hair germ: the trichoepitheliomas and milia develop from hair follicle, the cylindromas from apocrine glands, the leiomyomas from pilar cells, and the syringomas from sweat glands. A related (hair matrix-derived) tumour is the calcifying epithelioma of Malherbe
Blue rubber bleb nevus syndrome	Medulloblastoma, leukemia, renal cell carcinoma	Vascular nevi mainly on upper body; but also on leg, mucous membranes, and gi tract
Cowden syndrome	Adenomas and adenocarcinomas of breast and thyroid; and widespread angiomas, and lipomas	A striking hamartomatous condition involving also virginal hypertrophy of the breast, widespread cysts, oral papillomas, colon polyps, and hair follicle hamartomas
Ectodermal dysplasia	Cancers of tongue, and cervix	Atrophic skin, absent skin appendages
Familial polyposis coli	Adenocarcinomas of colon and rectum; many other tumours	Polyps may be restricted to colon or to colorectum, or they may be widespread in gi tract when gastric polyps may be malignant. May be part of Gardner's syndrome
Gardner's syndrome	Adenocarcinomas of colon and rectum	Classic diagnostic criterion is triad of colon polyps, epidermoid cysts, and cutaneous fibromas, but many associated tumours variously reported, e.g. lipoma, leiomyoma, melanoma, and tumours of thyroid, ovary, duodenum, bone, adrenal, bladder, brain, ampulla of Vater, and parotid
Keratoacanthoma (one type)	Mainly spontaneously regressing tumours of skin, and nonregressing visceral tumours, e.g. of duodenum, colon, and other sites	Associated skin lesions resemble squamous cell tumours, e.g. those associated with hereditary disorders such as albinism, epidermolysis bullosa dystrophica, hereditary porphyria, epidermodysplasia

...verruciformis, porokeratosis, ectodermal dysplasia, and dyskeratosis congenita

Condition	Tumours	Associated changes
Multiple endocrine neoplasia I (Werner's syndrome)	Mainly carcinomas of pituitary, parathyroid, pancreas, and adrenal	Lipomas, sometimes in association with various carcinoids, may also be present
Multiple endocrine neoplasia II (Sipple's syndrome)	Medullary thyroid carcinoma and phaeochromocytoma	Associated tumours rarely described include gliomas, glioblastomas, and meningiomas
Multiple endocrine neoplasia III (mucosal neuroma syndrome)	Medullary thyroid carcinoma, phaeochromocytoma and neuromas	Associated neoplasms are those of parathyroid, CNS, and other sites
Multiple leiomyomas	Multiple cutaneous leiomyomas, uterine leiomyomas or sarcomas	Cutaneous leiomyomas are of pilar origin; hypernephroma may be associated
Multiple nevoid basal cell carcinoma syndrome	Multiple basal cell carcinomas	Skin changes include multiple nevoid appearing basal cell carcinomas, benign cysts, hypokeratinizations of palm, 'palmar pits', and soles. Other changes include jaw cysts, intracranial calcifications, and vertebral, ophthalmologic, and neurologic anomalies
Neurofibromatosis (von Recklinghausen's syndrome)	Malignant neurilemmoma; also phaeochromocytoma, astrocytoma, acoustic and spinal neuromas, meningiomas	Widespread cutaneous neurofibromas, axillary 'freckles', giant nevi, and cafe-au-lait spots; oral papillomatous lesions, multiple congenital anomalies
Peutz-Jehger's syndrome	Colonic, duodenal, gastric, and ovarian carcinomas	Polyposis of gi tract except esophagus, melanin pigmentation of mouth, lips, nose, face, and digits
Sclerotylosis	Carcinomas of tongue, breast, and uterus	Skin changes include hyperkeratosis of hands and feet, atrophy elsewhere
Tuberous sclerosis	Mixed tumours of CNS (astrocytomas, glioblastomas); also kidney tumours	Skin changes include hypopigmented macules, shagreen patches, adenoma sebaceum, subungual fibromas. Other features include epilepsy, mental retardation, and hamartomas in kidney, heart, and brain
Tylosis (keratosis palmaris et plantaris)	Esophageal cancer; also carcinoma of larynx, lung, and stomach	Hyperkeratosis of palms and soles of

Table 6.3:   Some Cancer-associated Conditions Showing Autosomal Recessive Inheritance

Disorder	Associated neoplasms	Other associated features
Albinism	Basal and squamous cell carcinoma of skin	Partial or total absence of pigmentation of skin, hair, and eyes; premature ageing of skin denoted by actinic chelitis, telangiectasia, keratosis, and cutaneous horns; stunted growth, and impairment of vision and hearing
Bloom's syndrome	Acute leukemia; rarely, carcinoma of tongue	Stunted growth, fine-featured face, and dolicocephaly; in skin, congenital telangiectatic erythema, photosensitivity, occasional cafe-au-lait spots, ichthyosis, and lichen pilaris
Chediak-Higashi syndrome	Lymphoma, including Hodgkin's disease	Partial albinism, hyperpigmentary response to sunlight, excessive sweating
Fanconi's panmyelopathy	Acute leukemia; rarely, carcinomas of skin, esophagus, and liver	Abnormal skin pigmentation, dyskeratosis, pancytopenia, bone marrow hypoplasia, and congenital abnormalities including hypoplasia of thumbs and absent radius
Louis-Bar syndrome (ataxia telangiectasia)	Acute leukemia, lymphoma; rarely cancers of ovary, stomach, and brain, and basal cell carcinoma	Telangiectasia of eyes, ears, and anticubital fossa; cerebellar ataxia, mental and growth retardation, lymphopenia, IgA deficiency, and recurrent sino-pulmonary infection
Rothmund-Thomson syndrome	Squamous cell carcinoma	Juvenile cataract, congenital bone defects, saddle nose, and hypogonadism; in skin, atrophy, pigmentation, telangiectasia, and disturbance of hair growth
Turcot's (glioma-polyposis) syndrome	Brain tumours, mainly glioblastoma multiformae; rarely, colorectal adenocarcinoma secondary to polyposis coli	Cafe-au-lait spots

Heredity and Cancer: Human Aspects 219

Werner's syndrome (adult progeria)	Sarcoma, meningiomas; rarely, acute leukemia, and tumours of breast, thyroid, and liver	Premature ageing of skin, with sclerodermoid changes, loss of subcutaneous fat, greying of hair and baldness, and leg ulcers; juvenile cataract, diabetes mellitus, hypogonadism, arteriosclerosis and short stature
Xeroderma pigmentosum	Basal and squamous cell carcinoma of skin; also malignant melanoma; rarely, acute leukemia and carcinoma of tongue	Multi-system involvement; skin changes alone include dryness, scaling, hyperpigmentation, freckling, hyperkeratosis, telangiectasia, and ultraviolet light hypersensitivity

Table 6.4: Some Cancer-associated Conditions Showing Sex-linked Recessive Inheritance

Disorder	Predominant cancer	Skin changes and/or other features
Bruton's agammaglobulinemia	Leukemia, lymphoma	Defective humoral immunity associated with multiple recurrent infections; skin changes include pyoderma, furunculosis, cellulitis, and conjunctivitis
Dyskeratosis congenita	Carcinomas of oropharynx, nasopharynx, esophagus, lung, cervix; rarely, leukemia	Skin changes include reticulate hyperpigmentation, leukoplakia of mucosae, nail dystrophy, hyperkeratosis of palms and soles, atrophy of skin of extensor surfaces; pancytopenia
Wiscott-Aldrich syndrome	Leukemia, lymphoma	Thrombocytopenia, IgM deficiencey, recurrent (often fatal) infections; skin changes include purpura, chronic eczema, erythroderma, petechiae, furuncles

Table 6.5: Some Miscellaneous Cancer-associated Disorders with Mixed or Unknown Modes of Inheritance, or with Unknown Heritability

Disorder	Associated neoplasms	Comments
Acanthosis nigricans	Gastric and other adenocarcinomas; rarely, undifferentiated or squamous carcinoma, lymphoma	Extensive skin pigmentation defects, involving mainly the axilla, groin, umbilicus, and nipples. The disorder may also have non-malignant causes, e.g. obesity, Cushing's syndrome, acromegaly, and Stain-Levanthal syndrome; its pre-pubertal appearance may be genetic
Dermatomyositis	Visceral adenocarcinomas	Inflammatory changes of skin and muscle, erythema, edematous swelling of eyelids, 'heliotrope bloating' minute telangiectasia. Raynaud's phenomenon may precede serum enzyme and electromyographic changes
Giant pigmented (bathing trunk) nevi	Melanomas in childhood	Extensive, variable cutaneous nevi
Kaposi sarcoma	Angiosarcomas, particularly of extremities, stomach, intestine	Inheritance possibly autosomal dominant. Disorder associated with an unusual racial predilection (Ashkenazi Jews, Northern Italians, Bantus); cell source unknown
Klippel-Trenaunay-Webber syndrome	Hemangiomas, ? Wilms' tumour	Disorder not known to be genetic
Maffuci syndrome	Hemangiomas, chondrosarcoma, ? pituitary tumours	Disorder not known to be genetic
Neurocutaneous melanosis	Melanomas of CNS	Inheritance possibly autosomal dominant. Skin changes mainly giant hairy nevi

Scleroderma	Bronchiolar carcinoma, malignant carcinoid, possibly esophageal	Associated manifestations include skin 'stiffness' with loss of lines of normal facial expression, and esophageal dysfunction. Esophageal cancer rarely reported in association with the CREST syndrome (Calcinosis, Raynaud's phenomenon, Esophageal mobility dysfunction, Sclerodactyly, and Telangiectasia)
Sebaceous nevus of Jadassohn	Widespread and multiple, include basal cell and sebaceous epitheliomas, salivary gland adenocarcinoma, and keratoacanthoma	One of the more striking of the hamartoma syndromes. Hamartomas, mainly of scalp, face, and neck may be present at birth. Features include linear verrucose plaques on skin, neurological and other abnormalities such as ocular epidermoids and colobomas, hemangiomas, congenital heart disease, and nodular (often bilateral) nephroblastomatosis
Sjögren's syndrome (keratoconjunctivitis sicca)	Lymphoma	Associated manifestations include rheumatoid arthritis, dryness of skin and mucous membranes, hyperpigmentation, cafe-au-lait spots, and purpura and telangiectasia of lips and fingertips
Squamous cell carcinoma	Squamous cell carcinomas	Can be due to diseases with multiple modes of inheritance, e.g. to the autosomal dominant or autosomal recessive epidermolysis bullosa dystrophica, the autosomal dominants ectodermal dysplasia and porokeratosis, and the X-linked recessive dyskeratosis congenita (Schimke, 1978)
Systemic lupus erythematosus	Leukemia, lymphoma, thymoma	Associated features include intermittent fever, arthritis, arthralgia, arteritis, phlebitis, CNS and renal disease, and skin changes such as malar erythema and macules

ondary function. In lung cancer, genes of the arylhydrocarbon hydroxylase locus have been implicated (Chapter Five, Section 5.3.2; Chapter Nine, Section 9.5.2). Breast cancer has been linked with the glutamate pyruvate transaminase (GPT-1) locus (King *et al.*, 1980). Interestingly, these cancers (of the stomach, nasopharynx, lung, and breast) are precisely those with which modern cancer epidemiology has associated a variety of environmental factors (Chapter Nine, Sections 9.3.2 and 9.4).

Finally, a large variety of inherited genetic disorders has been associated with increased risk of practically every type of human cancer. Of these disorders, several are thus associated with colon cancer alone (Table 6.1). As already mentioned (Section 6.1), they include some 200 mendelian disorders. In Tables 6.2, 6.3 and 6.4, representative examples of these and their prominent features are shown, respectively displaying autosomal dominant, autosomal recessive, and sex-linked modes of inheritance. Some of the disorders display mixed or unknown modes of inheritance, as represented in Table 6.5. Also, among the recessively inherited disorders are ataxia telangiectasia, Bloom's syndrome, Fanconi anemia, and xeroderma pigmentosum. Since these are associated with chromosome-breakage, their discussion is deferred to the next chapter, where their prominent features are summarized in Table 7.4. Expert reviews of these various neoplasia-predisposing inherited conditions are available (e.g. Schimke, 1978; Purtilo *et al.*, 1978; Lynch and Lynch, 1979; Harris *et al.*, 1980; Strong, 1981; Harnden *et al.*, 1984).

6.4 Some Specific Cancers

6.4.1 Skin Cancer

In its overall incidence, skin cancer is one of the commonest of human cancers. It is of two types. These are non-melanoma skin cancer (NMSC), which consists of the basal cell carcinomas and squamous cell carcinomas; and malignant melanoma (MM), of which the lentigo maligna (LM) subtype, constituting some 10 per cent of all MM, is notable. Of the two types, by far the more common is NMSC which, unlike the usually fatal MM, but somewhat like LM, is highly responsive to treatment. For this reason, most cases of NMSC are successfully treated in local surgeries and are rarely recorded, so that all reported incidences of

NMSC are likely to be gross underestimates. None the less, some indication of the relative incidence rates can be gleaned from the results of two studies in New Zealand. Per 100,000 population, the first study (Eastcott, 1963) gave the incidence rates for basal cell carcinoma as 113, for squamous cell carcinoma as 38, and for MM as 5.5. In the second study, a comprehensive NMSC survey (Freeman, 1981), the corresponding incidence rate for basal cell carcinoma was 316, and that for squamous cell carcinoma was 165. These figures illustrate two worldwide features of skin cancer incidence: its rising trend, and the predominance of NMSC over MM.

It is a widespread notion that the prime cause of skin cancer is sunlight, particularly the latter's UVB radiation. While NMSC and, to a lesser extent, LM are significantly associated with UVB radiation (cf. Section 6.1), this is not true for MM (for reviews, see Emmett, 1974; Urbach, 1983). For instance, the incidence rate, per 100,000 population, is less than 2 for all skin cancers among the Johannesburg Bantus and the Negroes of Soweto and Uganda, but 579 and 408 respectively for male and female albino Bantus (Oettle, 1963). Similar studies in several other countries, e.g. Brazil, India, Japan, Taiwan, and the United States, have pointed to the existence of marked sunlight-independent ethnic and male/female differences in predisposition to skin cancers of all types, but particularly to MM. As variously reviewed (e.g. Urbach, 1983; Holman and Armstrong, 1984), the incidence of MM in whites shows some consistent features which are independent of the geographical place of abode or of the degree or duration of exposure to sunlight. It is consistently three to four times higher in the white than coloured races, even when they share the same geographical place of abode and the same cancer registry. In countries as disparate as Finland and Australia, the incidence of MM rises sharply from adolescence to early adulthood, reaches a plateau through middle age, and then rises again. The disease also preponderates in young females, affecting mainly their lower legs but the trunk in males.

Such examples of ethnic and sex differences are not the only indications of inherited genetics as the basis of the variable predispositions to skin cancer. In MM, pigmentary traits, ethnic origin, benign nevi, and family history as risk factors have been reported to be independent of one another (Holman and Armstrong, 1984). Among the widely reported risk factors for MM are fair skin, red or blonde hair, blue or green eyes, Celtic ancestry, family history, and number of palpable benign nevi on arms. Also, MM is often associated with a peculiar lesion (the 'B-K' mole), which occurs at an early age and also sometimes in families. MM also occurs in families, in which it also presents at an early age, and with a higher frequency of multiple primaries and a better prognosis than in the nonfamilial MM cases.

A familiar indication of the genetic basis of skin cancer predisposition is xeroderma pigmentosum (XP) (cf. Section 6.1). XP is sometimes regarded as a major cause of skin cancer. However, the very rarity of XP and the commonness of skin cancer should dispel this notion. XP has also been associated with defective excision repair of sunlight-damaged DNA, and sometimes also as having its genetic basis in one of the prezygotic 'mutations' of the type proposed by Knudson for the heritable retinoblastoma and other 'mutant cancer genes' (Knudson, 1981). However, patients with XP rarely develop any malignancy other than skin cancer (German, 1979). This is despite the fact that the presumptive XP mutant gene, by virtue of its prezygotic existence, would be present equally in all of the normal nucleated somatic cells and would very likely have participated in the normal development of the XP patient. XP is also associated with genetic factors other than defective excision repair. Among these are consanguinity, the ABO blood group system, and different numbers of XP alleles, e.g. more in Caucasians than in the Japanese (Hashem *et al.*, 1980).

The importance of the genetic element in skin cancer predisposition among humans is underlined by the following fact. Like bronchogenic carcinoma and the many futile attempts at its experimental induction by tobacco smoke (Chapter Nine, Section 9.2.4), cutaneous malignant melanoma is a peculiarly human disease having no known naturally-occurring or inducible non-human counterpart.

6.4.2 Colorectal Cancer

Cancer of the colon and rectum together constitutes the second most common cancer in both sexes in most Western countries, i.e. next only to lung cancer in males and breast cancer in females. Almost traditionally, though not without controversy, its etiology has been associated with environmental factors as diverse as intestinal flora, bile acids and other cholesterol metabolites, fecal transit time, nitrosamines, certain occupations, parity, and a 'Western-type' diet (high in animal fat and protein, low in fresh vegetables and fibre) (for a recent review, see Miller, 1983). Two interesting features are evident from these results based upon literally hundreds of separate studies conducted practically world-wide over the past 50 years. First, the epidemiologically depicted etiology for colon cancer is not identical with that for rectal cancer. Multiparity, for instance, with its hormonal and other physiological changes, may protect against development of colon cancer without affecting that of rectal cancer (McMichael and Potter, 1980). Second, an 'Eastern-type' diet (one that is high in vegetables and natural fibre but low in animal fat and protein) is 'unlikely to be hazardous and will probably prove beneficial' (Miller, 1983), i.e. in protection against the development of colon cancer (see also Chapter Nine, Section 9.4).

Colon cancer shows some interesting inter-ethnic features. It is far commoner among Caucasians than among Asians or Africans, with some of its highest rates occurring among the Caucasians of New Zealand and Scotland (Miller, 1983). Also, it more commonly involves the distal colon in Caucasians than in Japanese. However, proximal colon cancer in both groups constitutes some 51 per cent of all their familial colorectal cancers, suggesting that the hereditary influences in colon carcinogenesis in both groups are independent of dietary or other environmental differences (Murata and Tanaka, 1983). This sub-site ethnic difference is apparently accentuated during colon carcinogenesis. For instance, different expressions of mucus-associated antigens have been found between proximal and distal human adenocarcinomas, but not between the normal sub-sites (Bara *et al.*, 1984).

Some 25 per cent of all colon cancers belong to at least two broad, heritable clinocogenetic categories. The first of these, comprising the familial gastric, gastrointestinal, Gardner's, Peutz-Jehger's and others of the polyposis syndromes (Table 6.1) accounts for about one per cent of all large bowel cancers. The second, which is not associated with polyposis, accounts for some 12 to 26 per cent of all such cancers (Anderson, 1980). Contributing to this second category are at least four subtypes, all hereditary and familial. These are hereditary colonic cancer, which is characterized by the occurrence of large bowel cancer as the primary malignancy; hereditary gastrocolonic cancer, by the occurrence of large bowel and stomach cancers as double primaries together and/or separately in relatives; hereditary adeno-carcinomatosis, by the occurrence of large bowel and uterine cancers, first described by Warthin in 1913 but now included in the 'cancer family syndrome' described by Lynch and his associates (Lynch, 1976; Lynch and Lynch, 1979); and 'Muir's syndrome'. Muir's syndrome, described by Muir *et al.* (1966) as 'multiple primary carcinomata of the colon, duodenum, and larynx associated with keratoacanthoma of the face' is also known as 'Torre's syndrome', or as 'Muir-Torre's syndrome' in recognition of Torre's description of a case of multiple sebaceous tumours in 1968.

Muir's syndrome has recently been characterized more fully by Anderson (1980). Its principal features are multiple skin tumours, i.e. sebaceous adenomas, keratoacanthomas, and basal and squamous cell carcinomas. These occur with polyps and adeno-carcinomas, mainly of the large bowel but also of the small intestine and stomach. Other neoplasms, such as uterine adeno-carcinoma, transitional cell carcinoma of the ureter or urinary bladder, squamous cell carcinoma of the larynx, esophagus, or vulva, and breast cancer, may also occur with the multiple skin tumours with or without malignant involvement of the intestines. The syndrome displays a dominant mode of inheritance with high penetrance, and with an expressivity that is variable, apparently more so in females than in males.

6.4.3 Lung Cancer

There can be no doubt that the most important achievement of modern cancer epidemiology is its clear demonstrations, repeated almost ad nauseam, that lung cancer incidence and mortality in most industrialized countries have been rising alarmingly over the past fifty years, and that the overwhelming cause of this rise is the habit of cigarette smoking (cf. Doll and Peto, 1981). The incidence of lung cancer was almost certainly low at all times before the habit became so widespread (Chapter Three, Section 3.4.2.6), and it is also low among non-smokers (Enstrom, 1979). It is declining among ex-smokers, and also among those Western male populations experiencing recent declines in the habit (Doll and Peto, 1981); but it is rising among those Western female populations and those developing nations where the habit is on the increase (World Health Organization, 1979; Taha and Ball, 1980).

However, several lines of evidence suggest that the smoking

habit, by itself, cannot be the cause of lung cancer, as distinct from that of the increasing incidence of the disease. In addition to the evidence already discussed above (Section 6.1), the habit is strongly associated with squamous cell carcinoma of the lung but not with lung adenocarcinoma. In the etiology of the latter there is some evidence that heritable factors are more important than smoking (Schimke, 1978). Among the Chinese of Hong Kong, lung adenocarcinoma is prominent, showing a rising trend, a predominance in females, a decreasing incidence with age, and an independence of smoking habits (Kung *et al.*, 1984).

Published data on the synergism between heritable and environmental factors in lung cancer genesis and development are sparse. However, Tokuhata and Lilienfeld (1983) compared lung cancer mortality among relatives of lung cancer patients and controls. They showed that smoking and heritable factors are not independent of each other, neither by an additive nor a multiplicative model. Among the heritable factors may be those related to the inducibility of arylhydrocarbon hydroxylase and sister chromatid exchanges (Section 6.3).

Lung cancer sometimes occurs in families, usually in association with other cancers, e.g. as part of the 'SBLA' syndrome (see Section 6.4.4). It has also been shown to share a familial component with disorders such as chronic obstructive pulmonary disease (COPD) and chronic nonspecific lung disease (CNSLD). Thus Lynch *et al.* (1977) described an association between COPD frequency and increasing genetic relationship (co-ancestry) to lung cancer probands in twelve pedigrees. Orie *et al.* (1977) found that 89 per cent of patients with lung cancer had a personal history of CNSLD, and that 77 per cent had a family history of CNSLD as compared with about 34 per cent in neighbourhood controls. These results, and others from comparative pulmonary-function tests on first-degree relatives of cases (patients with lung cancer and COPD) and controls (Cohen, 1978), suggested the shared familial component, but with the ultimate clinical manifestations being dependent upon one or more cofactors. However, little is known about the nature and relative roles of the familial component, of the cofactor(s), and of the pulmonary impairment in lung cancer genesis and development.

At clinical presentation, lung cancer represents a well-nigh hopeless situation. Over 90 per cent of the presented cases are doomed to fatality, and over half are even unfit for resection. That 'prevention is better than cure' is hence particularly relevant to this disease. The latter, fortunately, is potentially the most preventable of all cancers since, more than any other, the specific cause of its mounting incidence worldwide is known. However, the proven difficulties of abandonment of the smoking habit only serve to underline the vital importance of prevention at the biochemical level. To this end, the indispensable prerequisite is appropriate understanding of the molecular genetics of lung cancer predisposition. This, unfortunately, represents largely uncharted territory.

6.4.4 Breast Cancer

In contrast with lung cancer, preventive oncology based upon current epidemiological data has little to offer in breast cancer, the major cause of cancer mortality among women of most Western countries and of the Bombay Parsis. These data have associated breast cancer with one of the most bewildering sets of endogenous and exogenous extragenetic factors known to modern environmental oncology. Other than their component endogenous hormones such as estrogens and prolactin, these factors may well function secondarily, i.e. through their varied influences upon such hormones that, finally, influence gene expression (Chapter Four, Sections 4.2 and 4.4). Among these factors are early menarche, late menopause, late first parity, low parity, nulliparity, endogenous and exogenous hormones, high frequency of ovulation failure, body height and weight, certain mammographic features, hypercorticoidism, and many others including dietary fat, cosmetic talc, cold climate, and even the mouse mammary tumour virus (for reviews, see Herity, 1983; Kodama and Kodama, 1983; Brisson *et al.*, 1984; also Chapter Nine, Section 9.4). Among the more important of these factors are those, such as parity, dietary fat, and abode in cold climate, which are controllable. However, even these may show a marked dependence upon the peculiarities of host genetics. For instance, in comparative studies, early first parity and multiparity may reduce the breast cancer risk among women; but this risk is significantly higher among breeders than virgins in C3H, AKR, and some others strains of mice which are naturally predisposed to the disease (Chapter Five, Section 5.2.1.2). Also, breast cancer is rare among some (e.g. Eskimo) women who habitually consume large amounts of animal fat, and who may also live in a cold climate

(Shaefer, 1969). It thus seems that dietary and other (e.g. endogenous hormonal) environmental factors may operate conjointly with genetic factors to account for some of the well-established incidence patterns of women's breast cancer. These patterns include the consistently four to six times higher prevalence of the disease among Caucasians than Africans and Asians, and the 'Clemmeson's Hook', i.e. the slight fall in its incidence in the 50 to 54 age group (cf. Herity, 1983).

A genetic base for breast cancer is suggested by a variety of ethnic, hormonal, and familial factors. For instance, the lower risk of breast cancer experienced by Japanese women in comparison with their Caucasian counterparts compares with the earlier age of onset of the oriental disease. This situation seems consistent with aspects of ovarian estrogenic activity among the Japanese, but with those of adrenocortical and/or other (e.g. adipose tissue) non-ovarian estrogenic activity among the Caucasians (Lynch and Lynch, 1979). As reviewed by these authors, breast cancer can occur in families in association with a variety of breast cancer genotypes that include site-specific breast cancer marked by early age of onset and excess of bilaterality. They also include breast cancer co-occurring with neoplasms of the ovary and endometrium; with gastrointestinal cancers; with sarcoma, leukemia, brain tumours, and carcinomas of the larynx and adrenal cortex; and with cutaneous malignant melanoma and other malignancies. In some instances, breast cancer also occurs as part of the 'SBLA' syndrome, which is characterized by an excess of *s*arcoma, and cancers of the *b*reast, the *l*ung and larynx, and the *a*drenal cortex (Lynch *et al.*, 1981).

The complexity of the genotypes associated with heritable breast cancer predisposition is further illustrated by the growing list of inherited conditions with which the disease is associated often in co-occurrence with other types of neoplasm. Among these conditions are Klinefelter's syndrome, Cowden's disease, and possibly Sipple's syndrome (Lynch and Lynch, 1979), as well as Peutz-Jehger's syndrome. For instance, in phenotypic males with Klinefelter's syndrome, which is the most common cause of male hypogonadism, the breast cancer risk is some 66 times that in normal men; and this neoplasm may co-occur with others, particularly primary mediastinal embryonal carcinoma and other germ-cell neoplasms (McNeil *et al.*, 1981). An analogous situation, predominant in females, is provided by the Peutz-Jehger's syndrome. This, characterized by nasal and intestinal polyps, carries a high risk of gonadal neoplasms in women usually, in whom Sertoli-cell tumours constitute the main threat; but gonadal neoplasms may also develop in men. This syndrome also occurs, familially, in association with breast cancer (Riley and Swift, 1979).

Sipple's syndrome (MEA-11) is the less prominent of the two multiple endocrine neoplasia (MEA) syndromes. It usually involves the triad of thyroid medullary carcinoma, pheochromocytoma, and parathyroid neoplasia but, as indicated above, also breast cancer rarely. There is little support for the commonly encountered hypothesis that these MEA syndromes are due to hyperfunction of the parathyroid, pancreas (islets of Langerhans), and pituitary. These organs are usually involved in MEA-I (or Werner's syndrome), which is often associated with carcinoid neoplasms, mainly in the lung. The MEA syndromes may be genetically linked to some pleiotropic gene locus showing an essentially dominant mode of inheritance and variable degrees of expression, or they may represent dysplasia of neuroectodermal tissues.

A strong genetic component is evident for a particular type of 'precancerous' lesion of the breast, i.e. lobular carcinoma *in situ*. Generally, the study of precancerous lesions is a highly controversial and inexact discipline. There is no certainty that any such lesion, if left untreated, will not disappear, remain unchanged, or progress to frankly invasive carcinoma. However, the occurrence of lobular carcinoma is unusually high among first-degree female relatives in breast-cancer-prone families. In such women, it has been calculated that the probability of developing clinical breast carcinoma is some 14 times higher than the expected rate (Lattes, 1980). Moreover, this familial association is the only known risk factor for lobular carcinoma (for a review, see Koss and Greenebaum, 1983).

The complex ecogenetics of cancer causation and development is well exemplified by the breast cancer experience of the Parsi women of Bombay. On the one hand, biochemical studies have implicated various environmental causes, most curiously the murine mammary tumour virus or some antigenically related agent, for the remarkable fact that breast cancer alone accounts for almost half (49 per cent) of the total cancer experience of these women (Paymaster and Gangadharan, 1970). On the other hand, as an ethnic group, the Bombay Parsis have remained genetically isolated for centuries. They have maintained a high level of inbreeding, which has been suggested (Moore *et al.*, 1971) to be the basis of their peculiar proneness to the disease inherited recessively. Yet, the high proportion, rather than the rate of incidence or the inbreeding association, is the unique feature of their disease. Among most Western women, for instance, the overall rate (per 100,000 of the population) of breast cancer tends to be higher than that (34.8) among the Parsi women, e.g. it is 51.6 in Iceland, 64.8 in Norway, 69.6 in Scotland, and 72.0 in New York, but the proportion is about 25 per cent (Waterhouse *et al.*, 1976). Further, this rate is low (11.3) in Japan, where inbreeding is also common, but the proportion (about 10 per cent) like the rate, is among the lowest known anywhere (Jussawalla *et al.*, 1970). Breast cancer is also rare among the Tamils of South India, among whom consanguinity practices are centuries-old (Rao and Inbaraj, 1979).

Thus the factors contributing to breast cancer risk of the Parsi women are likely to be multiple, involving complex ecogenetic interactions. The implicated genetic factors may include consanguinity, dominant or recessive inheritance, ethnic peculiarities, and interindividual and interfamilial genetic differences. This is suggested by the unique susceptibility of these women to cancer of the breast rather than of another body site, somewhat analogously to the susceptibility of XP patients almost exclusively to skin cancer (Section 6.4.1). Also, the Parsi women have, for centuries, lived in a city marked by breast cancer occurrence, overall, at a low rate (about 11 per 100,000 population), and also at a low proportion (about 17 per cent) of the total female cancers (Waterhouse *et al.*, 1976). Moreover, the non-Parsi Indian women have a preponderance of uterine cervical cancer, which is almost unknown among the Parsi women.

For any conceivable environmental factor to exercise such drastic differences in the cancer experiences of the Parsi and non-Parsi women of India, it must be a factor of unparalleled importance to the etiology of human cancer.

6.4.5 *Nasopharyngeal Cancer*

Cancers of the nasopharynx are of two types: nasopharyngeal squamous-cell carcinoma (NPC), and malignant neoplasms of either glandular epithelium or soft tissue. Regardless of race or geography, by far the commoner of the two types is NPC. This occurs in three distinguishable subtypes: keratinizing (differentiated) squamous carcinoma; non-keratinizing carcinoma; and undifferentiated carcinoma.

Many environmental factors have been variously associated with the etiology of NPC. These include the Epstein-Barr virus (EBV); prior history of ear and nose disease; traditional Chinese nasal medication; exposure to smoke and fumes, particularly during food preparation; and nitrosamines and other carcinogens in food, especially dried, salted, and/or fried fish (for reviews, see Ho, 1972; Henderson and Louie, and other authors in de-Thé and Ito (eds.), 1978; Hirayama and Ito, 1981; Yu *et al.*, 1981; McMichael, 1983). Cigarette smoke has also been implicated, though mainly for differentiated NPC (Balakrishnan and Gangadharan, 1982). Ho (1972) proposed a combination of EBV and food-derived carcinogens interacting with genetic predisposition to NPC. A complex interaction involving EBV, bacterial fatty acids with EBV activation effects, and ingested vegetable-derived 'promoter' substances such as croton oil (cf. Chapter Nine, Section 9.5) was proposed by Hirayama and Ito (1981).

Thus, the implicated environmental factors centre largely upon food. Certain major features of NPC suggest a complex ecogenetic etiology for the disease. Among these is the fact that NPC is rare in Northern China, Japan, and most parts of the world, but is almost a disease peculiar to certain Southern Chinese sub-ethnic groups, mainly those of Kwangtung (Canton), but also of Kwangsi and Fukien. These groups have maintained their high rates of NPC incidence (10 to 20 cases per 100,000 population) even after migration to Southeast Asia and North America. Armstrong *et al.* (1979) reported that, in Malaysia, these rates remained unchanged between 1968 and 1977 among the various Chinese sub-ethnic migrant groups. They were highest in the Cantonese, intermediate in the Kheks, and lowest in the Hokkiens and Teochius. Also, per 100,000 population, the rates were, respectively, 16.5 and 7.2 among the Chinese males and females, but 2.3 and 0.7 among Malay males and females, and 1.0 among Indian males. Many other studies (cf. the reviews cited above) have confirmed these inter-ethnic differences, and also the two-to-three times higher incidence of NPC in males than in females in all countries and in all races, Chinese or non-Chinese. These implications of the involvement of genetic factors in NPC etiology, including intersexual (hormonal?) differences, are further supported by certain HLA-associated features of NPC. The HLA haplotype A2-Bsin2 is significantly associated with NPC in the Chinese but not in the Tunisians or Malayans; while Malayan NPC and the A9-B18 haplotype are significantly associated (cf. Dausset and Svejgaard, 1977).

In contrast with such clear indications of a genetic role in NPC etiology, the extant epidemiological data as outlined above do not define any environmental etiology for NPC sufficiently clearly to direct any primary preventive measure. Thus, among the Southern Chinese, women compared with men eat the same food, are more exposed to cooking fires and fumes, but still maintain their lower risk; and the 'boat people' of Hong Kong, who cook in the open air, nevertheless have high rates of NPC (Ho, 1972). Also, both in mainland China and Malaysia, the Cantonese have remained genetically isolated from the Kheks. However, they have continued to share the same cultural background, including herbal and other medicinal practices, methods of food preparation, and type of food with a preference for dried, salted, and fried fish (Armstrong *et al.*, 1979).

6.5 Summary and Outlook

For mainly traditional and methodological reasons, a significant inherited basis for the genesis and development of most human cancers remains to be widely accepted among modern oncologists (Section 6.1). Instead, the still prevalent trend is the traditional regard of cancer etiology as almost exclusively environmental (Chapter Five, Section 5.1; Chapter Nine, Section 9.3). Yet, were this so, effective approaches to cancer prevention would hardly have remained as elusive as they are. It seems unlikely that cancer of *any* type would disappear even if all of the major implicated environmental causes of the disease were removed, e.g. if cigarette smoking and alcoholism were totally abandoned, the Western-type dietary practices were replaced by the Eastern-type, and all women had single or very few sexual partners and many babies starting soon after puberty. This scenario almost perfectly matches the traditional lifestyles of many religious groups, some small such as the Seventh Day Adventists of California, and others counted in hundreds of millions such as the Buddhists and Hindus of Asia. Yet, they too are afflicted with cancer, in some ways almost as much and as severely as other groups. The Japanese Buddhists, for instance, are thus afflicted with stomach cancer and some forms of leukemia, and the Indian Hindus with cervical and oral cancers. Although at usually lower incidences than in the general human populations, the Seventh Day Adventists suffer from all types of cancer, and non-smokers from lung and other cancers.

Another reason for the widespread reluctance to accept the inherited basis as fundamental is interpretative. The usual interpretation of an observed change in the incidence of a given type of cancer with a change in environment, e.g. among second or third generation migrants or among ex-smokers, is that the old environment was the cause of the cancer itself. However, there is an alternative interpretation. Since the inherited factor is a genetic predisposition to the cancer and not the cancer itself, each individually variable predisposition would remain a constant quantity in any environment. A change in the latter, however, would correspondingly influence the rate of expression of the genetically fixed predisposition, even negatively in some instances. The recent worldwide declines in the rates of some cancers, e.g. of the uterine cervix and stomach, are illustrative. This alternative explanation can thus readily accommodate even those epidemiologically established features which the former interpretation cannot, e.g. features such as the individually variable carcinogenic responses among similarly exposed groups such as those of heavy smokers, of non-smokers, or of any shade in between.

From ancient times, many types of cancer have been known to run in families. In modern times, cancers associated with ethnic groups, families, and inherited conditions are being increasingly documented. With the recent growth of molecular genetics, some of the genes associated with cancer etiology are also being increasingly discovered. These include the so-called oncogenes which, however, appear to be normal cellular genes of vital importance in biological evolution and development (Chapter Nine, Sections 9.2.6 and 9.6.3).

Certain types of chromosomal characteristic are also being increasingly associated with cancer etiology. These are considered next.

7 CHROMOSOMES AND CANCER: GENERAL PRINCIPLES

7.1 Introduction

Certain of their generalized features make chromosomes the ideal discursive transition from the basically genetic to the basically environmental aspects of cancer. On the one hand, chromosomes display certain relatively constant, essentially genetically-determined features. Among the latter are the streamlining of chromosomes in prokaryotes in contrast with their redundancy and higher-ordered packaging in eukaryotes; their species-specific shape, size, number, and banding pattern; and their individual-specific combinations of relatively common phylogenetically and mitotically stable subunits contained in specific gene pools. On the other hand there are variable features, many of which can be induced by suitable environmental agents. Among these are features reflected in meiotic nondisjunctions giving rise to monosomies and trisomies of whole chromosomes; and in chromatid breakages which may or may not be viable, be repaired, be repaired faithfully, or be followed by aberrations such as fragmentations, deletions, duplications, exchanges, trans-locations, and ring formations. Indeed, it was the observations of some of these chromosomal instabilities that led Boveri, significantly during the year the First World War started, to pro-pose his somatic mutation hypothesis of tumorigenesis. This hypothesis was born in a state of healthy controversy that still, some seven decades later, characterizes the turbulent world of cancer theories and their practical implications (cf. Chapter Nine). Today, this controversy has developed beyond the fondest dreams of Boveri. Proponents of the hypothesis now rely for support upon evidence showing or purporting to show the monoclonal origin of neoplasms, and the capacity of mainly experimental carcinogens to combine with DNA and alter its chemical structure, and to be mutagenic in bacterial and other systems, mainly *in vitro*. Most importantly, this evidence includes certain neoplasia-predisposing human conditions, such as xeroderma pigmentosum, which are

235

usually associated with pronounced chromosomal instability and defective DNA repair. In contrast, dissidents rely mainly upon one all-encompassing feature of practically all neoplasms. This is that the latters' properties are non-qualitative aberrations of the normal developmental capabilities of inherited genomes.

In this chapter and the next, the question of chromosomal relationships with mainly human neoplasia is critically appraised.

7.2 Boveri's Hypothesis and the Birth of a Continuing Controversy

Around the closing decades of the nineteenth century, the phenomenal growth in the use of the light microscope for visualization of stained chromosomes and some features of their gross infrastructure all but supplanted the reliance of the resurrected mendelian 'classical' genetics upon observations of genetic behaviour. One predictable consequence of this development was the attempts to correlate chromosomal structural changes first with evolutionary phenomena, as initiated by the Dutch botanist, Hugo de Vries, and then, as an extension, with neoplastic and other diseased states.

It is a curious fact of history that the most remembered of the contemporaneous geneticists preoccupied with the neoplasia-chromosome correlations was the German, Theodor Boveri, who, himself, had never examined tumours cytogenetically. Boveri's cytogenetic studies were confined to those of normal and abnormal mitosis mainly in sea urchin eggs but also in *Ascaris*. This endeavour led him, early in his career (in 1887), to attempt a correlation of Mendel's theory of independent segregation of unit characters with aspects of the chromosomal reduction phenomenon at meiosis. In this, he received much support from Sutton and others of his contemporaries.

Boveri's major contribution to oncology was his hypothesis of a cancer-causative role for unbalanced chromosomal constitutions. This hypothesis, which he published in 1914 in his now classic *Zur Frage der Entstehung maligner Tumoren*, has remained, to this day, an issue of central significance to most of the theoretical and many of the practical aspects of oncology, but also one of much controversy. Indeed, as it has since been extended under the generic 'somatic mutation' hypothesis, it has effectively divided modern oncologists into two opposing factions, the most ardent disciples and the equally ardent dissidents, with the remaining oncologists assuming various intermediate or 'fence-sitting' postures. Some of the proponents feel that the hypothesis is so obvious that it should not even be questioned; whereas some of the opponents regard the hypothesis as a useless and even stultifying introduction into the oncologic dictionary. For instance, Peyton Rous, the Nobel Laureate and discoverer of the chicken sarcoma virus, wrote in 1959 that the introduction of the hypothesis resulted in 'no good thing but much that is bad' and in 'fatalism to blast many a hope and effort'.

It is hence important to underline the essential features of Boveri's hypothesis. These are, first, that all cancer cells have chromosomal abnormalities; and, second, that all cancers are directly caused by such abnormalities or by agents or events which produce them. He also advanced a number of supporting concepts which are still among the cornerstones of the hypothesis. These include the concepts of chromosomal factors enhancing or suppressing cell division; of those imbalances which favour the former and/or disfavour the latter factors precipitating malignant genesis; of what would now be called nondisjunction and pseudodiploidy (although meiosis and chromosome numerology were then very inexact sciences) as some of the causes of malignancy; and of the monoclonal origins of malignancy, as exemplified by his statement that 'typically each [malignant] tumour takes its origin from one and a single cell'.

Some of the basic features of the hypothesis, including its controversial nature, were by no means new in 1914 when Boveri published his *Zur Frage der Entstehung maligner Tumoren*. After Arnold (1879a,b) described the chromosomes of several human neoplasms, other workers reported asymmetrical karyokinesis (abnormal mitosis) in neoplastic cells. Notable among the latter was Von Hansemann who, in 1890, proposed that asymmetrical karyokinesis with its unequal distribution of chromosomes in daughter cells is the cause of all carcinomas. However, mounting dissenting evidence led Von Hansemann, two years before his death in 1920, to a retraction of his proposal. The dissent began in 1892, just two years after Hansemann's proposal, when Stroebe showed that asymmetrical karyokinesis is not restricted to carcinomas but is also present in sarcomas, benign tumours, and regenerating normal tissues. Through the efforts of many workers (cf. Heiberg and Kemp, 1929; Kemp, 1929, 1930), it then gradually developed that quantitative chromosomal changes such as those in nuclear size and in number of chromosomes are neither universal nor exclusive attributes of cancer cells.

Boveri's hypothesis, despite these early developments which seem to have threatened its very birth, has persisted to this day. This is because of factors such as the mounting observations of chromosomal anomalies in cancer cells and of the capacity of many tumour inducers to cause such anomalies in susceptible cells; and, mainly, the reliance of the hypothesis not only upon quantitative chromosomal changes, but also upon qualitative changes in chromosomal structure capable of causing corresponding changes in chromosomal function. Indeed, because of the all-embracing and largely unspecified or unknown nature of these hypothesized qualitative changes, it seems likely that the hypothesis will continue to persist, in one form or another, at least until appropriate comparative aspects of gene mapping and gene control in the normal and neoplastic genomes of man are properly understood.

A desirable prelude to the discussion of the role of chromosomes in cancer-predisposing conditions and cancer might be a brief consideration of three pertinent aspects of chromosomes. These are aspects of their instability and uniqueness, of their spontaneous and induced changes and anomalies, and of their heritability. Extensive reviews of these and other aspects of chromosomes are available, e.g. in the recent books: *Chromosomes and Cancer*, by German (ed.) (1974); *The Eukaryotic Chromosome*, by Bostock and Sumner (1978); and *The Chromosomes in Human Cancer and Leukemia*, by Sandberg (1980).

7.3 Chromosomal Instability

7.3.1 Chromosomes in Comparison with Their Structural Subunits

The reality of meiotically and mitotically stable chromosomal subunits, the basic building blocks of eukaryotic chromosomes, can hardly be doubted. Were this not true, the RNAs, enzymes, structural proteins, and other genome-specified cellular and extracellular components would not possess their recognizable structural and functional identities; nor, presumably, would cells, tissues, individuals, and species maintain their characteristic morphology and function. Indeed, this stability might also extend to those subunits which are not themselves transcribed but which may control transcription. Thus, overall, a certain degree of orderly arrangement of both the structural and control subunits within chromosomes would be essential for proper organismic development to proceed. The control function itself would be dependent upon maintenance of this orderly arrangement as well as upon the nature of the subunits themselves. Finally, the meiotic recombinations which generate individual uniqueness and diversity would be other than haphazard or of limitless range.

These considerations suggest that chromosomes are characterized by a degree of substructural stability and uniformity upon which is superimposed a high degree of inherent instability and uniqueness.

Within the human genome, the subunits would include the various 'genes' or 'transcription units' which have been sequenced either directly or through deduction from the known primary structures of their corresponding transcription (RNA) or translation (protein) products. One outcome of such endeavours, based upon interspecific structural comparisons, is the molecular clock which, at present, constitutes an intriguing area of some controversy. This is that the rate of evolutionary fixation of mutations within proteins of various classes is constant for each class, is dependent upon evolutionary time rather than upon generation time, is slower for functionally important proteins such as histones than for functionally less important proteins such as fibrinopeptides, and is measurable in terms of millions of years even for proteins of the latter class (for discussions, see Hartl and Dykhuizen, 1979; Dykhuizen and Hartl, 1980; Van Valen, 1980; Wilson *et al.*, 1977). These indications of biochemical evolution being essentially slow, clocklike, independent of species-lifespan, and subject to functional constraints would imply that, for all practical purposes, the subunits are also evolutionarily stable.

The subunits would also include the list of some 100 genes which have already been mapped at specific chromosomal regions within the human genome. To this list, new additions or confirmations are constantly being made. Some examples are the α-globin gene (Sanders-Haigh *et al.*, 1980) and the catalase gene (Wieacker *et al.*, 1980) to the short arm of chromosome 11, the peptidase A gene to 18q23 (Junien *et al.*, 1980), and the guanylate kinase-1 gene to 1q32-q43 (Dallapiccola *et al.*, 1980a). A partial listing, for illustrative purposes both here and later (Chapter Eight, Section

Table 7.1: The Gene Map of Human Chromosomes 1 and 17

Chromosome	Most consistent smallest region	Gene marker	Gene symbol
1	p32–pter	Enolase–1 (EC 4.2.1.11)	ENO
	p32–pter	Rhesus blood group	Rh
	p32–pter	Adenyl kinase–2 (EC 2.7.4.3)	AK_2
	p32–pter	Uridine monophosphate kinase (EC 2.7.4.4)	UMPK
	p21–p33	Phosphoglucomutase–1 (EC 2.7.5.1)	PGM_1
	p32–p34	α–L–Fucosidase (EC 3.2.1.51)	αFUC
	p34–pter	Phosphogluconate dehydrogenase (EC 1.1.1.44)	PGD
	p36–pter	Adenovirus–12 chromosome modification site–1p	AdV–12–CMS–1p
	1p	Amylase (salivary) (EC 3.2.1.1)	AMY_1
	1p	Amylase$_2$ (pancreatic) (EC 3.2.1.1)	AMY_2
	1p	Elliptocytosis	EI_1
	q21–q23	UDP Glucose pyrophosphorylase (EC 2.7.7.9)	$UGPP_1$
	q32–qter	Guanylate kinase (soluble) (EC 2.7.4.8)	GUKs
	q32–qter	Fumarate hydratase (soluble) (EC 4.2.1.2)	FHs
	q41–qter	Peptidase–C (EC 3.4.11.–)	PEPC
	q42	Adenovirus–12 chromosome modification site–1q	AdV–12–CMS–1q
	q42	5S RNA locus	RN5S
	1q	Duffy blood group	Fy
	1q	Zonular pulverulent cataract	Cae
		Scianna blood group	Sc
		Retinitis pigmentosa–1	Rp_1
		Glucose dehydrogenase (EC 1.1.1.47)	GDH
		Dombrock blood group	Do

17		
	Antithrombin III	AT3
	Aniridia type II	AN–2
	Cholinesterase (serum)–1 (EC 3.1.1.8)	E_1
	Nail–patella syndrome	NPa
	Transferrin (provisional)	Tf
	Hemoglobin–β (also on No 4 and ? No 21)	Hbβ
q21	Thymidine kinase (soluble)(EC 2.7.1.75)	TKs
q21–q22	Galactokinase (EC 2.7.1.6)	GALK
q21–q22	Adenovirus–12 chromosome modification site–17	AdV–12–CMS–17q
	Acid α–glucosidase	α–GLU
	Collagen–1	COL_1
	SV40 integration site	SV40–I
	SV40 transformation site	SV40–T
	Surface antigen	SA–17

8.3.3), is given in Table 7.1 (for more comprehensive listing, see De Grouchy and Turleau, 1977; Shows and McAlpine, 1978; Sandberg, 1980). Comparative data from population genetics, especially of the HLA gene system, indicate that some of these genes occur on chromosomes as more-or-less independent subunits; whereas others occur in linked groups showing, evolutionarily, either marked stability or various degrees and types of linkage disequilibria (for reviews, see Bodmer, 1978).

The gene mapping, currently achieved mainly by use of somatic cell hybrids in conjunction with pedigree analysis, shows that one of the genes may be confined to a specific locus on a particular human chromosome, but that another may occur on two or more loci and/or chromosomes. For example, just the structural gene for but one type (type 1) of the collagens occurs on at least two chromosomes (chromosomes 7 and 17). In contrast, the genes (HLA genes) of the astoundingly diverse major histocompatibility complex (MHC), or of the various blood group systems, are located at single chromosomal regions. Thus, the genes for the HLA antigens are located at region p12-p22 of chromosome 6, for the ABO blood group antigens at region p12-p22 of chromosome 9, for the Rhesus blood group antigens at region p32-pter of chromosome 1, and for the Duffy blood group antigens at region 1q of chromosome 1. This apparent distinction, i.e. of genomic localization of individual-specificity genes, e.g. of the HLA and blood group types, and of genomic delocalization of widely shared genes, e.g. of the collagen type, is deceptive. For instance, widely shared genes such as those for α-L-fucosidase, β-glucuronidase, lactate dehydrogenase-A, and mannose phosphate isomerase are also localized, i.e. respectively on chromosomes 1, 7, 11 and 15.

The phenomenon thus displayed is one of great complexity in genomic subunit arrangements and interrelationships. It is further illustrated by an opposite effect, that of the close functional coordination and interdependence of gene loci which may be widely separated physically within the genome, even occurring on different chromosomes. For instance, $\beta_2$microglobulin is an integral part, the light chain, of the structure of HLA antigens found on perhaps all cell surfaces, where it occurs exclusively in this combination (for a review, see De Wolf *et al.*, 1980). Its occurrence in blood and other body fluids, e.g. in elevated amounts in some neoplastic and other diseases (Hallgren *et al.*, 1980), may be due to breakdown of the cell surface-bound HLA antigens or to factors such as unbalanced cellular synthesis of the antigens marked by β_2-microglobulin overproduction. Yet, the HLA locus is on chromosome 6, the β_2-microglobulin locus is on chromosome 15, and the chromosomal location of the MHC-microglobulin genetic control system remains to be found. Operationally, the MHC system is associated with the control of many functions. Among these are functions necessary for evolution, and for self-maintenance and other physiological features ultimately involved in neoplastic and other disease processes, e.g. immune regulation, cancer susceptibility, transplantation, development, and ageing (Dausset and Svejgaard, 1977; De Wolf *et al.*, 1980).

The ascription of meiotic, mitotic, and evolutionary stability to chromosomal subunits might, at first glance, appear to contradict the fact that some genomes can undergo heritable adaptive changes quite rapidly in evolutionary terms. An important example of this is provided by the influenza virus, various new and sometimes recurring types and subtypes of which have been causing, at least since 1889 and perhaps for centuries, the truly international influenza pandemics that have been occurring at irregular intervals. As recently reviewed by various authors in Schild (ed.) (1979), evolution of the virus has been characterized by the rapidly changing antigenicity of two of its surface glycoproteins, its hemagglutinin in particular and its neuraminidase less often. These rapid changes, which constitute the major obstacle to effective control of the viral disease by vaccination, are characterized by two distinct components: 'antigenic drift', which results apparently from immunologically-mediated selection pressure; and 'antigenic shift', which results from more radical antigenic alterations (Ward and Dopheide, 1979; Verhoeyen *et al.*, 1980).

The genetic basis of these changes is not properly understood. However, the balance of current evidence, including evidence from gene sequencing (Verhoeyen *et al.*, 1980), indicates it to be recombination, rather than mutation, of the stable chromosomal subunits, i.e. between types or subtypes of the human virus or between these and their counterparts in birds or non-human mammals (Pereira, 1979; Laver and Webster, 1979). Presumably, by analogy with viral evolution in other virus-host systems such as the sarcoma virus-mouse system (Dulbecco, 1980), the recombinations might also involve suitable viral and host genetic elements. Even resistance to the viral action or sensitivity to the antiviral effects of interferon, both of which are individually variable among humans, seems to be selectively influenced by host genes (Bang, 1978; Haller *et al.*, 1980). The mechanism of interferon's antiviral activity is not properly understood, but the agent induces the activities of several cellular enzymes (cf. Kimchi *et al.*, 1979). One of the latter, an oligoisoadenylate synthetase, becomes incorporated into the ribonucleoprotein core of at least two viruses, the Moloney murine leukemia virus and the vesicular stomatitis virus (Wallach and Revel, 1980).

Indeed, it is becoming increasingly evident that Nature's organisms possess, both within their own genomes and within the latters' variable capacities to recombine (or pair) with other suitable genomes, all of the information necessary to generate their natural variants without the necessary intermediacy of structurally mutated genes. Thus, participants in the above-discussed genetic recombinations also include those 'mobile' genes or transposable elements which, when they first became recognized many years ago, were widely regarded as genetic curiosities of little significance to general molecular biology. Nowadays, however, gene mobility is being increasingly documented, and is rapidly assuming the status of one of the major dogmas of the discipline. Already, the known list of such transposable elements includes those of *Zea mays*, the insertion elements and transposons of bacteria, and the mating-type elements of yeast which seem to fit the cassette model in their reshuffling movements into new sites (Kamp *et al.*, 1978; Strathern *et al.*, 1979, 1980). Others include the transposable elements in immunoglobulin coding sequences. These are known to operate in both B-cells (Sakano *et al.*, 1979; Early *et al.*, 1980) and T-cells (Forster *et al.*, 1980), and even to be involved in selective deletion of certain immunoglobulin heavy chain genes from the expressed but not the unexpressed allelic chromosome (Yaoita and Honjo, 1980). Transposable elements also occur in the coding sequences for the wide repertoire of surface antigens of the trypanosomes and their continually-generated immunologically distinct variants (Williams *et al.*, 1979; Hoeijmakers *et al.*, 1980). These variants, analogously to the above-discussed influenza variants, are confounding both the immunological defences of their hosts and the efforts at their control by immunological means. Through a sojourn in their tsetse fly vectors, they are continuing to create much havoc in man and beast across a wide belt of Africa (Turner, 1980).

Genetic material is thus increasingly being shown to exist in a surprising state of flux. Chromosomes rearrange and recombine; they swap homologous pieces of DNA during mitotic and meiotic crossing-over that may be equal or unequal; and stretches of DNA, with their mobility often aided by transposons, hop about the genome like monkeys on a tree. Indeed, the phenomenon of mobile genetic elements is becoming so well documented that it almost certainly has many more surprises in store. Among the latest surprises are the 'orphons' described by Childs *et al.* (1981) (see also Lewin, 1981) from studies of histone genes that become switched on late during sea urchin development, i.e. shortly after hatching. In this later stage, Childs *et al.* found the same quintuplet (H1, H2A, H2B, H3 and H4) of histone genes that, in earlier stages and generally, occur in orderly tandem repeats, hundreds of times on the genome, rather like that other well-known tandemly repeated multigene family — the ribosomal genes. However, the later genes occurred in fewer copies; they were not clustered as neat quintuplet multiples; and they were scattered all over the genome. As such, these orphaned histone genes appeared to become free to develop their own control system, and perhaps to diverge, eventually to encode information for an entirely new product. As speculated by Childs *et al.*, 'there may no longer be a clear distinction between tandem and dispersed multigene families'. Genetic mobility rather than gene mutation appears to be Nature's mode of creating not just diversity but also the types of alteration in gene control that may, sometimes, lead to neoplastic transformation.

7.3.2 The Role of Recombination and Related Processes

Genetic adaptation, whether rapid or slow in evolutionary terms, appears to share an essential basis with diversification. This is selective recombination and related processes (e.g. duplication, deletion and motility) that involve the basically stable chromosomal subunits or building blocks contained in specific 'gene' pools. The mechanisms of the recombinations are not well understood. They may be variable among species of organisms; and model studies show that homologous pairing can occur both after (Holliday, 1964; Meselson and Radding, 1975) and before (West *et al.*, 1981) strand unwinding and heteroduplex formation.

Chromosomes cannot be investigated in fossils or extinct species, only in living organisms. This means that the chromosomes of, say, *Homo erectus*, the major direct ancestor of modern man, cannot be known. Yet, comparative chromosomal studies of living organisms are increasingly showing a remarkable preservation of chromosomes and their banding patterns within closely related species. For instance (cf. Seuanez, 1979), every human chromosome has a recognizable counterpart in each of the four species (gorilla, orang-utan, and the two species of chimpanzee) of great apes but not in species (e.g. rat and mouse) of rodents. Between the chromosomes of apes and man, banding patterns are remarkably similar. Differences which are recognizable involve reorganization of pre-existing genetic material, mainly through pericentric inversions, and through one major fusion resulting in the 46 chromosomes in man in contrast with 48 in apes. In the different primate species, certain highly repetitive genes, such as those for ribosomal RNA, may be distributed differently. For instance, rRNA genes occur on nine pairs of acrocentric chromosomes in the orang-utan, on five (different) pairs in man and the chimpanzee, and on two (or three) pairs in the gorilla. Counterparts of one or more genes on practically every human chromosome are found in the great apes, and even in the rhesus and African green monkey, particularly in a chromosome 1 segment which thus seems to have conserved its banding pattern for perhaps 35 million years. In their non-repeated DNA, man and chimpanzee share at least 98 per cent homology, as indicated by DNA hybridization studies, i.e. sufficient similarity to suggest the possibility of a viable hybrid (Lovejoy, 1981). Conservation of chromosome complements and morphology of even more ancient ancestry, over 100 million years, has been described, e.g. for the ratites including the New Zealand kiwi (de Boer, 1980) and the ostrich, the emu, the Australian cassowary, and the common and Darwin's rhea (Sasaki *et al.*, 1968).

Genetic diversification in Nature thus seems to be based largely upon various redeployments, within highly conserved chromosomal complements, of pre-existing chromosomal subunits. That structural mutations within these subunits may play a secondary role in the diversification process is indicated by major observations such as those of the slow rate of fixation of such mutations and the generation of even some 'mutant' gene products independently of such mutations. For instance, unusual immunoglobulin light chains can arise through nonmutational processes such as aberrations in subunit arrangement, in splicing of primary transcripts, or during or after mRNA translation (Choi *et al.*, 1980; Seidman and Leder, 1980).

In their broad morphology and banding patterns, species-specific chromosomes are thus remarkably stable structures, both evolutionarily and developmentally. This contrasts sharply with the temporariness and uniqueness of the individually specific chromosomal recombinants which, most likely, neither pre-existed nor will ever exist again. These chromosomal features are designed to last only during the individual's lifetime to characterize his pro-genitor zygote and all of the latter's nucleated progeny cells, and to be disassembled with but one half of the resultant subunits being used for engendering new recombinants with every new generation. Together with few others, such as subunit selection and pairing of heterogametic meiotic chromosomes during fertilization, these features of chromosomes represent, rather than evolutionary weaknesses, the major recourses of evolution for the generation of diversity among species and individuals.

7.3.3 The Role of Extrinsic Agents

A recurrent theme in biology is that the role of extragenetic (including extracorporeal) agents in influencing biological phenomena such as tumour genesis, development, expression, and therapeutic response is variable in accordance to the dictates of the selectively evolved genomic structures and substructures. It is hence not surprising that any one or various simultaneous or sequential combinations from a great multitude of environmental agents can, in suitable circumstances, exacerbate the inherent capacity of chromosomes to undergo aberrations. As recently reviewed by Sandberg (1980), these agents include ultraviolet, gamma, X and other types of ionizing and non-ionizing radiation, and a host of chemicals such as benzene and the alkylating agents used in industry, experimental tumorigenesis or clinical cancer therapy. These two types of the agents (radiation and chemicals) have already given rise to much public fear of induced chromosomal damage, as exemplified by the 'ban the bomb', the 'Three Mile Island' anti-nuclear, and other campaigners, including residents of Niagara's 'Love Canal' (a chemical waste-dumping area) and the dioxin-exposed personnel and populace of Seveso and Vietnam. Some of these fears may have been unfounded (cf. Holden, 1980), but it cannot be unwise to guard against agents that can seriously damage an individual's chromosomes.

The known chromosome-damaging agents also include a variety of viruses. Among these are human viruses of the DNA type, such as adenoviruses types 2, 7, 12, 18 and 31, and herpesviruses such as herpes simplex types 1 and 2, herpes zoster, the Epstein-Barr virus, and the poxviruses; and RNA viruses such as the paramyxoviruses of mumps and measles. The known chromosome-damaging viruses also include a large number of myxoviruses, arboviruses and picornaviruses of man and animals, and the oncornaviruses associated with sarcomas in mice, chickens, and cats.

Thus, various chromosomal aberrations might also be induced in analytical specimens fortuitously contaminated by any of these agents. This suggests that methodological vagaries can sometimes exacerbate the intrinsic instability of chromosomes.

7.3.4 The Role of Methodology

7.3.4.1 The Pre-modern era: Enumeration of Human Chromosomes. Current appreciation of the large spectrum of changes and anomalies which human and other eukaryotic chromosomes so readily undergo (Section 7.3.5) would, retrospectively, underline the magnitude of the difficulties faced by pre-modern cytogeneticists in their heroic attempts to isolate and characterize these structures. This is aptly illustrated by the confusion which surrounded the task, which is nowadays quite routine, of simply counting the complement of human chromosomes accurately. This is despite the many signal discoveries of the pre-modern era of cytogenetics, which may be dated from the days of the light microscopes of Anton Leeuwenhoek (1632–1723) to the year 1959. This year may be said to mark the inception of the modern era, for it saw the discoveries of trisomy 21 in Down's syndrome (Lejeune *et al.*), monosomy X in Turner's syndrome (Ford *et al.*), and extra X-chromosomes in Klinefelter syndrome (Jacobs and Strong).

Among the older discoveries were those of various mitotic events, made around a century ago, largely through studies of animal cells. This is exemplified by the descriptions of 'karyokinesis' by Schleicher in 1879; and of 'mitosis', 'chromatin', and 'equatorial plate' by Flemming in the 1880s. In 1882, Flemming also depicted and described the structures which were first named 'chromosomes', by Waldeyer in 1888.

Despite all this, enumeration of human chromosomes, until

1956, varied between 16 and 48, the latter figure remaining popular from 1921. Thus, the haploid chromosome number (n) was given during the 1880s by Flemming as 20 to 24, and variously by Wieman and others during the first two decades of the present century as 16, 24, 32, 34, 38, or 40. From 1912 onwards, Winiwarter in Liège and Oguma in Hokkaido, and subsequently both workers together in Liège, gave the diploid chromosome number as 47 for males (2n = 46 + XO) and 48 for females (2n = 46 + XX) (Makino, 1973). In the United States, Painter (1921) and Evans and Swezy (1929) gave the diploid number as 48 (2n = 46 + XX in females, and 46 + XY in males). What now appears to be the correct diploid number, i.e. 46 (2n = 44 + XY in males, and 44 + XX in females), was first reported in 1956, by Tjio and Levan. This result was quickly confirmed during the 1950s (Ford and Hamerton, 1956; Kodani, 1958; Makino and Sasaki, 1959), and it has, since then, been repeatedly reconfirmed.

This story of human chromosome numerology, which has been thoroughly recounted by Makino (1975), illustrates the principle that advances in genetics, as in science generally, are at the mercy of methodology. The earlier cytogenetic studies were based mainly upon light microscopic examination of testicular tissue specimens obtained from patients with tuberculosis of the epididymis or from executed criminals. The specimens were then fixed with Carnoy-Flemming's solution or one of its variants, embedded in paraffin sometimes under high temperature conditions, and stained with iron-hematoxylin. Thus, the variability of the chromosomal counts in these earlier studies could have been due to methodological inadequacies, in addition to other factors such as the diseased status and postmortem changes of the specimens used.

7.3.4.2 The Modern Era: Cell Culture and Chromosome Banding.
Modern cytogenetic analyses are based upon an increasing array of methodological improvements and innovations. For instance, the new tissue culture techniques, colchicine-mediated mitotic arrest, and hypotonic treatment are now serving, respectively, to increase the number of cells available for examination; to increase the number of metaphases available for counting; and to facilitate dispersion and visualization, within the swollen cytoplasm, of the metaphase chromosomes, thus counteracting the natural tendency of mammalian chromosomes to crowd together.

Problems with the modern methods stem from various sources.

These are related to the intrinsic morphology of chromosomes, the paucity of metaphases in most analytical specimens, the selectivity and other difficulties of the necessary tissue culturing systems, and the uncertainties of banding analyses.

7.3.4.2.1 Chromosomal Morphology. Microscopically, chromosomes are transient structures which become clearly visible only briefly during the lifespan of the cell, i.e. during metaphase when they are at their most contracted and condensed state. At practically all other times, whether in or out of the cell cycle, they appear as chromosomally formless, tangled threads maintaining, none the less, the complex chromatin (e.g. nucleosomal, solenoidal, and super-solenoidal) organization seen at interphase. It is for this reason that chromosomal studies are practically confined to metaphase cells. Operationally, chromosomes are thus a metaphase phenomenon, just as chromatin is an interphase phenomenon.

7.3.4.2.2 Metaphase Paucity: The Direct and Indirect Methods, and the Use of Mitogens. Except in rare instances, usually in some specimens from bone marrow, lymph nodes, and spleen, analytical specimens from normal or neoplastic tissues do not contain metaphases sufficient for 'direct' chromosomal analysis, i.e. without pre-culturing. In these latter instances, resort is made to the 'indirect' method, based upon cell culturing in the presence of mitogens, as indicated above, to increase the number of cells and metaphases available for analysis. This method is applied particularly to cells such as peripheral blood lymphocytes which are usually mature and are hence capable of limited or no division.

The technique of mitogenic stimulation of cells in culture stemmed from the original discovery, by Osgood and Brooke in 1955, of the capacity of phytohemagglutinin (PHA) from *Phaseolus vulgaris* (the red kidney bean) to agglutinate erythrocytes in gradient cultures of normal or leukemic leukocytes. Currently, the principal mitogens found useful in human studies are either PHA or sodium metaperiodate for stimulation of T lymphocytes, pokeweed mitogen (PWM) or the calcium ionophore A23187 for both B and T lymphocytes, and the Epstein-Barr virus for B lymphocytes. All of these mitogens, as well as concanavalin A (Con A), have also found use in animal (especially murine) systems, e.g. PHA and Con A for lymph node cells and thymocytes and PWM for spleen cells and B and T lymphocytes in the mouse, and the ionophore for B and T lymphocytes in the pig. (For a review, see Sandberg and Abe, 1980.)

It is generally felt that many of the cultured cell populations are inducible by the appropriate mitogens to form more primitive blast-like cells capable of re-entering the cell cycle and hence of increasing the number of metaphases. However, it now seems likely that only selected cells, forming perhaps a small minority of the total lymphocyte population, are thus inducible. Recently, leukemic cells from the peripheral blood and bone marrow of patients with acute non-lymphocytic leukemia were separated by centrifugal elutriation to yield major kinetically quiescent and minor kinetically active fractions, and the clonogenic potentials in agar *in vitro* of these fractions were compared (Preisler, 1980). Only the minor fraction was found to be significantly clonogenic. This suggested to the author that the quiescent cells may be incapable of resuming active proliferation, and also that the usual growth-kinetic models based upon re-entry of such cells into cycle to account for the apparent discrepancy between observed proliferative rates of leukemic cells and the expansion of the leukemic cell compartment may be questionable. It is also known that the numbers of erythroid and myeloid precursor cells in the peripheral blood of humans are variable both temporally and individually (Grilli *et al.*, 1980).

7.3.4.2.3 Problems Intrinsic to the Indirect Method. Selectivity is a widespread phenomenon in tissue culture studies, and hence a central problem in related aspects of experimental neoplasia (Easty and Easty, 1976). Conceptually, the problem stems from the remarkable cell-type heterogeneity of most neoplasms, and from the variable responses of the component cell types attempting to adapt to the artificial culture conditions. Whether *in vitro*, or *in vivo* in nude mice or other systems, the culturing process remains highly selective and may itself be accompanied by new cytogenetic changes in one or more of the cell types adapting in the interest of their own survival within their new environments (Becker, 1979; Stuttman, 1980). For example, one of the *in vivo* techniques, ascites tumour formation in rodent peritoneal cavity, has been described by Becker to display unnaturalness to 'the nth degree'. This technique became extremely popular during and since the 1950s after its introduction, as the mouse system, by Ehrlich and Apolaut in 1905, and by Yoshida in 1949, as the rat system. Particularly in the hands of workers such as the Kleins (Klein and Klein, 1956), Yoshida (1952), Hauschka (1952, 1953), and Makino (1957), the technique began to show some distinct advantages. Mainly, it provided metaphases in numbers which could be increased by judicious intraperitoneal administration of mitogens and colchicine, and it afforded the opportunity to remove suitable study specimens of ascitic fluid at convenient time intervals.

Despite these advantages, the indirect method in any of its forms can yield spurious results, particularly in studies of human neoplastic cells. In culture, whether *in vivo* or *in vitro*, such cells show a pronounced tendency to die off. Among those that manage to survive, some often fail to divide significantly and hence to accumulate metaphases sufficient for chromosomal analysis. Others may succeed, but only through development of presumably adaptive karyotypic changes, particularly in lines established by long-term serial culture.

Such difficulties constitute a serious source of error in the indirect method. They belie the not uncommon belief, stemming from the early successes with transplantation of animal tumours such as the Walker rat carcinoma and L1210 mouse leukemia, that artificial propagation is necessarily easier for tumour cells than for their normal counterparts, presumably because of the apparent proliferative advantage displayed by the former over the latter (cf. Broxmeyer *et al.*, 1978). In fact, until about a decade ago, such propagation had proved almost impossible with human tumour cells. In culture, these cells generally died or, at best, grew into fibroblasts when they were from epithelial sources, as most human tumours are. In contrast, some normal human cells passing a 'crisis' phase at which most died, survived in culture, as did others that were non-neoplastically transformed, e.g. by the Epstein-Barr virus. Even today, successful culturing of most human epithelial tumours depends largely upon use of various immunoincompetent animal culture media, such as the cheek pouch or eye chamber of the hamster and the nude or antilymphocyte serum (ALS)-treated mouse. For the mesenchymal counterparts, some success began to be achieved after the introduction, in 1970, of the 'soft agar colony' technique (Pike and Robinson, 1970). Significantly, this technique, which is based upon use of a semi-solid agar underlay containing a 'feeder layer' of normal human peripheral lymphocytes, was devised by Pike and Robinson for the growth of normal maturing myeloid colonies of human bone marrow cells. Unmodified, the technique is generally associated with severe depression of colony growth of acute leukemic cells and with variable growth of blast crisis cells (for references, see Lowenberg *et al.*, 1980).

The technique is now widely used with various modifications. These include use of an irradiated feeder layer, of PHA or some other mitogen in the liquid overlay, of hydroxyurea 'suicide' (Morardet and Parmentier, 1977), and/or of feeder cells depleted of E-rosette-forming (i.e. T) cells (Lowenberg *et al.*, 1980). By such means, various successes with the *in vitro* culturing of leukemic or normal leukocytes from human blood or bone marrow have been reported (e.g. Dresch *et al.*, 1980), but not always concordantly. For instance, leukemic clonogenic cells have been claimed to respond to PHA by forming colonies (Dicke *et al.*, 1976; Buick *et al.*, 1977), with PHA showing some selectivity for leukemic colony formation (Dicke *et al.*). This contrasts with claims that PHA is a potent stimulator of colony formation by normal T-lymphocytes (Claesson *et al.*, 1977) and by normal and leukemic lymphocytes equally (Lowenberg and De Zeeuw, 1979). Some of these discrepancies might have been due to the source (blood or bone marrow) of the cells under investigation, since chromosomal aberrations detectable in the bone marrow metaphases of leukemic patients (such as Ph' in CML patients) do not always remain uniform (Hagemeijer *et al.*, 1979), and are not always detectable in their PHA-stimulated blood cells (Rowley, 1975; see also Chapter Eight).

Other sources of error relate to cloning in soft agar, e.g. of colony forming units (CFUs) in bone marrow. As a general rule, cloning is expressed in relation to the number of nucleated cells plated, i.e. colonies and clusters per 10^5 nucleated cells. Various workers have discussed the shortcomings of the method due, for instance, to the influence of dilution of marrow samples by peripheral blood or other sources of nucleated cells, and have suggested improvements based upon methodology and upon mode of expression of results from the cloning studies (Parmentier *et al.*, 1978a, b; Blackett and Gordon, 1978; Coiffier *et al.*, 1980).

7.3.4.2.4 Banding and its Problems. Almost certainly the most outstanding and most useful of the modern methodological innovations is chromosome banding. This was introduced and initially developed over a decade ago, by Caspersson and his colleagues (Caspersson *et al.*, 1969, 1970). An appraisal of the importance of this innovation can be fairly made against the background of the state of cytogenetic analysis in the pre-banding era. In this era, analysis of human chromosomes was restricted to studies of the length, arm ratio, secondary constrictions, and autoradiographic labelling patterns of chromosomes. None the less, this proved sufficient for a number of notable achievements. These include the proper enumeration of human chromosomes (Tjio and Levan, 1956); classification of chromosomes into seven autosomal groups (from A to G) and two pairs (XY and XX) of sex chromosomes (the 'Denver' classification of 1960); and the discoveries of 1959 already referred to, and of what are now known as heterochromatinized X-chromosomes or 'Barr' bodies (Barr and Bertram, 1949), and as the Philadelphia chromosome (Ph') in chronic myelogenous leukemia (Nowell and Hungerford, 1960).

The banding techniques, whose prototype is the quinacrine mustard-based 'Q' banding of Caspersson and his associates, are being multiplied and improved with great regularity. At the Paris Conferences of 1971, 1972 and 1975, five (Q, C,G, R and T) types of banding became recognized and standardized. The G and Q types have proved particularly useful for general identification of homologous pairs and substructural details, the C type for heterochromatin identification and for characterization of 'marker' (abnormal) chromosomes with multiple and/or abnormal centromeres, and the R and T types for revealing telomeric details which can include translocations. (For recent detailed reviews of the various modern techniques, see Yunis and Chandler, 1977; Yunis *et al.*, 1978; Sandberg, 1980; Sandberg and Abe, 1980.)

However, as touched upon in the above discussion of the indirect method, even these modern techniques tend to fall significantly short of the ideal requirement, i.e. that the microscopic picture should mirror the cytogenetic state *in vivo*. Thus, a standard practice, prior to banding analysis (e.g. with Giemsa), is the culturing of the specimen cells for two generations in the presence of the halogenated thymidine analogue, 5-bromodeoxyuridine (BUdR), for the detection of sister chromatid exchanges (SCEs). However, BUdR itself can induce SCEs, which are symmetrical interchanges of segments between sister chromatids. Such interchanges were first demonstrated in

1957, by Taylor *et al.*, who used an autoradiographic technique in plant chromosomes; but the use of BUdR as an improved method for SCE detection was introduced by Latt in 1973 (for reviews, see Kato, 1977a, b). Among the many effects, in addition to SCE induction, of BUdR on mammalian cells are cytotoxicity, mutagenesis, and suppression of differentiation. These effects are generally felt to be due largely to BUdR incorporation into cellular DNA during the *in vitro* growth of the cells, but some recent evidence would indicate otherwise. For instance, it has been shown that both mutagenesis (Kaufman and Davidson, 1978) and SCE induction (Davidson et al, 1980) by BUdR are much more dependent upon the concentration of BUdR in the culture medium than upon the BUdR incorporation into DNA.

7.3.4.2.5 Other Problems, and an Appraisal. The D_o (a measure of the slope of the clonogenic survival curve) for the same human diploid fibroblast cell strain (the FA1B1 strain from a case of Fanconi anemia) has been reported to be 160 ± 16 rads of X-rays (Weichselbaum *et al.*, 1980) but 69 ± 5 rads of Y-rays (Arlett and Harcourt, 1980). It remains uncertain whether methodological variation alone is responsible for such a discrepancy. For several other cell strains, the same methodological variation used by these two groups of workers failed to produce similarly discrepant results.

Another methodological variable (in type, degree, use, or non-use) capable of yielding markedly variable results is washing of blood cells with culture fluid or saline prior to incubation of pretreated cells during assay of SCEs, other exchanges, breaks and related types of lesion. For instance, in a recent study of the cytogenetic effects of the direct-acting clastogen, bleomycin, on human lymphocytes, the *in vitro* exposed G_o lymphocytes, but not the lymphocytes from cancer patients pretreated with the agent, were washed before culturing (Dresp *et al.*, 1978). By such techniques, various chromosomal lesions are increasingly being reported in cultured peripheral blood cells of people exposed to a variety of industrial and other mutagens, e.g. to pesticides and herbicides (Yoder *et al.*, 1973). These lesions are usually thought to be present in the circulating (G_o) cells. Indeed, detailed theoretical mechanisms for the production of such lesions in cells at various cell-cycle stages have been proposed (Kihlman, 1971; Bender *et al.*, 1974). However, the true mechanisms remain unknown and are under active investigation (cf. Natarajan *et al.*, 1980; Geard *et al.*, 1980; Marshall *et al.*, 1980). Recently, Dufrain *et al.* (1980) studied the influence of washing upon the chromosomal effects of streptonigrin, an antitumour antibiotic acting at all cell-cycle stages, on the lymphocytes of rabbits pretreated with the agent. They found the same levels of chromatid breaks, and no chromatid exchanges, in both the test and control samples when washing preceded incubation. In contrast, when the washing was omitted, the test samples developed elevated levels of breaks and significant exchanges. This effect of washing, however, has not been universally observed, e.g. in cyclophosphamide-treated rabbits or mitomycin-treated humans (Littlefield *et al.*, 1980). Also, elevated levels of SCEs have been reported in melanoma patients up to four months after cessation of therapy with cyclohexylchloroethyl nitrosourea (CCNU) (Lambert *et al.*, 1979).

It thus seems that, in some instances, the cytogenetic changes observed by even the best of the modern techniques and interpreted to have occurred *in vivo* might have, in fact, been at least partly due to inadequacies of the techniques themselves or of the latters' usage. This would appear particularly relevant to studies of tumour cytogenetic changes, because of the exaggerated fragility and instability of most types of tumour-cell genomes.

7.3.5 Spontaneous Changes and Anomalies

7.3.5.1 Cyclical Changes. The evolution-designed features of considerable instability and uniqueness have conferred upon chromosomes an unrivalled intrinsic capacity to undergo a vast array of morphological and structural alterations. Thus, during much of the cell cycle, which lasts about 30 hours in most human cells, the chromosomes, as visualized microscopically, appear as indistinct, formless and nuclear membrane-encapsulated threads. These threads remain single during the highly temporally-variable G_1 phase (sometimes distinguished from G_0, the non-cycling phase) (cf. Lajtha, 1963) but double during the G_2 phase (Johnson and Rao, 1970). The spatial organization of the structures does not seem to be random. For instance, the 'telophase configuration', characterized by the telomeres and the centromeres occupying opposite sides of the nucleus, is maintained throughout interphase (Fussell, 1975). However, the structures display significantly lower packing ratios than the 28.3:1 ratio of a typical 250 Å metaphase mammalian chromatin fibre (DuPraw and Bahr, 1969; Pardon and Wilkins, 1972). Only during certain phases (from the end of prophase to the beginning of telophase) of the relatively short mitotic stage do the chromosomes condense sufficiently, with shortening and thickening, to become clearly structured and visible in their familiar forms, most prominently during metaphase. Thus, in practical terms, 'chromatin' and 'chromosomes' are operational descriptions of nuclear DNA complexes seen, respectively, during interphase and metaphase.

Also, during mitosis, chromosomes undergo complex movements about the mitotic spindle, when they may become involved in various aberrant segregations. Among the latter are nondisjunctions, wherein two homologous chromosomes fail to separate during anaphase. This results in their co-migration to the same pole along the spindle and production of an unequal chromosomal distribution between the two daughter cells eventually formed after cytokinesis at telophase. That such aberrations may be quite common is suggested by the findings of some 20 per cent of the thousands of aborted or live fetuses already studied by amniocentesis for biochemical anomalies turning out to carry trisomies, monosomies, and/or other chromosomal anomalies (Galjaard, 1978; Golbus, 1978; Polani *et al.*, 1979).

7.3.5.2 Anomalies Involving Entire Chromosomes: The Role of Nondisjunction. Nondisjunction (failure of bivalents to separate at anaphase) is generally regarded to be the mechanism behind the chromosomal trisomies and monosomies found in progeny of ageing mothers in particular. However, Hassold *et al.* (1980) suggested that true nondisjunction might be largely independent of increasing maternal age and, instead, be influenced by the presence of large blocks of heterochromatin ('constitutive heterochromatin', or 'surplus' or 'repetitive' DNA). They found the maternal age effect, which was first noted for trisomy 21 some half a century ago (Penrose, 1933), in most trisomic abortuses, particularly those involving the small chromosomes, but with the trisomic 16 abortuses showing, comparatively, a higher frequency of occurrence and a lower dependence upon maternal age. They thus hypothesized that an alternative or supplementary mechanism to nondisjunction for generation of the maternal age-dependent trisomies might be precocious disjunction of the bivalents and random segregation of the resulting univalents. This process, they reasoned, would affect chromosomes with the fewest chiasmata, and might be predominant in the oocytes of older women.

However, whether or not heterochromatin plays a role in the causation of trisomies or spontaneous abortions is controversial. Interindividually, human heterochromatin, like many other parts of the genome, is highly polymorphic due to factors such as duplications, deletions and inversions. Heterochromatic polymorphism in chromosomes 1 and 9, for example, has been described by various workers to bear a relationship to features such as recurrent abortions, fetal wastage, and abnormal phenotypes (for references, see Hemming and Burns, 1979). However, Hemming and Burns found no significant difference in the heterochromatic regions of chromosomes 1 and 9 in a comparative study of two groups of 50 couples each, one group with a history of spontaneous abortions and the other with normal pregnancies.

The alternative mechanism proposed by Hassold *et al.* is not concerned with paternal contribution to the generation of the trisomies. Since 1973, when Uchida, and also Sasaki and Hara, independently demonstrated that paternal nondisjunction can also contribute to trisomy 21 in offspring, this phenomenon has become well documented (Mattei *et al.*, 1979; Mikkelsen *et al.*, 1980). Thus, in a study of 110 Danish families, Mikkelsen *et al.* found the paternal contribution to the trisomy 21 cases to be variable, i.e. to be 11 per cent and 23.5 per cent in two different parts of Denmark. They also found a predominance of paternal nondisjunction failure of first meiotic division among the DS patients. This contrasts with the predominance of the maternal counterpart among trisomic spontaneous abortuses compared with trisomic live births (Niikawa *et al.*, 1977; Lauritsen *et al.*, 1979).

Consecutive nondisjunction has also been proposed. Rinaldi *et al.* (1975) described a glucose 6-phosphate dehydrogenase (G6PD) mosaic 22-years-old male in Sardinia, where the incidence of G6PD deficiency of the Mediterranean type can be as high as 30 per cent among males. The propositus, whose mother and father were both karyotypically normal but were, respectively, heterozygous and hemizygous for the Gd^{Med}gene, displayed a 48,XXYY karyotype in all ten of the metaphases from his peripheral blood culture examined by Q-banding. These findings suggest that the propositus developed from an XXYY zygote derived from a consecutive meiotic nondisjunction during paternal gametogenesis. At least two other similar cases (De la Chapelle *et al.*, 1964; Pfeiffer *et al.*, 1964) from a total of 36 XXYY propositi (Sanger *et al.*, 1977) have been described.

Thus, the cytogenetic mechanisms which generate anomalies of entire chromosomes during gametogenesis are complex and, as yet, poorly understood.

7.3.5.3 Anomalies Involving Parts of Chromosomes. The phenomenon of an apparently higher incidence of partial than total monosomy would suggest two important generalizations. Firstly, of the two fundamental processes of meiosis, reduction division and recombination, the latter might be more error-prone than the former. Although the opposite of total monosomy, i.e. total trisomy, is by no means uncommon, recombination is the major natural source of interindividual heterogeneity and is hence apparently more variable and more error-prone than the separation of homologues involved in reduction division. The latter, or 'the two divisions of the nucleus in the course of which the chromosomes only divide once' is necessary to avoid the geometric increase in ploidy with eventual nuclear explosion which would otherwise ensue at successive fertilizations. However, by itself, reduction division cannot explain meiosis since, logically, a single division of a diploid nucleus is necessary to produce the haploid state. Moreover, the diploid state can be generated and maintained without the mediation of haploidization, i.e. conceptually by division of a tetraploid zygote formed at fertilization involving two diploid germ cells, as occurs analogously during somatic cell mitosis and during the first meiotic division. Indeed, haploidization, which occurs only during the second meiotic division and both before (in higher plants and animals) and after (in lower plants) fertilization is sometimes aberrantly absent in some protozoa (Cleveland, 1947). Also, modified meiosis is obviously necessary to maintain the haploid male honey bee (Sharma *et al.*, 1961) or the rare polyploid animals including some species of fish (Dingerkus, 1976), amphibians (Maxson *et al.*, 1977) and birds (Wang and Shoffner, 1980).

Secondly, the phenomenon suggests that chromosomal anomalies more commonly involve parts of than entire chromosomes. Considered in conjunction with the basic stability of the genetic subunits (Section 7.3.1), this implies further that the essential basis of the anomalies is error of recombination rather than of substructure of the subunits. The basis for this difference is presumably that most subunit structural (or 'gene') mutations, such as the various base modifications which can be induced randomly by diverse means, are essentially deleterious and are thus removed by selection or by the DNA repair mechanisms which are universal in the biosphere. Such a protective effect is particularly evident in the egg. For example, the so-called 'Hertwig effect', first described by Hertwig in 1911 in frogs, has now been observed in several avian, mammalian and other species. In this effect, eggs fertilized by sperms treated with high doses of ultraviolet radiation, ionizing radiation, or one of a variety of mutagenic chemicals give rise to embryos which survive better than those developing from the lower-dose counterparts. It now seems that the egg is more protected from genetic damage than the sperm, due partly to the greater prominence of photo-reactivating and perhaps other repair systems in the egg than in the sperm (Rupert, 1975). At the high doses, the sperm chromatin is completely inactivated or destroyed, the sperm acts as a parthenogenesis-like stimulus, and embryogenesis proceeds in a gynogenetic haploid condition. This condition seems to be far less detrimental to development than the aneuploid condition which results from fertilization of the egg by the sperm having its chromatin only partially inactivated at the low doses (reviewed by Ijiri and Egami, 1980).

A somewhat analogous observation is the capacity of many mutagens to induce sperm head abnormalities in mice (Topham, 1980). However, although eggs appear to be more naturally shielded from damage than sperms, the protection is far from extensive. Dominant lethals, for instance, have been induced in immature oocytes mainly of *Drosophila*, e.g. by X-rays at least since the 1950s. (For references and the effects of single or fractionated X-ray exposures, see Sankaranarayanan and Volkers, 1980).

Chromosome anomalies involving parts of chromosomes are widespread and varied. Not uncommon are single or multiple breaks, with the latter sometimes resulting in chromosome fragmentation even down to 'pulverization', occurring in one or both of the sister chromatids held together at the centromere. These aberrations are either of the chromosome-type, in which both chromatids are affected at the same location; or of the chromatid-type, in which only one chromatid is affected at a given location. Achromatic lesions or gaps which, strictly, are not structural changes also may occur, affecting either one or both chromatids, and varying in size from a small nick to an area occupying the whole width of the chromatid (Scheid and Traut, 1971).

The mechanism of aberration production is poorly understood. This is aptly illustrated by the continuing controversy between the breakage-and-reunion hypothesis (reviewed by Evans, 1974) and the primarily breakage-independent exchange hypothesis (reviewed by Revell, 1974). However, important factors appear to be the intrinsic fragility of chromosomes, and their 'stickiness' particularly of their broken ends when breaks occur.

By these and other (unknown) means, chromosomes may undergo a large variety of structural and morphological changes. They may clump together, as is often seen in tumour cell metaphases. They may also undergo rejoining at the broken ends, before or after inversion of presumably separated segments, and either within a single chromosome (intrachanges) or between different chromosomes (interchanges). They thus often display aberrations such as sister chromatid and other exchanges, paracentric or pericentric inversions, various (e.g. reciprocal, Robertsonian, symmetrical, and asymmetrical) types of translocation, interstitial or terminal deletions, and fusions to form ring chromosomes that, with duplication, may assume a figure 8 appearance. Of the chromosome-type aberrations alone, the asymmetrical intrachanges can produce acentric fragments, minutes, and centric or acentric rings; the symmetrical intrachanges can produce pericentric or paracentric inversions; the asymmetrical interchanges can produce dicentric or polycentric and acentric fragments; and the symmetrical interchanges can produce reciprocal translocations. To the previously known types and subtypes of these aberrations, new additions are constantly being made, e.g. the (p25q21) subtype (Duckett and Roberts, 1980) to the previously known (p2q2) (Lamm *et al.*, 1974), (p21q15) (Emanuel, 1978), and (p21q25) (Pearson *et al.*, 1979) subtypes of pericentric inversion of chromosome 6. (For recent reviews of this subject, see Bostock and Sumner, 1978; Sandberg, 1980.)

7.3.5.4 Anomalies Involving Sex Chromosomes and Autosomes: A Comparison. A curious phenomenon is that a type of developmental abnormality which would be logically associated with an autosomal or a sex chromosomal anomaly can sometimes show the reverse association. A recently reported example of this (Sulewski *et al.*, 1980) is the case of a 19-year-old girl with a normal male karyotype in 75 per cent of her cells and a double autosomal trisomic (48,XY,+8,+21) karyotype in her remaining cells. She showed no detectable sex chromosome abnormality. Development appeared quite normal until puberty. After this, however, and despite the apparently normal sex chromosomes, the classic signs of gonadal dysgenesis (mainly amenorrhea and sexual infantilism) appeared.

Gonadal dysgenesis, usually, is one of the hallmarks of a group of sex chromosome anomaly syndromes, the discovery of which was pioneered by Ford *et al.* in 1959. These syndromes are now known to include various sex chromosome monosomies and trisomies that contrast with the autosomal counterparts in that they tend to be more compatible than the latter with survival to adulthood. Their archetype is Turner's syndrome with its predominantly 45,XO karyotype but sometimes also with mosaic (e.g. 45,XO/46,XX and 45,XO/47,XXX) and other (e.g. X isochromosomal) karyotypes. Affected individuals are phenotypic females. In the more extreme cases, they present with 'streak' gonads, i.e. ovaries replaced by fibrous tissue resembling ovarian stroma but devoid of follicles, and with primary amenorrhea, infantile genitalia, failure of secondary sexual characteristics at puberty and obvious congenital abnormalities including short webbed neck, low hairline, dwarfism, and, sometimes, cardiovascular and renal defects.

An analogous condition occuring in males is the Klinefelter syndrome. This, with its predominantly 47,XXY karyotype, was first described by Jacobs and Strong in 1959. Affected individuals are azoospermic, and they have testes which are widely believed to be devoid of germ cells, except in those rare instances when mosaicism may be present. However, growing oocytes have sometimes been observed in testes or ovotestes, e.g. in a 16-year-old human hermaphrodite (Overzier, 1964) and in a substantial proportion of genetically sex-reversed male mice (McLaren, 1980).

Among the various other sex-chromosome anomaly syndromes, four which are also associated with abnormalites of gonadal anatomy and function are the Klinefelter-syndrome-like (i.e. extra sex chromosome-containing) 47,XXX and 47,XYY syndromes, and two others, both of which are associated with the female phenotype. These are the 'testicular feminization' and the 'pure gonadal dysgenesis' syndromes. In the first of these syndromes, females with a normal male (46,XY) karyotype can present with an attractively feminine appearance, e.g. with good figure and breast development, but they fail to menstruate. Very rarely, this syndrome is associated with other karyotypes, usualy mosaicism and the 47,XXY karyotype (Gerli *et al.*, 1979). In the second, the characteristic congenital abnormalities of Turner's syndrome may be absent, and either a 46,XY or 46,XX karyotype may be present; but the invariant features are streak gonads, primary amenorrhea, and sexual infantilism (Chandley, 1979).

7.3.5.5 Anomalies and Viability: Loss, Gain, and Mosaicism. However they may arise (cf. Section 7.3.5.2), aberrant chromosomal segregations are characterized by loss, gain, or mosaicism involving entire chromosomes in various pathological (and some physiological; see below) states (Berger, 1971; De Grouchy and Turleau, 1977; Sandberg, 1980).

The relative viability of these anomalies is difficult to quantify. In mice, autosomal trisomies usually result in failure of fetal development; and short postnatal survival is associated with trisomies 13, 16, and 19 only, but some of the trisomic cells themselves are quite viable. Thus, hemopoietic stem cells from mouse fetuses trisomic for chromosome 12 or 19, but not 13 or 16, can, in radiation chimeras, restore hemopoiesis, including lymphopoiesis, without showing any undue signs of cytogenetic instability (Herbst *et al.*, 1981). In man, the karyotypes of spontaneous abortuses can show monosomies, trisomies, double trisomies, triploidy of sex chromosomes, tetraploidy, and hypodiploidy/hyperdiploidy mosaicism, in addition to the anomalies involving parts of chromosomes (Creasy *et al.*, 1976; Chandley, 1979; Hassold *et al.*, 1980). However, the losses appear to be less viable than the gains, since total autosomal monosomies are extremely rare among viable humans, in contrast with the less rare trisomies and partial monosomies. Among the viable partial monosomies number the partial deletions of group B chromosomes as in the 'cri-du-chat' syndrome, the partial deletion of the long arm of chromosome 13 (the 13q-deletion) associated with heritable retinoblastoma (Knudson and Strong, 1972; Knudson,

1977), and the ring chromosomes. Ring chromosomes, which may be formed from autosomes such as chromosome 21 or from the Y chromosome (Chandley, 1979), may fail to pair during cell division, thus producing features such as maturation arrest and cellular (e.g. spermatocyte) death (Burgoyne, 1979).

That autosomal monosomies may be less viable than autosomal trisomies would suggest that human life is more compatible with an excess than a deficiency of the normal chromosomal complement. The arch example of the viable autosomal trisomies, and also the best and oldest known, is trisomy 21 in Down's syndrome (DS, or 'mongolism'). Although DS is compatible with survival (Rosner and Lee, 1972), it does reduce normal life expectancy. The reduction has been estimated to be about 53 years per 1,000 total live births, according to a study conducted in the United States (Jones, 1979). However, most of the other viable autosomal trisomies, which involve mainly the smaller chromosomes largely of groups D, E and F, are known only in children as the affected individuals rarely live beyond the first year postnatally (Magenis *et al.*, 1968). In rare instances, however, survival beyond five years has been reported (cf. Hodes *et al.*, 1978), a rather unusual case being that of a 9-year-old boy with trisomy 13 (Patau's syndrome) (Cowen *et al.*, 1979). Moreover, viable cases of double autosomal trisomies are exceedingly rare; and, when they do occur, they are associated with severe physical defects (Grosse and Schwanitz, 1977). Viable partial autosomal polysomies can be quite complex, e.g. partial tetrasomy qp (Moedjono *et al.*, 1980).

It seems that survival in the case of the autosomal trisomies is aided by mosaicism. For instance, three cases of group E triple mosaicism in surviving patients have been described (for references, see Frydman *et al.*, 1979), including one case, described by these workers, with the 45,XY,−18/46,XY/47,XY,+18 mosaic karyotype. Other examples are the 45,X/47,XY,+21 mosaicism, and three analogous cases involving trisomy 21, i.e. three cases displaying the 45,X/46,XY/47,XY,+21 triple mosaic karyotype (Edgren *et al.*, 1966; Konstantinova, 1978; Sparagana *et al.*, 1980). The case described by Sparagana *et al.* seems to be an apt illustration of the typical features of the autosomal trisomic mosaicisms. The subject was a 48-year-old Negro male who, physically, was muscular, non-eunuchoidal, and well virilized with normal external genitalia. He was also of normal intelligence, and he married and believed that he fathered two normal male children. He showed none of the physical stigmata of Turner's syndrome, although his biopsies showed testicular immaturity with a predominance of Sertoli cells in rather small and sparse seminiferous tubules. A somewhat analogous case is that of the already mentioned (Section 7.3.5.4) 19-year-old girl described by Sulewski *et al.* (1980). She showed none of the dysmorphic features of either of her trisomies (8 and 21). This, however, contrasts with the situation in most other reported double trisomic patients, who tend to display the signs of at least one of their trisomies, e.g. of the Patau (trisomy 21), Edward (trisomy 18), or Down (trisomy 21) syndrome in appropriate instances (Grosse and Schwanitz, 1977).

While loss compared with gain of genetic material appears to be less compatible with human survival, this may not be equally applicable to cellular survival. Since Kessous and colleagues (Kessous and Colombies, 1975; Kessous *et al.*, 1975) described the first known case of a near-haploid ALL cell line, three other related cases have been reported. This first case was that of a cell line, from a 5-year-old girl, which showed only 27 chromosomes in 58 per cent of the bone marrow cells, and only 4 normal pairs (X,10,18 and 21) of chromosomes. During remission, the line disappeared, only to be replaced, at relapse, with an exact duplication of the 27 line, i.e. with a 54 line. In 1977, Oshimura *et al.* reported an almost identical situation, involving a 12-year-old girl with ALL, but which showed the four normal pairs to involve chromosomes No 10, 14, 18 and 21, and also a 7p+ anomaly. In 1978, Prieto *et al.* described a 26-chromosome-containing leukemic cell line in a 14-year-old boy with ALL, but they performed no banding analysis although their regular Giemsa-stained preparation showed chromosome pairs in only groups D and G. In the fourth example (Kessous *et al.*, 1980), a 61-year-old woman with the Philadelphia (Ph') chromosome-positive type of chronic myelogenous leukemia showed, during lymphoid blast crisis, 55 per cent of her blast cells to have 28 chromosomes and 36 per cent to have the exact duplicate of this near haploid chromosome complement. Karyotypic analysis by R-banding revealed the near haploid cells to have only four chromosome pairs (Nos 13, 14, 18 and 21) retaining normal morphology. The G 22 pair contained a Ph' chromosome, the C6 pair was totally absent, one of the C11 pair was structurally modified, and all the other pairs including the X pair were haploid.

From just four cases currently available, only tentative conclusions can be drawn regarding the essentiality of particular chromosomes to cellular survival. On this proviso, a comparison of the available results (Table 7.2) suggests that survival requires at least one normal chromosome from each pair, with the exception of the C-group chromosomes Nos 6 (totally deleted in the example of Kessous *et al.*, 1980) and 7 (involved in a translocation in the example of Oshimura *et al.*, 1977), an intact X-chromosome, and two normal pairs, i.e. 18 and 21. This entire situation may be compared with the viable haploid gametes, which contain one normal chromosome from each pair inclusive of one normal X or Y chromosome.

7.3.5.6 Variants and Anomalies in Physiological States. The capacity to undergo a great variety of morphological, structural, and even numerical changes is clearly intrinsic to chromosomes. Not only is this capacity largely responsible, through meiotic recombination, for such natural marvels as the almost certain genetic individuality of each of the millions of sperms normally contained in a single human ejaculate despite their common paternity, but it also appears to remain expressible in various ways throughout the chromosomal lifetime. It would thus be quite surprising were the capacity not expressed in normal tissues subject to the dynamics and the wear and tear of a normal lifetime.

In man, as in other species, chromosomes are heteromorphic, even by the gross criteria of length, centromere position, and banding pattern available to modern cytogenetic analysis. Also, their normal diploid number as well as their morphology can show some variations, with the exact type and extent of the variations being dependent upon factors such as tissue source of the cells under examination, and the age and sex of the individual donor. For instance, it has been known for some time (Court-Brown *et al.*, 1964; Jacobs *et al.*, 1964) that the proportion of 45X cells increases with age in men and women. In blood, this becomes most clearly evident in men around age 65 years and in women about 10 years earlier, with the proportion of the affected blood cells reaching about 2 per cent in women and about 7 per cent in men. Later studies have shown that the marrow of perfectly normal males can lack the Y chromosome in from a few to almost all of their marrow cells; and that aneuploidy of various types, but mainly involving loss or gain of single chromosomes, can occur in

Table 7.2: Chromosomal Distribution in the Four Near-haploid Human Leukemic Cell Lines Which Are Currently Known

Cell line	A			B		C							D			E			F		G		Sax		Reference
	1	2	3	4	5	6	7	8	9	10	11	12	13	14	15	16	17	18	19	20	21	22	X	Y	
1	1	1	1	1	1	1	1	1	1	2	1	1	1	1	1	1	1	1	1	1	2	1	2	0	Kessous *et al.*, 1975
2	1	1	1	1	1	1	1[a]	1	1	2	1	1	1	2	1	1	1	2	1	1	2	1	1	0	Oshimura *et al.*, 1979
3	1	1	1	1	1	0[b]	1	1	1	2[b]	1	1	3	2	1	1	2	2	1	1	2	2[c]	1	0	Kessous *et al.*, 1980
4[d]	3 chrs.			2 chrs.		7 chrs.							4 chrs.			3 chrs.			2 chrs.		3 chrs.		1	1	Prieto *et al.*, 1978

Notes: a. Chromosome 7 involved in an apparently minor translocation. b. The C6 pair is absent, but a segment of C6 origin might have been translocated to the deleted end of a C11 chromosome. c. One of the G22 chromosomes is the Ph′ chromosome. d. The chromosomes in this line were not identified by banding analysis.

both the marrow and blood of healthy humans (Sandberg *et al.*, 1967; Golloway and Buckton, 1978). Not unusual findings are loss of the Y chromosome in males and of an X chromosome in females, a metacentric or an unusually long or short Y chromosome morphology, and a variety of ploidy changes in bladder and other epithelial tissues undergoing normal development or normal healing or other types of regeneration (Geraedts *et al.*, 1975; Soudek and Laraya, 1976; Sandberg, 1980). As discussed above, in some of the chromosome anomaly syndromes (e.g. the Turner, the Klinefelter, the XYY, the triple X, and various mosaic syndromes), affected individuals sometimes appear quite normal with or without displaying unusual gonadal features (Sparagana *et al.*, 1980; Sulewski *et al.*, 1980).

Such intraspecific displays of variable chromosomal constitution are widespread in nature. For instance, there is the well-known phenomenon of 'alternation of generations' which is most evident in ferns, mosses, and other ancient organisms, but it also occurs in higher organisms, in the less obvious form of haploid gametes and diploid somatic cells. Also, changes in chromosome number, size, and organization can occur during normal life cycles, even in a single tissue such as the root-tip meristems of the lily *Puschkinia libanotica* (Das, 1980). Further, some species are natural mosaics. In *Planaria*, for instance, the somatic cells are triploid in both sexes, but the germ-line cells are diploid in the male and hexaploid in the female; and cells of more than one of these ploidy levels become actively involved during processes of regeneration from a blastema (Gregmigni *et al.*, 1980a, b). Functionally, all human females are mosaics, in the sense that inactivation of one or the other of the X chromosomes in every somatic cell is a random process.

7.4 Heritability

Despite their protean properties (e.g. morphologic and structural changes), human and other eukaryotic chromosomes display a not inconsiderable array of essentially constant features, suggesting that chromosomes are significantly heritable structures. These features include the recognizably species-specific numerology and certain morphological (shape, size, centromere positions, and banding pattern), biochemical (localizations of subunits, allowing gene-mapping), and behavioural (e.g. movements about the mitotic spindle) aspects of chromosomes.

These, however, are features of normal chromosomes. They do not seem to apply to aberrant chromosomes, whose aberrations seem to be exaggerations of the inherent instability of chromosomal arrangements whether within or between themselves or within the genome. This raises some doubt as to whether chromosomal aberrations of any description can be, in themselves, truly heritable. Thus, in familial studies, different types of chromosome aberration can occur in different members of the same family, suggesting that the heritable basis of the anomalies may be in peculiarities of the more stable heritable subunits than in the aberrations themselves. Among some recent examples are the chromosome mosaicism found in parents of children with trisomy 18 (Holmes-Siedle *et al.*, 1980). Also, Williamson *et al.* (1980) described occurrence of the pericentric inversion 46,XY,inv(13)(p11q22) in a father, the normal chromosomal complement in one of his daughters, the rec(13)dup q,inv(13)(p11q22) recombinant in another daughter and a son, and a similar recombinant in a first cousin. Analogously, Berg *et al.* (1980) found a reverse dicentric tandem translocation involving 2 chromosomes 21, i.e. 46,XX,−21,+dic(21;21)(pter→q223→pter)tan, in a daughter of a karyotypically normal father and a mother whose only detected karyotypic anomaly was an atypically long secondary constriction extending into both arms of chromosome 9.

Familial segregations of a variety of other chromosomal anomalies have been described. These anomalies include about 25 per cent of the unbalanced interchange trisomies which are associated with G21 or D21 Robertsonian translocations and which account for some 3 to 6 per cent of all Down's syndrome (DS) cases (Kikuchi *et al.*, 1969; Hamerton, 1971). However, the frequency of DS increases, but that of DS occurring in association with the inherited translocation decreases, with increasing maternal age (Albright and Hook, 1980). Also, development of the stigmata of DS has been variously observed to require trisomy of chromosome 21, at least of the long arm distal region of the chromosome (for references and a further confirmation, see Daniel, 1979). However, Sulewski *et al.* (1980) described a patient with trisomy 21 co-occurring with trisomy 8, but who displayed none of the usual clinical signs of DS. Also, this patient developed a teratoma at age 13 years and gonadoblastomas at age 18 years;

whereas DS is associated mainly with acute leukemia which, in turn, spares inordinately more DS patients than it afflicts (Miller, 1970; Rosner and Lee, 1972). In contrast, most other cases of double trisomies display the clinical features of at least one of the trisomies (Wilson *et al.*, 1974; Grosse and Schwanitz, 1977).

Reports of familial chromosome anomalies are numerous. However, they rarely provide much information or significant clues that may aid discernment of a genetic or chromosomal basis of the inheritance. Some recent examples (Table 7.3) include familial segregations of X chromosome anomalies spanning three generations (Priest *et al.*, 1975); an X ring chromosome spanning two generations (Dallapiccola *et al.*, 1980); and the translocations t(7;10)(q11;q22) and t(14;21)(14qter→cen→21qter) spanning three generations (Bass and Sparks, 1979), as well as others occurring in association with Turner's syndrome (Kondo *et al.*, 1979). Other familial chromosome anomalies which have been described include pericentric inversions involving the autosomes 1 (Taysi *et al.*, 1973), 13 (Hauksdottir *et al.*, 1972; Williamson *et al.*, 1980) and 19 (Jordan *et al.*, 1980); the above-discussed inverted tandem translocations described by Berg *et al.* (1980); partial trisomy 14 (Miller *et al.*, 1979); and trisomy 21 mosaicism (Parke *et al.*, 1980).

Table 7.3: Some Recent Examples of Chromosomal Anomalies Occurring in Families

Anomaly	Reference
Triploidy and D and G trisomy	Brennan and Carr, 1979
Trisomy 16q from material 15p; 16q translocation	Ridler and McKeown, 1979
Partial trisomy 7p	Berry *et al.*, 1979
Balanced t(1;2)(q32;q21)	Kondo *et al.*, 1979
Unbalanced G21 or D21 (Robertsonian) translocations	Albright and Hook, 1980
Partial X duplication	Bernstein *et al.*, 1980
X ring chromosome	Dallapiccola *et al.*, 1980b
Pericentric inversion 13	Williamson *et al.*, 1980

Some inkling of the nature of the genetic involvement in inherited chromosome anomalies has been provided by associated studies of gonadal differentiation. Historically, in

1902, McClung described a possible sex-determining 'accessory chromosome' in insects. Since then, the mammalian equivalent, the Y chromosome, has become widely implicated in the control of differentiation of the primordial gonad which, in the absence of the Y chromosome, appears to become an ovary (reviewed by Wachtel and Ohno, 1979). It now seems that this control is at the level of the H-Y gene locus. However, the expression of the H-Y genes is itself under control of other genes not necessarily located on the Y chromosome. Thus, Bernstein *et al.* (1980) found a partial X chromosome duplication, i.e. dup(X)(p21→pter), to occur in a family in association with the H-Y negative Y chromosome in phenotypic females with the male karyotype. The anomalous segregation of the Xg^a allele in these women suggested to the authors that meiotic crossing-over had occurred or that the Xg locus was involved in some non-random inactivation of the abnormal X chromosome.

The basis of inheritance of chromosome anomalies is clearly complex. The complexity illustrated above is increased by the well-established observations of phenotypic males possessing karyotypes that seem to lack any Y material, e.g. the 46,XX (de la Chapelle *et al.*, 1972) and, in at least one known case, the 47,XXX (Bigozzi *et al.*, 1980) karyotypes. In contrast, total absence of X chromosomes is not known in viable humans, suggesting that at least one X chromosome is vital to human existence. Presumably, only one X chromosome is ever necessary for cellular viability, since heterochromatinization (apparently inactivation in the form of Barr bodies) is the fate of any additional X chromosomes that may be present. However, the validity of this simple concept is marred by the fact that cells with just one X chromosome are characteristic of Turner's syndrome.

7.5 Anomalous Chromosomes in Cancer-predisposing Human Disorders

7.5.1 The Disorders

An increasing number of human disorders is being shown to be associated with chromosome anomalies, congenital and/or induced, and with enhanced susceptibility to neoplasia of, usually, more than one type in each disorder. Like xeroderma

Table 7.4: The Principal Chromosome-breakage Neoplasia-predisposing Syndromes, All Autosomal Recessive, and Their Major Associated Neoplasms, Anomalies, and Sensitivities (with Related Features)

Syndrome	Neoplasms	Anomalies				Sensitivities and related reactions
		CtB	CtE	HoE	SCE	
AT	Hodgkin's disease, ALL, CLL, RCS, lymphosarcoma, other lymphomas, and less often, gastric adenocarcinoma, ovarian dysgerminoma, cerebellar medulloblastoma, mixed glioma, and uterine, pyloric, colonic, and breast carcinomas	?+	?+	−	n	Ionizing radiation, cells defective in repair of X-ray-induced DNA damage; induction of SCE difficult
BS	Acute leukemia, lymphoma, and carcinoma of tongue	+	+	++	++	Ethyl (or methyl) methane sulfonate, which can increase SCE frequency in BS cells. Latter display slow rate of fork motion during DNA replication

FA	Acute leukemia, hepatoma, and esophageal (squamous cell) and skin carcinomas	++	++	–	n	Agents causing DNA cross-links, which are difficult to repair by FA cells; induction of SCE difficult
XP	Basal cell and squamous cell carcinomas, malignant melanoma, and, less often, ocular malignancies, ALL, carcinoma of tongue, and testicular sarcoma	–	–		n	UV radiation, which can increase SCE frequency in XP cells. Latter show variable defects in repair of UV-induced DNA damage (mainly pyrimidine dimers)

Abbreviations: AT, ataxia telangiectasia; BS, Bloom's syndrome; FA, Fanconi's anemia; XP, xeroderma pigmentosum; CtB, chromatid breakage; CtE, chromatic interchange; HoE, homologous exchanges; SCE, sister chromatid exchanges; ALL, acute (CLL, chronic) lymphocytic leukemia; RCS, reticulum cell sarcoma.

Source: Abstracted from tables by Schimke, 1978; Kidson, 1980; Sandberg, 1980.

pigmentosum (XP), these disorders may be significantly or entirely heritable; partly or vaguely heritable, like some rare cases of Down's syndrome (Sections 7.3.5.2 and 7.3.5.5); or, like most cases of Down's syndrome and perhaps all of Klinefelter's syndrome (Section 7.3.5.4), acquired congenitally, e.g. by non-disjunction during parental gametogenesis (Section 7.3.5.2).

The better known of the heritable conditions, with their associated neoplasms and major sensitivities to the anomalous inductions, are shown in Table 7.4. A notable feature of these conditions, their autosomal-recessive mode of inheritance, represents a departure from the dominant inheritance usually displayed by most of the neoplastic and preneoplastic disorders known to be inherited in mendelian fashion (Chapter Six).

There is also a growing list of mainly heritable disorders showing, in variable type and degree, chromosomal hyper-sensitivity to radiation and/or mutagenic chemicals, high predis-position to neoplasia, and immunodeficiencies (e.g. Wiscott-Aldrich syndrome) or premature ageing (e.g. Werner's syndrome). This list includes dyskeratosis congenita, incontinentia pigmenti, retinoblastoma, progeria, prokeratosis of Mibelli, Kostmanni agranulocytosis, the nevoid basal cell carcinoma, Rothmund's, Thomson's, Werner's, Chediak-Higashi, and Wiscott-Aldrich syndromes (Kidson, 1980; Sandberg, 1980), and possibly also Gardner's and Peutz-Jehger's syndromes (Sasaki, 1978). Down's syndrome represents a special example. Though rarely inherited, it has been associated with defects of humoral (Seger *et al.*, 1977) and cellular (Schlesinger *et al.*, 1976) im-munity, with chromosomal hypersensitivity to ionizing radiation (Holmberg, 1974) or chemical mutagens (Kaina *et al.*, 1977), with defective UV-induced DNA repair synthesis (Lambert *et al.*, 1976), and with increased risk of leukemia (Rosner and Lee, 1972).

7.5.2 The Associated Anomalies

The chromosomal anomalies or instabilities associated with these various disorders show no consistent pattern (Table 7.4). For instance, in XP, chromosomal aberrations are as rare a feature (German, 1972) as are sister chromatid exchanges (SCEs) (de Weerd-Kastelein *et al.*, 1977), despite the marked hypersensitivity of XP patients to UV radiation. Ataxia telangiectasia (AT) is associated with a normal model karyotype and, in some cases, with chromatid breaks (Hecht and McCaw, 1977) or translocations involving 14q (Jean *et al.*, 1979). The frequency of SCEs is usually high in Bloom's syndrome (BS) (Chaganti *et al.*, 1974), but it can be variable in different lymphocyte populations of even the same patient (German *et al.*, 1977). In Fanconi's anemia (FA), it is at or below normal levels (Hecht and McCaw, 1977); and at normal levels in both XP (above) and AT (Galloway and Evans, 1975). When cells from patients with these disorders are irradiated or treated with chemicals, SCE frequency can be increased in BS cells and in some strains of XP cells (Wolff *et al.*, 1977) but not in AT (Galloway, 1977) or FA (Latt *et al.*, 1975) cells. DS cells, which are radiation hypersensitive, show no significant increase in spontaneous SCE (Lezana *et al.*, 1977). Non-patterned SCEs, spontaneous or induced, are also seen in the leukemias with which most of the disorders are mainly associated (Chapter Eight), e.g. acute leukemias (Abe and Sandberg, 1980).

7.6 Summary and Outlook: The Question of Causality

Like the human body itself and, indeed, practically all others of the major temporary structures (e.g. cells, tissues, organs, and their arrangements) in biological Nature, chromosomes, in evolution and development, display much diversity upon a background of uniformity. All cells that are capable of division display chromosomes, operationally defined as metaphase structures, and certain chromosomal characteristics (e.g. size, shape, number and banding pattern) which are, broadly, uniform intraspecifically but diverse interspecifically. Among the primates, for instance, the characteristic chromosome number is 46 in humans and 48 in the great apes, with the former due to a fusion having occurred in the latter during human evolution. Between the two groups, certain banding patterns (e.g. in chromosome 1) have been retained for perhaps 35 million years, while others have diverged due mainly to pericentric inversions (Seuanez, 1979). Other characteristics are intraspecifically (e.g. interindividually) variable. These can be chromosomal (e.g. in the whole monosomies and trisomies); but they are predominantly subchromosomal, due mainly to the specificities of meiotic recombinations. The recombinational processes such as exchanges, translocations, and inversions may occur between rather than within the stable chromosomal subunits. They may involve the types of breakage and rejoining which are involved in other major cytogenetic processes, e.g. DNA repair essential for maintenance of the integrity of chromosomes and DNA structures, and splicing of immunoglobulin genes and primary RNA transcripts. The capacity to undergo breakages and reorganizations is thus intrinsic to chromosomes. Presumably, it is genetically determined, variably on the basis of the specific chromosomal subunit inheritances of species and individuals. Presumably also, this capacity determines the nature and extent of the chromosomal anomalies which are displayed, variably, by cells in their peculiar microenvironments.

It thus seems unlikely that the chromosome anomalies which occur in neoplastic cells or in the various chromosome-anomaly including neoplasia-predisposing syndromes, are, necessarily, themselves direct causes of the associated clinical manifestations, neoplastic or otherwise. DS, for instance, can occur in the presence of a trisomic chromosome 21 as well as of various translocations such as the inverted tandem translocation described by Berg *et al.* (1980); whereas a similar translocation (Hagemeijer and Smit, 1977), or even the 21 trisomy (Sulewski *et al.*, 1980), can occur in the absence of a characteristic DS phenotype. Analogously, the primary amenorrhea associated with Turner's syndrome is also found with the X;3 and other X;autosome translocations (Carpenter *et al.*, 1980). Also, most or all of the male sexual anomalies associated with Klinefelter's syndrome can occur in the presence of a variety of anomalous chromosomal constitutions including not only the usual XXY or the rare constitution 47,Xi(Xq)Y (Ponzio *et al.*, 1980) but also constitutions lacking the male-determining Y chromosome. Among the latter are the 46,XX (de la Chapelle *et al.*, 1964) and 47,XXX (Bigozzi *et al.*, 1980) constitutions mentioned above. Proffered explanations of this latter phenomenon have included selective loss of an initially present Y-chromosome-containing stem line (de la Chapelle, 1972); translocation, to another chromosome, of the male-determining genetic component of the chromosome (Madan, 1976); failed inactivation of male-determining genes presumed to be present on the X chromosome (Rios *et al.*, 1975); and mosaicism involving a not readily detected but extremely circumscribed Y cell line (Miro *et al.*, 1978).

Similar apparently haphazard associations are seen in relation to the associated neoplasms. Thus, not all individuals with the chromosome 13 deletion anomaly associated with heritable retinoblastoma develop the disease, neither do all patients with the disease possess the anomaly (Knudson and Strong, 1972). The same considerations apply to the chromosome 11 deletion anomaly and nephroblastoma (Wilm's tumour), a disease which is also associated with the triad of aniridia, genito-urinary abnormalities, and mental retardation (for detailed discussions, see Schimke, 1978; Kolata, 1980). They also apply to the mainly quadriradial formations seen in association with BS, to the chromosomal breaks and gaps with FA, to the chromosomal breaks and rearrangements with AT, and to the chromosomal rearrangements with XP (Sandberg, 1980).

In all of these four conditions (BS, FA, AT, and XP), the chromosomal picture may appear normal and/or anomalous. In addition to the examples of SCEs and other anomalies discussed above (Section 7.5.2), both normal and aberrant chromosomal constitutions have been described in XP (Reed *et al.*, 1969; German, 1973; German, 1974b). Also, of the about 250 known cases of AT, at least three have been subjected to bone-marrow cytogenetic analysis. One patient showed a normal karyotype (Hecht and Case, 1969), the second showed chromatid breaks in 33 per cent of the metaphases (Lisker and Cobo, 1970), and the third showed an unusually small G-group chromosome in 40 per cent of the metaphases (Lampert, 1969). In this third case, who also had leukemia at the time of analysis, it remains unclear whether the anomaly was associated with AT or was due to the leukemic process. Further, as in the other conditions, peripheral lymphocytes in AT lack sufficient metaphases; and, in culture they neither grow well nor respond well to mitogenic stimulation. This complicates attempts at cytogenetic analysis by the direct or indirect method. However, the peripheral lymphocytes of some 30 of the 250 known cases of AT have been analyzed indirectly. Of these, chromosome anomalies of one type or another were found in 9 patients, and various gaps, breaks, and rearrangements in 6, in frequencies ranging from 0 to 40 per cent (Sandberg, 1980). As in the other conditions, the anomalies are irregular, and unpatterned findings in AT.

Whether spontaneous or induced, or inherited or acquired, chromosome anomalies in the various neoplasia-predisposing disorders are hence heterogeneous. In different patients with the same disorder, or in different cell populations from the same patient, the anomalies may or may not be present; and, when they are present, they vary considerably in type and severity. This suggests that the essential basis of the anomalies, or of the disorders themselves, reflects the genetic (structural and functional) individuality of each patient. A not uncommon notion is that the basis of either feature is genetic mutational. Xeroderma pigmentosum, for example, is the arch example of a defined inherited defect (in DNA repair capacity) that is believed to encourage persistence of further genetic mutations and thus to enhance cancer susceptibility and development (cf. Knudson, 1980). Yet, in different XP patients, the disease may or may not develop. When it does, it affects mainly skin cells, and, even then, very few of these, rather than other body cells. This is despite the fact that the genetic defect, due to its inherited and hence pre-zygotic nature, is present in all the nucleated somatic cells of the affected individual. Since the molecular basis of development is differential expression of a constant genome, this basis of the intracellular differences in the individual is phenotypic and differentiational. That is, it is basically functional and, as such, it is the same for every individual, whether or not the latter is an XP patient. Both the capacity for DNA repair and the variability of this capacity are as evident among XP patients as they are among normal individuals. The difference thus appears quantitative rather than qualitative. Accordingly, skin cancer occurs among both XP patients and other (including normal) individuals; and neither its variability nor its identity shows any qualitative specificity in either group.

Overall, therefore, susceptibility to cancer of the skin, as of other body sites, is variable among patients with cancer-predisposing conditions, and among the different phenotypes of the single patient. This variability is not fundamentally different from that which is evident in the normal human population on an individual, familial, or related (e.g. ethnic) basis. Neither is it fundamentally different among those cancer patients whose neoplastic cells themselves display chromosome anomalies, as the next chapter documents.

8 CHROMOSOMES AND CANCER: HUMAN ASPECTS

8.1 Introduction

Chromosome anomalies constitute one of the more commonly observed of the morphologic features of clinical neoplasms. Overall, they represent all known and some remarkably bizarre types, and display a generalized aneuploidy that tends to increase with tumour progression. This has several implications. First, by back extrapolation of the tendency, the anomalies are rare or nonexistent during the earliest stages of oncogenesis; second, malignant progression is partly through increasing genomic instability; and third, aneuploidy can aid in clinical staging of some malignancies. All too rarely, certain specific anomalies occur in a largely nonrandom manner, and they are then also diagnostic and, sometimes, prognostic aids.

In general, as discussed in the preceding chapter, occurrence of the anomalies in neoplastic cells can be influenced by various intrinsic and extrinsic factors, and their actual observation by various methodological inadequacies. In addition, there are certain confounding variables which are peculiar to cytogenetic analysis of neoplasms. These variables, operating singly or in various combinations, would theoretically and/or practically confound attempts at accuracy in detection of the anomalies and in definition of their role, if any, in oncogenesis in particular. These variables include the heterogeneity of, and progressive structural and functional changes in, the genotypic and phenotypic components of the neoplasms; the long (latency) period which precedes appearances of the clinical neoplasms, the usual sources of the analytical specimens, during which cytogenetic anomalies may or may not develop, change, and be selected as perhaps secondary aids in malignant progression; the cytogenetic effects of therapy of the clinical neoplasms with chemicals and/or radiation; and certain methodologically induced (or inducible) karyotypic variations.

The first and the last of these variables, together with the random and nonrandom anomalies, the latter represented in particular by the Philadelphia chromosome, constitute the subject matter of this chapter.

8.2 Confounding Variables

8.2.1 Naturally Occurring Cellular Heterogeneity

Despite the fact that the origin of many established human neoplasms appears to be monoclonal, they rarely display cellular homogeneity, karyotypic or otherwise. Usually, even the single neoplasm is a complex mixture, e.g. of stromal elements, of normal cells inclusive of tissue-specific cells and of the infiltrating macrophages and lymphocytes upon which tumour growth and survival may well depend, and of a variety of dead, dying, and viable neoplastic cells. The neoplastic cells may themselves be heterogeneous, e.g. in karyotype, in hormonal and other physiological dependence, in resistance or susceptibility to therapeutic agents, and in growth and metastatic potential (Eccles and Alexander, 1974; Underwood, 1974; Wood and Gollahon, 1977; see also Chapter Nine, Sections 9.6.4 and 9.10.2). For instance, acute lymphocytic leukemia (ALL) can show immunological features of T-cells, B-cells, null (non-B, non-T) cells, and cells displaying the common-ALL antigen with or without behaving like T-ALL cells (Chessels *et al.*, 1977; Roberts *et al.*, 1978; Foon *et al.*, 1981). In the widely used French-American-British (FAB) system, ALL is subclassified cytochemically and morphologically into the relatively homogeneous L^1 subgroup found generally in childhood ALL, the more heterogeneous L^2 subgroup in adult ALL, and the B-derived L^3 subgroup in Burkitt's lymphoma (Gialnik *et al.*, 1977). Such protean features of single types of malignancy are also exemplified by metastatic properties, e.g. by the capacity of bronchogenic carcinoma to metastasize from lung to leg, via the arterial or venous circulation, not only as single cells or microemboli but also as macroscopic emboli large enough to cause frank ischemia at the point of lodgement (Starr *et al.*, 1981).

The cell-type heterogeneity of single neoplasms may itself give rise to selection *in vivo*, e.g. in metastatic, clonogenic, and related features. Metastases, once established, have been reported to grow more rapidly than their primaries (Spratt *et al.*, 1977), perhaps reflecting selections of the metastatically more proficient cell populations from the kinetically heterogeneous primary neoplasms. In human acute leukemias, for instance, which comprise a majority of kinetically quiescent cells and a minority of actively proliferating cells (Clarkson, 1969), only the latter cells, constituting the 'growth fraction', show significant growth in soft agar (Preisler, 1980). The growth fraction is controlled by the extremely complex immunological, feedback, and related homeostatic mechanisms of the host organism, and it can undergo significant alterations only when these mechanisms fail sufficiently due to essentially intrinsic factors that may be subject to various extrinsic influences. For example, in human infectious mononucleosis, it is increased in the circulating lymphocytes which have been infected with the Epstein-Barr virus (EBV) (Robinson *et al.*, 1980). However, the increase is significantly more prominent *in vitro* than *in vivo* (Klein *et al.*, 1976; Katsuki *et al.*, 1979), probably because of the stricter operation and greater extent of the homeostatic mechanisms in the latter than the former situation.

The great complexity of these mechanisms is indicated partly by the large variety of cellular and humoral factors already known to exert control over cellular growth (and differentiation). These include factors with various types of colony stimulating activity (CSA) (Metcalf *et al.*, 1974; Burke *et al.*, 1977; Koeffler and Golde, 1978), and others that can variously stimulate growth of selected cell populations. Among the natural body mitogens are unfractionated serum (Sivak, 1977); plasma, platelet-derived growth factor, fibroblast growth factor, a factor with multiplication-stimulating activity, and epidermal growth factor or EGF (Frantz *et al.*, 1979); fibroblast-derived growth factor, and insulin; retinoids (Dicker and Rozengurt, 1979); and anti-tubulin agents and the neurohypophyseal hormone vasopressin (Dicker and Rozengurt, 1980). (See also Downward *et al.*, 1984; Sanes, 1984.)

Further, the activities of this complex array of natural body factors can themselves be influenced by exogenous agents, but apparently only in ways which are dependent upon the intrinsic mechanisms. In various experimental systems such as the mouse skin and 3T3 cell systems, for instance, 12-0-tetradecanoyl-phorbol-13-acetate (TPA) and other phorbol ester 'promoters' in tumorigenesis have been shown to exert variable and even opposite effects which seem to depend upon the intrinsic properties of the target cell populations. In mouse systems, TPA enhances cellular transformation by two oncodnaviruses, an adenovirus (Fisher *et al.*, 1978) and EBV, but it stimulates synthesis of the murine mammary tumour virus (Arya, 1980). It also reversibly inhibits differentiation in Friend mouse erythroleukemia cells (Rovera *et al.*, 1977) and mouse myeloid leukemia M1 cells (Kasukabe *et al.*, 1979); but it induces differentiation in other mouse erythroleukemia cells (Miao *et al.*, 1978) and mouse myeloid leukemia cells (Lotem and Sachs, 1979). In human promyelocytic, myelocytic, and myelomonocytic leukemia cells, TPA-induced differentiation seems irreversible, in contrast with the reversibility in the mouse systems, and it occurs in the absence of DNA synthesis (Rovera *et al.*, 1980). (See also Chapter Nine, Section 9.10).

The mechanisms involved in these various growth and differentiational effects of the experimental tumour promoters are poorly understood. However, they seem to operate, presumably primarily at cell surfaces, through both the hormonal and non-hormonal homeostatic mechanisms that are intrinsic to the host organisms. Thus, in the 3T3 cell system, TPA acts synergistically with almost all known mitogens to stimulate DNA synthesis, but not with vasopressin to stimulate the synthesis of DNA, the uptake of 2-deoxyglucose, or the activity of ornithine decarboxylase (Dicker and Rozengurt, 1980). Its mechanism of action thus seems to converge with that of vasopressin and perhaps other hormones but not with the mechanism(s), perhaps based upon non-selective influences on cellular sensitivity to growth factors (Weinstein *et al.*, 1977), utilized by the other mitogens.

The growth fraction is only one of the many variables of which a particular property of neoplasms, their doubling time, is a result. Among these variables are the composition and fate of the stromal and cellular elements of the neoplasm; and the size, the rate of growth, division, retention, and loss (e.g. by death or desquamation), and the degree of compaction of its cellular components. Differences in doubling time hence provide a useful, if somewhat crude, measure of the heterogeneity of different neoplasms of the same histogenesis. The histologic type-specific doubling times vary considerably, e.g. those of different human breast carcinomas have been reported to range, in days, from 23 to 209 in one large series and from 23 to 1,869 in another (Fournier *et al.*, 1980).

The heterogeneity is also evident in other ways. Thus, in several instances of tumour cell types successfully examined by banding, e.g. in both lymphocytic (Oshimura *et al.*, 1977a, b; Cimino *et al.*, 1979; Whang-Peng and Knutsen, 1980) and nonlymphocytic (Killmann, 1968; Abe and Sandberg, 1980) leukemias, the initially observed tumour karyotypes can disappear at remission only to be replaced at relapse with different karyotypes. Relapse can also be associated with alterations reflective of new epigenetic adaptations, i.e. in patterns of gene control. For instance, this has been noted for antigenic phenotype, e.g. relative to the leukemia-associated cell surface glycoprotein antigen, gp100 which is shared by blast cells from the common (or 'non-T, non-B') subtype of acute lymphoblastic leukemia and from a variety of Ph'-positive and Ph'-negative leukemias (Greaves *et al.*, 1980a, b).

In experimental studies also, such phenotypic diversity has been widely observed. It has been observed in rodent hepatocellular carcinomas, for instance, through studies of parameters such as chromosomes (Becker *et al.*, 1971; Wolman *et al.*, 1973), biochemical and histochemical properties (Morris, 1975; Pitot, 1978; Pugh and Goldfarb, 1978; Ogawa *et al.*, 1980), biological behaviour (Morris, 1975), antigenicity (Baldwin, 1973; Becker *et al.*, 1973), and cell composition and structure at light and electron microscope levels (Farber *et al.*, 1979). Ogawa *et al.* (1980) have shown that such phenotypic diversity can be selectively established as an early property of putative preneoplastic cell populations. Other considerations suggest that the diversity might then persist throughout all stages of tumour development, leading eventually to component phenotypes with different invasive and metastatic properties that, in turn, may depend upon karyotypic and biosynthetic differences. Thus, in the murine B16 melanoma system, different cell lines of variable karyotypes exhibit a 10-fold difference in metastatic proficiency (Fidler and Kripke, 1977). This difference has been correlated with the capacity of the lines to synthesize proteases capable of degrading type IV collagen (Liotta *et al.*, 1980). The latter is a major structural protein of the basement membranes which delimit both *in situ* carcinomas and blood vessels (Kefalides, 1973), and which must be ruptured to facilitate local invasion and metastatic spread by the more proficient of the tumour phenotypes (Roos and Dingemans, 1979). It seems unlikely, however, that the tumour-elaborated proteases differ qualitatively from the normal counterparts present in, for example, normally, turning-over basement membranes (Liotta *et al.*, 1979) or healing vasculature.

Such a diversity of tumour-cell types, including their changing patterns with tumour evolution and their individual features representing overlaps or nonqualitative aberrations of normal features, has a further confounding consequence. This is that the inadequacies of tumour classification, which is an evolving discipline based largely upon growth of understanding of normal phenotypic characteristics and is still an inexact science, are making somewhat uncertain the ascription of an anomaly observed in a given metaphase to a particular class of neoplasm. This is clearly evident in the hematologic neoplasms, which are currently the major objects of cytogenetic analysis. One example is chronic myelogenous leukemia (CML) in which, as is discussed later (Section 8.4), both myeloid and lymphoid differentiation can occur, particularly during transition from the chronic to the refractory ('acute') phase of the disease (cf. Martin *et al.*, 1980). Analogously, acute lymphoblastic leukemia (ALL) during its terminal blast crisis, can show both lymphoid and myeloid differentiation (cf. Rowley, 1980). Such relatively unrestricted behaviour of specific neoplasms makes some of their conventional class distinctions rather arbitrary. An example is the usual distinction between 'lymphoma' and 'leukemia', i.e. on the basis, respectively, of growth as a discrete mass and involvement of the bone marrow (the intravascular compartment); and between, in consequence, 'lymphoma therapy' and 'leukemia therapy'. Thus, lymphoblasts in acute B-cell leukemia can sometimes resemble Burkitt's lymphoma (BL) cells (Catovsky and Galton, 1977; Gralnick *et al.*, 1977), suggesting that the former disease is a rare manifestation of the latter. Further, the two cytogenetic anomalies (a 14q+ and an 8/14 translocation) which are thought to be characteristic of African BL have also been found in some cases of 'American' or non-African BL as well as of undifferentiated non-BL and acute B-cell leukemia (Berger *et al.*, 1979; Mitelman *et al.*, 1979; Douglass *et al.*, 1980). Analogously, aneuploidy and the Epstein-Barr virus (EBV), which are characteristics of African BL, occur also in some cases of non-African BL; and aneuploidy in some 50 per cent of ALL. Indeed, no known parameter, whether based upon karyotype, morphology, bone-marrow involvement, a cell surface marker (e.g. an immunoglobulin or SI_g, an F_c receptor, a complement receptor, or E-rosette formation), an enzyme (e.g. the p23,30 Ia-like antigen, a phosphatase, or a terminal deoxynucleotidyl transferase), or a particular therapeutic response, is capable of differentiating accurately between the lymphomas and leukemias. In a recent review of this topic, Magrath and Ziegler (1980) showed that the human lymphomas share one or more of the various features usually thought to distinguish one type of lymphoma from another (Table 8.1).

Conceptually, the phenomenon of cell-type heterogeneity of even single primary neoplasms is not surprising. It might be expected to be especially marked in the case of neoplasms derived from tissues such as bone marrow and gonads which contain stem cells, i.e. partly differentiated cells possessing the dual capacity to replenish themselves and to undergo alternative modes of differentiation (cf. Section 8.5).

8.2.2 *Methodologically Induced Karyotypic Variations*

The confounding factors are not restricted to those which, as exemplified above, are applicable mainly to the natural situation *in vivo*. They include others which stem largely from the fact that most human neoplasms lack enough metaphase cells to make cytogenetic analysis by the 'direct' method feasible. Consequently, the 'indirect' method must be employed, i.e. the neoplastic cells must first be artificially grown *in vivo* or *in vitro*, with use of various devices, in order to accumulate sufficient metaphases (Chapter Seven, Section 7.3.4). Contrary to the expectation from experiences with animal neoplasms, most of these cultured cells neither grow well nor respond well to mitogenic stimulation. Although culturing has been achieved in numerous instances, with varying success, this has been predominantly for certain types of leukemias and lymphomas and rarely for epithelial cancers, the latter being by far the commoner malignancies in man. According to one estimate (Mitelman, 1980), for example, the myeloproliferative disorders alone account for about 65 per cent of all the human neoplasms which have thus far been analyzed by banding with some degree of success, and only about 50 epithelial cancers have been so analyzed.

In most instances, as discussed earlier (Chapter Seven, Section 7.3.4.2.2), the resort has been to the indirect method. For tumour cells, this method has involved, since the early 1970s, one of the various guises (cf. Lowenberg *et al.*, 1980) of the basic soft agar colony technique introduced by Pike and Robinson in 1970, i.e.

Table 8.1: Various Non-Hodgkin Lymphomas Showing Significant Morphological Similarities

Lymphoma types	Other names	Features
1. African BL	Undifferentiated[a] or lymphoblastic[b,c] lymphoma; Burkitt type; Burkitt lymposarcoma;[e] endemic BL	EBV DNA often present, SIg positive; jaw involved often, bone marrow rarely; uniform cell size
2. Non-African BL	As above [a,b,c,e], but excluding endemic BL and including non-endemic BL	EBV DNA rarely present; SIg positive; jaw involved rarely, bone marrow and gut often; uniform cell size
3. Diffuse, undifferentiated non-Burkitt type lymphoma	? Stem cell lymphoma; unclassified[b] or non-Burkitt type[c] of lymphoblastic lymphoma	Similar to, but differentiated from 2 by subjective criteria such as 'less' uniformity of cell size and 'more' cells with single nucleolus
4. Small, non-cleaved follicle-centre-cell lymphoma[d]	Apparently encompasses 2 and 3	
5. Lymphocytic, poorly differentiated (lymphoblastic) lymphoma[b,c]	Apparently encompasses 2, 3, and 6	
6. Lymphoblastic convoluted or non-convoluted lymphoma[a,b,c,e]	Convoluted T-lymphocytic,[d] convoluted cell mediastinal,[c] or lymphoblastic (acid phosphatase type)[b] lymphoma; lymphoblastic lymphosarcoma; Sternberg sarcoma	Lacks SIg; forms E and often EAC rosettes; similar to ALL in cytology
7. Large, non-cleaved follicle-centre-cell lymphoma[d]	Histiocytic,[a] centroblastic,[b] or follicle-cell (predominantly large)[c] lymphoma; ? prolymphocytic (centrofollicular) lymphosarcoma[e]	SIg positive; a diagnostic problem when presenting as a diffuse lymphoma. May be nodular, or may evolve from a nodular lymphoma of different (small-cell) morphology

8. Immunoblastic lymphoma[b,d]	Diffuse histiocytic[a] or undifferentiated (pleiomorphic)[a] lymphoma; ? immunoblastic lymphosarcoma[e]	Both positive and negative SIg types; negative type may or may not form E rosettes. Morphologically overlaps other (e.g. types 3 and 7) lymphomas
9. Undifferentiated large cell lymphoma[c]	Apparently encompasses types 7 and 8	
10. Diffuse histiocytic lymphoma[a]	Encompasses types 7, 8 and 9	Rarely of histiocytic origin. Includes many pathological entities

Source: Based upon the classification schemes of: a, Rappaport; b, Kiel; c, National Lymphoma Investigation of the UK; d, Lukes and Collins; and e, World Health Organization. Modified from Magrath and Ziegler (1980).

semisolid media impregnated with a feeder layer of normal cells. However, whether by this technique or another (e.g. growth in nude mice, hamster cheek pouch or eye chamber, chick chorioallantoic membrane, or as ascites in rodent peritoneal cavity), the tumour-cell metaphases which have been subjected to banding analysis would have represented highly selected cell populations. Further, the latter, in keeping with the propensity of progressing tumours, might have undergone selected karyotypic adaptations. Hence, even in the reported instances of tumour-cell lines maintaining their karyotypic identity inclusive of marker chromosomes over long periods of subculturing, there can be little certainty that the karyotype is truly representative of the respective parent neoplasms *in vivo*. At least some of the anomalies representing *de novo* adaptations to growth in the artificial surroundings may be behind the surface changes which have been observed in cultured neoplastic cells, e.g. changes in contact inhibition, in sialic acid content and sialyltransferase activity, and in an interesting glycoprotein that seems to be expressed in association with cell proliferation (Bramwell and Harris, 1979; Omary *et al.*, 1980).

Clearly, the significance to neoplasia of whatever cytogenetic anomalies happen to be detected in neoplastic cells must be evaluated against this considerable background of potential complications and uncertainty. The major components of this background pertain to the nature, distribution, and timing of the anomalies, i.e. whether they are truly representative of the neoplasms or only of their selected cells or cell lines in which they occur, and whether they arose before or after neoplastic transformation in the host organism, or only as selected adaptations to the conditions of artificial culture.

8.3 Random and Nonrandom Anomalies, and Their Significance

8.3.1 Nonrandom Anomalies

Despite these theoretical and practical difficulties, certain developments since 1959 have revived interest in the old concept, stemming from the days of von Hansemann and Boveri (Chapter 7, Section 7.2) of nonrandomness in the occurrence of chromosome anomalies in human and animal neoplasms. With the discoveries of the Down's syndrome trisomy in 1959, the anomaly now known as the Philadelphia chromosome (Ph') in 1960, and a variety of other nonrandom chromosomal anomalies in human neoplasia since the advent of banding, the resurgence of interest in the concept and of research activity aimed largely at its appraisal has reached an almost feverish crescendo. This is illustrated indirectly by the proliferation of the related review literature (some recent examples: German, 1974; Rowley, 1976, 1978a, 1980; Mitelman and Levan, 1976; Garson, 1980; Lawler, 1980; Mitelman, 1980; Sandberg, 1980, 1983; Whang-Peng and Knutsen, 1980; Rowley and Testa, 1982). Directly, it is also illustrated by the apparently nonrandom associations which have been found in both animal and human neoplasms.

In animals, the nonrandom associations are mainly with trisomy of one or more chromosomes, a finding which is not inconsistent with the already discussed phenomenon (Chapter 7, Section 7.3.5.5) of survival being apparently more consistent with gains than losses of chromosomes. Thus, trisomy of chromosome 15 has been found in spontaneous (Dofuku *et al.*, 1975), X-ray-induced (Chang *et al.*, 1977), radiation leukemia virus-induced (Wiener et al, 1978a), and arylhydrocarbon-induced (Wiener *et al.*, 1978b) mouse hematologic neoplasms of T-cell but not non-T-cell origin. In many rat neoplasms, chromosome 2 is often trisomic (Sugiyama *et al.*, 1978; Uenaka *et al.*, 1978).

In man, the nonrandom associations appear to be more varied than in animals, since they involve not only gains but also losses and translocations. The main associations are thus between chronic myelogenous leukemia (CML) and Ph' (Section 7.4), Burkitt's lymphoma (BL) and translocations involving the 14q+ marker chromosome (Mark, 1975); meningioma and partial or total deletions involving chromosome 22 (Mark *et al.*, 1972; Mark, 1973); retinoblastoma and interstitial deletions involving chromosome 13 (Francke, 1976; Yunis and Ramsey, 1978; Riccardi, 1978; Sparkes *et al.*, 1979); Wilm's tumour and partial deletions involving chromosome 11 (Riccardi *et al.*, 1978); renal cell carcinoma and translocations involving chromosomes 3 and 8 (Knudson, 1979); and certain 'preleukemias' or other conditions (e.g. polycythemia vera, refractory anemia without excess blasts, acute lymphoblastic leukemia, and lymphoma) and deletions involving the long arm of chromosome 20 (Reeves *et al.*, 1972; Lawler, 1980). However, at least some of the reported losses in human neoplastic cells may turn out to be no net loss. This phenomenon, which was first discovered for the Ph' chromosome (Chapter Six, Section 6.5.5; see also below, Section 8.4), has since been described for other cases, e.g. the 13qXp translocation recently found in retinoblastoma (Nichols *et al.*, 1980). Analogously, Wang *et al.* (1980) found the characteristic chromosomal lesions in testicular carcinoma to be partial trisomies involving chromosome 1. This is not to imply that net losses of genetic material cannot occur in viable neoplastic cells. In addition to the few nonrandom losses described above, chromosomal losses seen in such cells range from the types of small deletion that are sometimes associated with various birth defects (cf. Miller, 1980) to others of near haploidy (cf. Kessous *et al.*, 1980; also Table 7.2).

In general, the most significant of the nonrandom chromosomal anomalies seen in human neoplasms are translocations involving, apparently, no net quantitative change in genetic material. The most prominent of these are the 9/22, 8/14, and 8/21 translocations of, respectively, chronic myelocytic leukemia, Burkitt's lymphoma, and acute myeloblastic leukemia (cf. Sandberg, 1980; see also Hecht *et al.*, 1981).

8.3.2 Random Anomalies

Almost traditionally, the patterns of chromosome anomaly seen in human neoplasms have been viewed predominantly as random and epiphenomenal. Even today, in the era of chromosome banding, this view, but with few qualifications, remains basically unaltered (cf. Koller, 1947, 1960, 1972; Sandberg, 1980); although some workers feel that the patterns are predominantly or even 'strictly' nonrandom (cf. Mitelman, 1980).

It is hence important to consider at least five basic principles that are of direct relevance to this controversial state of affairs. *First*, the progenitors of all neoplasms are most probably normal cells with normal karyotypes. *Second*, such karyotypes most likely also characterize most if not all cells which have been newly transformed. *Third*, the anomalies which have been observed are almost exclusively in frank and hence highly advanced neoplasms, and, in support of the first two principles, practically never in any *de novo* neoplastically transformed progenitor cell. Together, these three principles suggest that the observed anomalies themselves are unlikely to be the cause of the initial transformation. The presence of an anomaly, such as in a cervical cell or a so-called 'preleukemic' or 'premalignant' cell, is usually indicative of a cell that is already cancerous or otherwise diseased.

This suggestion is further substantiated by the *fourth* principle, i.e. that many frank neoplasms, some highly malignant, contain no known chromosome anomaly. At present, because even the most sophisticated of banding techniques detect only gross chromosomal changes that may each involve many genetic components, it remains always possible that the apparently karyotypically normal neoplasms may contain micro anomalies which are undetectable by current methodology. Even further, as in the case of the usually diploid-looking endometrial carcinomas (Atkin, 1976) recently found to have subtle chromosomal alterations in some cases (Trent and Davis, 1979), such micro anomalies might be revealable by current available methodology. By this same token, however, such methodology has consistently failed to reveal chromosome anomalies in significant proportions of practically all types of human neoplasm which have been successfully analyzed by modern banding. These karyotypically normal-looking neoplasms include about 50 per cent of all non-lymphocytic leukemias (Garson, 1980); about 65 per cent of all 'pre-leukemias' (Pierre, 1974); over 50 per cent of all lymphocytic leukemias, whether the acute disease (ALL) which predominates in childhood or the chronic, predominantly adult disease (CLL) (Whang-Peng and Knutsen, 1980); and others. In the remaining cases, the anomalies which do occur tend to be varied in type, diffuse, and increasingly complex with advancing disease states. This is exemplified in Table 8.2 for the 'preleukemias' and acute lymphocytic leukemia.

As discussed earlier (Chapter 7, Section 7.3.4.2.4), banding analysis is difficult to perform in most cases. In CLL, it is hampered by the low mitotic activity of the neoplastic cells and by their poor response to antigenic or mitogenic stimulation; while in ALL, an additional difficulty is the ill-defined, blurred appearance of even the relatively more abundant mitotically active neoplastic cells. However, in one of the more successful of CLL banding attempts, Crossen (1975) found normal-looking karyotypes in 97 per cent (97 of 100) of the analyzed metaphases; and even the anomalous-looking karyotypes in the remaining 3 per cent, all from the same patient, appeared to have been induced by the chemotherapy of the patient.

Thus, although chromosome anomalies are certainly widespread

Table 8.2:   Some Karyotypes Found in Banding Studies of Preleukemias and Acute Lymphocytic Leukemia

Disorder	Predominant karyotypes in different patients
Pre-leukemias[a]	
Smouldering leukemia	+1; −5; −6; −7; +8; +8,multiples; +11,mar; −18; +18; −21; −A, Cq−
Refractory anemia and/or cytopenia	+1q; −6; −7; +8; +9; 17iq; 20q −−13; −C; +C; −D,mar; Dq+; −E; Ga−
Sideroblastic anemia	1q+; +8; +mar; −21; 20q−; 21q−; −B; Bq−; −C; Cq−; −D; polyploidy
Acute lymphocytic leukemia[b,c,d]	27,XX, −1to9, −11to17, −19, −20, −22,plus exact double of the 27 line: 43,XX,t(13;15),t(13;17), t(14q11;14q34),18q+,+3 small mar; 45,XX, −21/52, unknown;45,X, −X; 45,XY, −8; 45,XY,1q+, −6; 45,xy, −14/45,XY, −17/44,XY, −17, −21; 45,X, −X,dup(1)|(q31q41),del(5) (q22),del(17)|p11);45,XX, −9, −12,+t(9q;12q); 46,XX,t(4p+;4p−),t(11p+;14q−); 46,XY, 1q+(dup)(1)|q12q25); 46,XY,13q+,21q−; 46,XX,21q−; 46,XXp+,del(1)|q21),del(6)|q21), i(17q); 46,XY,t(4;11)|q21;q23); 46,XY,+2,6p+,+7, −12, −13,14q+,17p+; 46,XY,del(6) (q23−25); 46,XX,qp−,t(12;17)|p13;q12); 46,XX,del(9)|p21); 46,XY, −10, −11,+18, +mar/46,XY,2q+,6q−, −11, −C,+18, +mar/48,XY,+18,+mar; 47,XX,+8; 47,XX,+12; 47,XX,+19; 47,XX,+21; 47,XX,1q+,+13; 47,XX,+21,i(17q); 47,XX,+16; 47,XY,4q−,+17q−; 47,X, −X,del(6)|p23),+17p+,+18p−; 47,XX,+8/57,XX,+3,+4,+8,11p+,+14,+16,+17,+18, +21,+22,Xp+,+M1,+M2; 47,XY,+X,t(2;2)(q22;p22); 47,XX,+M1/50,X, −X, −11,+M1,+M2, +M3,+M4,+M5,+M6; 48,XY,t(1;22)|q21;p11),+5,+8,19p+; 48,XX,+13,+19; 49,XY,+7, +12, −13,+9p+,+del(13),t(1;13)|q12;p13),t(6;18)|p25,q21),t(11;14)|q23;q32)/50 same as 49 plus +20; 53,XX,+2,+5,i(7q),+8,+13,+21,+21+22; 55,XX,+4,+5,+6,+10,+17,+21,+3mar; 55,XY,+X,+3,+6,+10,+13,+14,+16,+21,+21; 57,XY,+X,+5,+6,i(7q),+10,+12,+13,+15, +18,+21,+21,+22; 58,XX,+4,+6,+7,+10,+14,+14,+C,+21,+18q−,+3mar; 61,XX,+X,+1,+2,+4,+5,+6,+6,del(6)|q21),+13,+14,+15,+16,+18,+21,+21,+22

Source: Culled from: a.Sokal *et al.*, 1980; b. Whang-Peng and Knutsen, 1980; c. Sandberg, 1980; and d. Lawler, 1980.

at least in clinical and hence highly advanced human neoplasms, they appear to be far from universal in such neoplasms.

The *fifth* and final principle can be pictured as occurrence of specks of nonrandomness within clouds of randomness. This principle becomes especially prominent, and perhaps even indicative of a certain measure of chance, when it is evaluated against the generalized background of the anomalies, when they do occur, involving practically every chromosome and every known type of aberration. The aberrations can range from partial to total chromosomal involvement, and from hypodiploidy (down to near-haploidy), through pseudodiploidy, to gross hyperdiploidy. They can occur differently in different metaphases from the same neoplasm, or from different neoplasms of the same histogenesis; and they can vary in the same neoplasm with progression of the disease.

One example is provided by a recent study of 914 patients with various Ph'-negative hematologic malignancies (Van Den Berghe *et al.*, 1979). Of these patients, only 222 (24 per cent) possessed abnormal karyotypes in their bone marrow, peripheral blood, lymph nodes, or spleen, as judged by results from three types (Q, RT, and C) of banding analysis. Of the 222 patients, 164 had anomalies evincing no discernible pattern. The remaining 58 patients showed 4 nonrandom patterns: an extra C chromosome, a missing C chromosome commonly involving a 7q deletion, an 8q deletion sometimes with loss of a sex chromosome, and a 5q deletion.

Another example is provided by acute monocytic leukemia (AMoL), a disease that accounts for about 7 per cent of all acute leukemias. Recently, Berger *et al.* (1980) carried out banding studies of ten cases of AMoL, seven of which were poorly differentiated and three well differentiated. They found rearrangements involving the long arm of chromosome 11 in five of the former group, but variably from case to case, and in none of the latter. Other reported anomalies in AMoL include a translocation, t(8;9), with an 8p-marker in one case (Brynes *et al.*, 1976); a 2p deletion (Weber *et al.*, 1979); and a translocation, t(11;17)(Van den Berghe *et al.*, 1979).

None of these anomalies is confined to AMoL. The rearrangements involving chromosome 11, for instance, have been found in other disorders including AML, preleukemia, blastic phase of CML, ALL, CLL, and various lymphomas. In malignant lymphomas, the chromosome 11 anomalies have included deletions (whole or partial), partial trisomies, inversions, and inter- and intra-chromosomal translocations. The break-points involved have included q12, q13 or q22, and q23. In AML, the chromosome 11 anomalies have included the translocations t(5;11), t(11;12)(q25:q13), t(11:22)(q23; p11 or p12), t)11;13) (q23−ter,q12−14), and t(6:11)(q,q13−qter); and the deletions del(11q), 11q−, del(11)(q23), and −11. In Ph'-negative CML, the chromosome has been involved in anomalies such as t(q;11)(q34;q13), t(11;18)(q23;q12), and 11p−q+. (For references, see Berger *et al.*, 1980.)

As a statistical probability, the larger of the chromosomes may be the more prominent repositories of the anomalies. Accordingly, anomalies of practically all known types have been found to involve chromosome 1 in a variety of hematological and other (e.g. cervical, vaginal, bladder) neoplasms and non-neoplastic disorders. These anomalies have included partial or total monosomies and trisomies, isochromosomes, translocations, pericentric and other inversions, and heterochromatin variants such as those with C-band size-heteromorphism (Atkin and Baker, 1977a,b,c, 1978; Rowley, 1978a; Wang *et al.*, 1980). Some of the reported translocations are shown in Table 8.3. Among the disorders found to be associated with total or partial trisomies or other structural anomalies of the chromosome are various lymphomas (Manolov and Manolova, 1972; Mark, 1975, 1977); melanomas (Kakati *et al.*, 1977); practically all types of hematological neoplasms (Hayata *et al.*, 1975; Hsu *et al.*, 1977; Gahrton *et al.*, 1978; Rowley, 1978a); neoplasms of the ovary (Atkin and Pickthall, 1977), cervix (Atkin and Baker, 1977a, 1979), testis (Wang *et al.*, 1980), vagina (Atkin and Baker, 1978), bladder (Atkin and Baker, 1977c), lung (Pickthall, 1976; Kakati *et al.*, 1975, 1976), colon (Pickthall, 1976), brain (Brodeur *et al.*, 1977), and breast (Sandberg, 1980). Sandberg has also reviewed occurrences of the anomalies in other disorders including melanoma, neuroblastoma, rhabdomyosarcoma, Wilm's tumour, polycythemia vera, myelofibrosis, and mycosis fungoides. Conversely, a single type of neoplasm can, in a single patient or in different patients, be associated with various anomalies involving several chromosomes. Some examples are shown in Table 8.2 for ALL.

Table 8.3: A Partial List Of the Known Translocations Involving Chromosome 1 in Some Lympho- and Myelo-proliferative Disorders

Disorder	Translocations
AML	t((1;4)(q22–25;p14–16); t(1;8)(p22;q24); tan(1;13); t(1;6;11)(q12;q23;p15); t(1;22)(q11;p11 or 12); t(1:9) (q22 or 23;p24); t(1;13)(p36;q14); t(1;x)(p1–q2;Xq); t(1;13); t(1;3)
CML	t(1;9)(q11;p11–13); t(1;9); t(1q;17q); t(1;3); t(1q–;1q+); t(1;8); t(1;20); t(1;8)(q25;qter)
ANLL	rcp(1;3); t(1p–;?)(1qter–1p22::?); rcp(1;17); t(1;1) (1pter–1q42::1q21–1qter); t(1;14)(14qter–14pter:: 1pter–1p22); t(1;15)(15qter–15pter::1pter–1p22); t(1;?) (1qter–1p3::?); t(1;2) (2qter–2cen::1q2–1qter)
Lymphoma	t(1;10)(q22;qter); t(1q;11p)(also 1q– and 1p–); 1q/i(17q) (also 1p+);
Histiocytic	t(1;7)(7pter–7q32::1p22–1pter); t(1;21)(21pter–21q22:: 1q22–1qter); t(1;18)(1qter–1p36:: 18q21–18qter); t(1q;17q)
Myelofibrosis	t(1:6)(q25;q25); t(1p+;4q–;7q–); t(1q;9p); t(1q+;3p–); t(1q;2q)

Abbreviations: AML, acute lymphocytic leukemia; CML, chronic
          myelogenous leukemia; ANLL, acute nonlymphocytic
          leukemia.
Source: Adapted from Sandberg (1980).

Although some of the larger chromosomes (e.g. chromosomes 1, 3 and 6) are frequently involved in the anomalies, chromosomal size alone can hardly be the sole criterion for the frequency. For instance, even the smallest of the autosomes (chromosomes 21 and 22) appear to be more often involved than some of the larger, e.g. chromosomes 2, 4 and 12. None the less, this conclusion remains tentative, since the great majority of human neoplasms, the epithelial cancers, remain to be properly analyzed cytogenetically, e.g. by banding.

A marked degree of randomness is displayed even by the two leading non-random anomalies, i.e. the Ph' (discussed in Section 8.4) and the 14q+ chromosomes. The 14q+ chromosome is most frequently associated with African Burkitt's lymphoma (ABL), as was first reported by Manolov and Manolova (1972). Since then, this finding has been widely confirmed, and also extended, initially by Mark *et al.* (1977), to include the related (8;14) translocation. However, as indicated above (Section 8.2.1), this anomaly, i.e.

14q+ or t(8;14), has been found in some cases of a considerable collection of unrelated disorders, including American and non-endemic BL as well as other presumably B-cell neoplasms such as histiocytic, Hodgkin's, mixed-cell, and malignant lymphomas, multiple myeloma, plasma-cell leukemia, and B-cell acute lymphoblastic leukemia (for review, see Rowley, 1980). It has also been found in presumably T-cell disorders such as T-cell chronic lymphocytic leukemia (Finan *et al.*, 1978), mycosis fungoides (Fukuhara *et al.*, 1978; J. Whang-Peng, quoted in Douglass *et al.*, 1980), and the types of 'adult T-cell leukemia' which are peculiarly prevalent among the Japanese (Takasuki *et al.*, 1979). Finally, it has been found also in disorders such as retinoblastoma, gastric cancer, ataxia telangiectasia, reticulum-cell sarcoma of brain, various acute leukemias, Ph'-negative chronic myelogenous leukemia, follicular lymphoma in transition, and EBV-genome-negative lymph node without malignancy in a patient with nasopharyngeal cancer and probable lymphoma (Mitelman *et al.*, 1979). (For other references, see Sandberg, 1980.)

Despite these varied occurrrences, chromosome 14 appears to have donor (q12) and receptor (q31) sites which, respectively, are commonly affected by deletions and by translocations in the associated neoplastic disorders. In those malignancies in which 14q+ is most frequent (mainly Burkitt's lymphoma, lympho-sarcoma, Hodgkin's disease, and multiple myeloma), a t(8;14) is usual; but other chromosomes (mainly chromosomes 1, 4, 5, 10, 11 and 14) have also been described to be involved with chromosome 14 in translocation in lymphomas (Sandberg, 1980).

Banding analyses, because they are usually performed on clinical and hence advanced neoplasms, give little clue as to the role of chromosome anomalies in tumori genesis. As indicated above, Mitelman *et al.* (1979) found a t(8;14) anomaly in an EBV-genome-negative lymph node of an African patient with EBV-genome-positive nasopharyngeal carcinoma, and postulated this finding as tentative evidence for the presence of the anomaly prior to actual development of the malignancy. However, in a recent study of eighteen patients with NABL and of nine of their derived cell lines, Douglass *et al.* (1980) found a t(8;14) in only ten of the patients and in seven of the cell lines, and either a t(8;14) or a 14q+ in fifteen of the patients and/or the cell lines. Analogously to the earlier report of Philip *et al.* (1977), who found a 14q+ anomaly in only 20 per cent of the abnormal cells of a patient with

NABL, Douglass *et al.* failed to find a 14q+ or a t(8;14) in every malignant cell they examined, except in two of their patients. However, they also found two normal-appearing chromosomes 14. A t(8;14), when it did occur, was rarely the sole karyotypic abnormality. In fact, practically every chromosome, in their eighteen patients considered together, was involved in one type of numerical or structural aberration or another.

8.3.3 Significance

Against this dense background of randomness in nature, occurrence, non-occurrence, and evolution, it might need an eye of faith to visualize a 'strict' non-randomness of occurrence of chromosome anomalies in human neoplasia. It is only after this background has been conceptually erased that a degree of nonrandomness of occurrence of the anomalies in certain (mainly hematological) types of human neoplasm emerges (Table 8.4; see also Section 8.3.1). There is then more frequent involvement, in comparison with their counterparts, of certain chromosomes (i.e. chromosomes 1, 3, 5, 7, 8, 9, 14, 17, 20, 21 and 22), parts of chromosomes (e.g. 5q in refractory anemia, 14q in lymphomas and 22q in CML), and anomalies (e.g. the partial or total trisomies of the long arm, isochromosomes, and heterochromatin variants of chromosome 1 in solid neoplasms, the 9;22 translocation in CML, the 22 deletion in meningioma, and the 8 trisomy in AML).

However they are manipulated, the available data consistently show that neoplasia exemplifies, perhaps second only to gametogenesis, the great diversity of viable karyotypes which can be constructed from a normal complement of chromosomes, or more accurately, of chromosomal ('genetic') subunits. The breakpoints in normal recombinations may well coincide with those involved in the great majority of the aberrations seen in neoplasms; and they may well differ from one individually specific chromosome set to another. Thus, chromosome anomalies have been found to be similar in identical twins with acute leukemia but not in paternal twins with AML (Sandberg, 1980). In identical twins also, only the twin developing CML showed the Ph' anomaly (Lawler, 1977). This suggests that the anomaly, with its breakpoint occurring at any one of the many possible points on 22q (Verma and Dosik, 1980), is acquired only by the suitably predisposed and presumably already neoplastically transformed cells. This anomaly, though clearly acquired, is unlikely to be induced by

Table 8.4: Chromosomes and Their Anomalies Showing Preferential Involvements in Various Human Neoplasms[a]

Neoplasms	Anomalies	Chromosomes
Myeloproliferative:		
Acute myelogenous leukemia	t(8;21)	5,7,8,21
Chronic myelogenous leukemia	t(9;22), i(17q)[b]	8,9,17,22
Polycythemia vera	20q−	1,8,9,20
Others		1,5,7,8
Lymphoproliferative:		
Lymphomas	t(11;14)	1,3,9,14
Burkitt's lymphoma	14q+, t(8;14)	7,8,14
Acute lymphocytic leukemia	6q−, t(4;11)	1,21,22
Chronic lymphocytic leukemia		1,14,17
Monoclonal gammopathies		1,3,14
Solid:		
Meningiomas		8,22
Benign epithelial tumours		8,14
Carcinomas		1,3,5,7,8
Sarcomas		13,14
Neurogenic tumours		1,22
Malignant melanomas		1,9

Notes: a. Each involvement shown can differ between patients with the same disease, or between affected cell populations in a single patient; it can be present and/or absent with or without other anomalies; and it can occur in other diseases (for details, see text). b. Mainly in refractory phase of CML.

Source: Based on tables by Lawler (1977); Mitelman and Levan (1978); and Sandberg (1980).

some exogenous carcinogenic agents, since the anomaly can occur in children (e.g. in Ph'-positive childhood leukemias), and no such agent in man is known to cause this anomaly or, with rare exceptions (notably benzene), to cause any type of chromosome anomaly as part of its neoplastic effect. Neither can the anomaly be regarded as causative of the neoplastic transformation, because of the phenomenon of clinically indistinguishable Ph'-positive and Ph'-negative CMLs, and of the *de novo* appearance of Ph' in CML presenting initially as Ph'-negative (Section 8.4.3). Further, in the neoplasia-predisposing chromosome breakage syndromes such as FA and BS (Chapter Seven, Section 7.5), susceptibility to chromosome breakage has been demonstrated, through *in vitro* studies, in the relatives of affected subjects but not in the subjects (propositi) themselves (Lieber *et al.*, 1972).

Practically all of the known major biological features of neoplasia reflect essentially non-qualitative aberrations or exaggerations of physiological propensities. The diversity of viable neoplastic karyotypes appears as no exception to this generalization. Although they range from normal to grossly abnormal appearances, they may reflect the natural propensity of the normal chromosomal subunits to undergo selective, controlled recombinations together with, sometimes, other changes such as deletions and duplications. The cytogenetic basis of the etiology, development, diagnosis and other aspects of the neoplasms may well be within the structural subunits and their arrangements within chromosomes, neither of which needs be structurally abnormal, rather than within the chromosomal anomalies themselves.

Consideration of the nature of the chromosomal segments most commonly involved in the nonrandom anomalies in neoplastic cells has led to certain speculations regarding the functional characteristics of genes in the subunits. For instance, consideration of gene-mapping data pertinent to the segments of human chromosomes 1 and 17 in particular, which are commonly involved in hematological and other malignancies, has led Rowley (1978a) to suggest that genes regulating nucleic acid synthesis and metabolism may be preferentially involved in the anomalies (e.g. by translocation) or, analogously, may be activated or suppressed by viral and other exogenous carcinogens.

At present, however, such speculations would appear to be premature. This is suggested by factors such as the above-discussed apparently non-causal associations between the anomalies and neoplastic transformation, the great heterogeneity and magnitude of the anomalies involved, the fewness (about 100) of gene loci which have thus far been mapped on the entire human genome, and the macro-determinations to which the current banding methods are limited. Thus, just over 30 gene loci have been mapped on chromosomes 1 and 17 (cf. Chapter Seven, Section 7.3.1 and Table 7.1). Also, these methods are incapable of detecting anomalies involving even up to one-third of the average chromosome band with its approximately 5 million base pairs which, theoretically, could contain well over one thousand structural subunits, even when due allowance is made for leader, insertion, and other sequences. Even the mouse myeloma im- munoglobulin light chain subunits, for instance, which are re- markably segmented in their germ-line DNA with its leader, variable, joining and constant regions, and which undergo com- plex recombinations and translocations during B-cell maturation into immunoglobulin-producing plasma cells, contain just over 3,000 base pairs (Sakano *et al.*, 1979; Steinheitz and Zachau, 1980; Altenburger *et al.*, 1980).

Clearly, there is much to be learnt about these subunits. Next to nothing is known about their arrangements, controls, functions, and inter-relationships within the genome in general and, in par- ticular, within the chromosomes or chromosomal segments that are more commonly involved in the anomalies. Until this has been sufficiently achieved, the question of the significance of the anomalies to neoplasia will doubtlessly remain highly controversial and any associated pronouncement equally conjectural. For in- stance, a not uncommon pronouncement is that of some survival advantage having been conferred upon the viable and, almost certainly neoplastic cells by their persisting chromosomal anomalies. Indeed, in many histological systems, tumour aneuploidy is a rough correlate of malignancy directly and of prognosis in- versely. However, significant exceptions to these features are known, e.g. the above-discussed examples of malignant neoplasms lacking any detectable chromosome anomalies, the examples of carcinomas of the uterine corpus and of the colon showing re- versals of the usual ploidy-prognosis relationships (Atkin, 1976) and the example of the Ph' anomaly being associated with a better prognosis than its absence.

Conceptually, the essential basis of the genesis, nature, and persistence of chromosome anomalies within viable and prospering neoplastic cells may be identical to that of the normal chromosomal complements of organisms and species during evolution and development. This basis is selective editing, with neutral or beneficial consequences to growth, survival, and reproductive fitness, of ecogenetically produced, largely random changes in composition and arrangement (e.g. by recombinations, gains and losses) of fundamentally stable chromosomal subunits (Chapter Seven, Section 7.3.1) and, to lesser extents, in substructure (e.g. by base substitutions and deletions) of the subunits. Developmentally, the basis is largely phenotypic-microenvironmental and largely genotypic-macroenvironmental evolutionarily; but, as stressed in a recent masterly exposition of modern evolutionary theory (Futuyma, 1979), the evolutionary significance of relationships between genotype and phenotype remains in deep obscurity.

Persistence of a chromosome anomaly in a given cell may be indicative of a genome having a peculiar propensity to develop that anomaly within the cellular-microenvironmental milieu. The propensity itself may be due to some peculiarity of the genome, e.g. the latter's subunit composition and arrangement and its state of differentiation. Thus, not all patients with CML develop the Ph′ anomaly (Section 8.4.3); and the rate of sister chromatid exchanges (SCEs) has been reported to be significantly higher in the bone-marrow cells than in the more differentiated peripheral blood lymphocytes of normal individuals (Knuutila *et al.*, 1978; Becher *et al.*, 1979a). Also, there may be non-identity of propensities to develop different types of anomaly. For instance, Ph′-positive bone-marrow cells or lymphocytes from patients with CML, in comparison with those from normal individuals, have been reported to have similar (Knuutila *et al.*, 1978; Kakati *et al.*, 1978; Cheng *et al.*, 1979) as well as significantly lower (Becher *et al.*, 1979b) propensities to develop SCEs. Furthermore, the anomaly, whatever its type, may persist without making a positive contribution to the cellular well-being, providing only that it is not detrimental to the latter. It is hence not necessarily causative of the neoplastic state itself. Indeed, this state, when it is associated with genomic instability, might lead to further anomalies, as in the case of bone marrow cells of Ph′-positive CML that tend to develop a variety of other anomalies, both structural and numerical, during progression of the disease (Prigogina *et al*, 1978; Lilleyman *et al*, 1978). Finally, because of the variability and complexity of the genome-microenvironmental relationships, the chromosome anomalies seen in neoplastic cells need not be uniform in the different cell populations of either the same neoplasm or the different neoplasms of the same histogenesis (cf. Tables 8.2 and 8.3).

With appropriate modifications, the major principles of normal evolutionary and developmental biology·may well be extendable to the cytogenetic and, indeed, general biology of neoplasia.

8.4 The Philadelphia Chromosome (Ph'): A Unique Anomaly

8.4.1 Introduction

Several references have already been made to this, the most interesting of chromosome anomalies in human neoplasia, i.e. the anomaly now known as the Philadelphia (or Ph') chromosome which was so named in honour of its city of discovery. The anomaly was first described in 1960, by Nowell and Hungerford, when they observed an unusually small G-group chromosome in cultured cells from blood and bone marrow of patients with chronic myelogenous leukemia (CML). To date, Ph'-CML represents the closest known approximation of a specific association between any chromosome anomaly and any human neoplasm. However, even for this association, which may be of some use in diagnosis and prognosis of the disease, there is increasing evidence for serious flaws in the once assumed near perfect specificity.

8.4.2 Structural Aspects

Initially, much confusion surrounded the structural aspects of the Ph' anomaly, i.e. its biochemistry and the identity of the chromosome involved. The anomaly was regarded as a deletion of almost one-half of the long arm of a G-group chromosome (Nowell and Hungerford) or of the Y-chromosome (Baikie *et al.*, 1960), or as a translocation of part of the long arm of chromosome 21 (Tough *et al.*, 1961), i.e. the chromosome that is trisomic in Down's syndrome. Banding studies by Caspersson *et al.* (1970) and others soon established that the Ph' anomaly and the Down's syndrome trisomy involved different pairs of chromosomes, with the consequence that the former became conventionally ascribed to chromosome 22 and the latter to chromosome 21. In 1973,

Rowley established that the Ph' anomaly was not a deletion but a translocation, i.e. of the missing 22q segment to the distal end of the long arm of chromosome 9. In its major form, the anomaly now appears to be a balanced reciprocal 9;22 translocation involving no net loss of genetic material (Mayall *et al.*, 1977). Thus far, this has been found in about 92 per cent of the over 800 Ph'-positive patients with CML that have been examined by banding (for a review, see Rowley, 1980).

Other studies have revealed that the anomaly is not as invariant as the above would suggest. In fact, practically every chromosome, with the possible exceptions of chromosomes Y and 18 only, is known to be involved in a simple translocation, or in a more complex translocation with participation of three or more different chromosomes (reviews: Mitelman and Levan, 1978; Sandberg, 1980; Rowley, 1980). In some cases, more than one translocation may be simultaneously present, e.g. a Ph' translocation to 6q26 and a t(1;9)(q21;q34), and a Ph' translocation to 17p and a t(X;9;6)(q13;q34;q21); or chromosomes in addition to nos 9 and 22 may be involved in the complex translocations, including 1p and 4q, 1q, 2q, 3p, 6p, 7, 8q, 10q, 11q, 13q, 14q, 15q, 17, 19, or Xq. (For references, see Rowley, 1980.) In different Ph'-positive cases, all of chromosome 22 may be translocated e.g. to chromosome 17 (Engel *et al.*, 1974); complex translocations to the end of the Ph' chromosome may occur (Lawler *et al.*, 1976); there may be no evidence of a translocation (Mitelman, 1974), thus bringing the initial observations of deletions (above) full circle; or an impression of an absent translocation may be replaced, through more careful banding studies, with evidence for a translocation (Hossfeld and Köhler, 1979). Although the Y chromosome is not known to be involved in a Ph' translocation, it has recently been found in a complex Ph'-like translocation involving chromosomes Y, 3 and 9, i.e. a t(3;9;Y)(q25;q34;q12), in a Ph'-negative case of classic CML (Verhest and Lustman, 1980). Finally, the breakpoint on chromosome 22, previously thought to be invariant (Watt *et al.*, 1977; Mayall *et al.*, 1977), is now known to occur randomly on different bands and at almost any point in the long arm of the chromosome (Verma and Dosik, 1980). Based upon the breakpoints and the relative size of chromosome 22, Verma and Dosik arbitrarily proposed four major types (very large, large, medium, and small) of Ph' chromosome having their break-points at bands q13.3, q13.1, q12, and q11.3, respectively.

Various anomalies other than the translocations are found in some 30 per cent of patients with CML (some reviews: Mitelman and Levan, 1978; Rowley, 1980; Sandberg, 1980). These, which assume particular prominence during the refractory phase of CML, include extra chromosomes, mainly nos 8, 9, 10, 17, 19 and 22q−, the extra 22q− occurring by duplication apparently without translocation; isochromosomes, mainly i(22q−) and i(17q); deletions, mainly of the Y chromosome but apparently not of the X chromosome; and translocations, e.g. t(1;20) and t(13;14). Changes in ploidy also occur, mainly hyperdiploidy represented by modal chromosome numbers from 47 to over 53, but sometimes also hypodiploidy down to near-haploidy (Kessous *et al.*, 1980), a state which has also been found in childhood ALL (Oshimura *et al.*, 1977b; Prieto *et al.*, 1978) in which hyperdiploidy is also common (Cimino *et al.*, 1979).

In summary, the Ph′ chromosome is structurally heterogeneous in several ways. It is heterogeneous relative to: the size of the translocated elements, which ranges from the entirety of chromosome 22 to variable segments of its long arm; the identity of the recipient chromosome (which is usually no. 9 but can be almost any of the other chromosomes inclusive of chromosome 22), or of the part of this chromosome which is involved in the translocations; and the type of the anomaly, e.g. a translocation, a deletion, a duplication, or an isochromosome. In addition, the Ph′ anomaly is associated with a variety of karyotypic changes occurring during progression of CML towards fatality. Finally, in view of the natural recombinant propensities of human and other eukaryotic chromosomes (Chapter Seven, Section 7.3.2), the Ph′ translocations, in one instance or another, might be expected to be balanced or unbalanced, and to occur with or without inversion.

8.4.3 Clinical Aspects

8.4.3.1 Association With Various Disorders. Clinically, the occurrence of the Ph′ chromosome in any of its forms is neither restricted to nor universal in cases of CML. On the one hand, about 15 per cent of all CML (Rowley, 1980) and over 96 per cent of childhood CML (Smith and Johnson, 1974) are Ph′-negative. Moreover, the Ph′-negative cases rarely display any chromosome anomaly, with some of the rare exceptions being loss of the Y chromosome, gain of a C-group chromosome, and the (6;14) translocation described by Mintz *et al.* (1979). On the other hand, the Ph' anomaly has been found repeatedly, but variably and usually in low frequency, in disorders other than CML (reviewed by Rowley, 1980). These include various acute non-lymphocytic leukemias (ANLL) such as acute myeloid leukemia (AML) and acute myelomonocytic leukemia (AMMoL) in which other anomalies such as the 8;21 translocation tend to be prominent (reviewed by Garson, 1980); as well as both chronic (CLL) and acute (ALL) lymphocytic leukemias (reviewed by Whang-Peng and Knutsen, 1980). Sandberg and Hossfeld (1970) and Hossfeld *et al.* (1971) reviewed pre-banding findings of the anomaly in AML, erythroleukemia, myeloid metaplasia with myelofibrosis, polycythemia, and thrombocytopenia. Banding studies have confirmed and extended these findings, so that polycythemia vera and a variety of other myeloproliferative disorders in addition to CML are now known to be both Ph'-positive and Ph'-negative (reviewed by Abe and Sandberg, 1979; Lawler, 1980). Occurrence of Ph'-like and/or Ph'-associated anomalies, particularly i(17q), has been reported in a variety of unrelated disorders including multiple myeloma (Van Den Berghe *et al.*, 1979), meningioma, eosinophilic leukemia (Ellman *et al.*, 1979) and erythroleukemia, malignant lymphoma, prostatic carcinoma, and mesothelioma (for detailed references, see Wurster-Hill *et al.*, 1979).

8.4.3.2 Association with Chronic Myelogenous Leukemia (CML): Individual and Tissue Variations, and Clonal Evolution. Certain karyotypes, particularly t(9;22), +8, 22q−, and i(17q), are consistently more frequent than others in patients with CML. Despite this, such karyotypes, when they do occur, are not necessarily uniform in the individual patients, in their affected tissues, or during evolution of the disease. For instance, of a total of 17 patients with CML subjected to simultaneous banding analysis of their spleen and marrow cells, 16 in the chronic phase showed only 46, Ph'+ cells. One patient in the blast phase showed only such cells in the marrow but 47,Ph'+,+8 cells in 31 per cent of the spleen cells. Yet others showed variable proportions of 46, Ph'+ cells in both bone marrow and spleen. One patient who showed 48,Ph'+,+17,+Ph' cells in spleen and 46,Ph'+ cells in marrow developed, five months later, cells with 48 chromosomes in both tissues. Another, initially with only 46, Ph'+ cells in both tissues, later showed a mixture of 46,Ph'+ and 49,Ph'+,+Ph',+8,+19 cells in marrow, and a mixture of 47,Ph'+,+Ph',48,Ph'+,+Ph',

+19, and 49 chromosome-containing cells in spleen (cf. Mitelman and Levan, 1976, 1978).

Such discrepancies in the aberrations seen in spleen and marrow suggest that both organs are sites of the clonal evolution. These sites may be quite complex, as is suggested by other data (e.g. Lawler, 1977) showing, for instance, the development of new anomalies long after splenectomy.

8.4.3.3 Role in Diagnosis and Prognosis. As discussed above, the Ph' chromosome and some of its associated anomalies occur with high frequency in patients with CML. For this reason, these anomalies are invaluable albeit, *per se*, insufficient diagnostic criteria in CML.

Particularly in its standard form, i.e. t(9;22), Ph' has some significance. Broadly, survival is better in CML cases presenting initially with than without the anomaly, and apparently even better still when some Ph'-negative cells are also present (Sakurai *et al.*, 1976). Significant reductions by aggressive chemotherapy of the proportion of Ph'-positive cells in CML patients presenting initially with 85–100 per cent of such cells have been associated with enhanced survival, but not with prevention of eventual development of the terminal refractory phase (RP) of CML (Cunningham *et al.*, 1979). Survival of Ph'-positive patients with CML has been reported to be uninfluenced by presentation with (Sonta and Sandberg, 1977) or development of (Sonta and Sandberg, 1978) the variant anomalies. In contrast, Prigogina *et al.* (1978) reported a correlation of such anomalous development during the RP with both the clinical course and the blast morphology of the RP.

This controversial state of affairs is only one example of the extremely complex and variable relationships which exist between CML, its RP, its genesis and differentiation, and its general response to therapy. This question is considered below after a brief discussion of the relevant background.

8.4.3.4 Survival, Blast Morphology and Ph': A Highly Complex Situation in CML. Survival in CML has not improved significantly since treatment of the disease by irradiation was first introduced about 60 years ago, or by busulfan and other chemicals some 25 years later (cf. Stryckmans, 1974; Canellos, 1979). This unfortunate state of affairs stems partly from the fact that the chronic disease, which belies its name by having a median survival of just about three years, usually terminates in the afore-mentioned refractory phase. The latter, which may be distinct from acute myeloid leukemia (Hayes *et al.*, 1974), is as poorly understood as is suggested by the plethora of strange-sounding names it has attracted. These include, among other names, 'blastic phase', 'blast crisis', 'acute transformation', and 'metamorphosis'. Regardless of the name, the phase is characterized by both myeloid and lymphoid differentiation, and by a degree of accelerated aggressiveness that is probably unmatched among the leukemias. In over 80 per cent of the affected patients, death ensues within three months (Canellos, 1979).

Various characteristics of the RP contribute to the great difficulties associated with clinical management of CML. The RP can precede, follow, or occur simultaneously with presentation of the disease. Its symptoms, which are many and are variable in occurrence and severity, include malaise, fever, night sweats, cachexia, and organomegaly indicative of extramedullary hemopoiesis. Hematologically, bone-marrow appearances are as variable as are those of the peripheral blood, and blast cells can range from less than 30 per cent to over 90 per cent. Cell variants may be myelomonocytic, monocytic, erythroblastic, megakaryoblastic, and/or lympoblastic. Unusual variants may be basophilic, hyperhistaminic, and indicative of systemic mast cell disease; or they may represent manifestations of subacute or chronic disease.

Cytogenetically, the blast cells can be positive or negative with respect to Ph' and/or its associated anomalies. In the Ph'-negative cases, other cytogenetic anomalies may or may not be present. Among 20 Ph'-negative adult cases of CML diagnosed from 230 consecutive CML admissions, for instance, Canellos *et al.* found aneuploidy in 7 cases. Of these 7 cases, 2 had hypodiploidy (44 chromosomes), one case in 100 per cent and the other in only 10 per cent of the examined metaphases. Of the remaining 5 cases, one case had pseudodiploidy (46 chromosomes, of which one or more showed some anomaly), and the remainder had hyperdiploidy (an extra C chromosome) but in 1, 2, 4, and 67 per cent of the metaphases. Many analogous examples, as well as others showing mixed karyotypes present initially and/or developing dependently or independently of therapy, are known (for reviews, see Canellos, 1979; Sandberg, 1980; Rowley, 1980).

It thus seems hardly surprising that the therapeutic response in

CML is highly complicated. Modern treatment protocols have relied heavily upon chemotherapy. In the RP, some welcome but rather unimpressive results have been achieved among responding patients by use of certain drug combinations. The latter include the so-called VP or 'ALL-type' therapy, i.e. a combination of vincristine and prednisolone (Hayes *et al.*, 1975; Canellos, 1979). They also include daunorubicin in various combinations with hydroxyurea, 6-mercaptopurine, and corticosteroids; and, more recently, just the latter combinations without daunorubicin (Coleman *et al.*, 1980). Coleman *et al.* reported an overall median survival of twelve weeks, with a median survival of thirty weeks among responders compared with seven weeks among non-responders. They also found no additional benefit from concomitant use of vincristine in induction and daunorubicin for consolidation.

Returning to the controversy mentioned above (Section 8.4.3.3), there are several reports of the Ph'-positive RP responding better to ALL-type therapy in cases with lymphoid blasts than with myeloid blasts (Marmont and Damasio, 1973; Beard *et al.*, 1976; Peterson *et al.*, 1976; Rosenthal *et al.*, 1977; Janossy *et al.*, 1979). However, the differential response is far from clear-cut. Rosenthal *et al.*, for example, found a favourable response to VP therapy in 9 of 18 patients with lymphoid blasts but also in 6 of 34 with myeloid blasts; and analogously, Janossy *et al.* gave corresponding figures of 14 of 15 and 4 of 25, respectively. In addition, other workers found no correlation between blast morphology and VP response, whether in adult or childhood cases of CML (Misset *et al.*, 1977; Marks *et al.*, 1978; Chessels *et al.*, 1979).

Even in responding patients, the clinical course is highly variable. For example, remission in eight of the patients investigated by Janossy *et al.* showed reappearance of the chronic phase. In four of the patients, there was elimination of the Ph'-positive cells with hypoplasia, followed by normal (Ph'-negative) marrow regeneration in two; but relapse, when it occurred, was of either the lymphoid or myeloid type. In addition, CML patients in the RP run a high risk of developing meningeal leukemias (Atkinson *et al.*, 1975; Schwartz *et al.*, 1975; Woodruff *et al.*, 1977). They also face a high risk of developing bone-marrow aplasia, which may be idiopathic or induced by chemotherapy with, for example, VP. In fact, aplastic anemia is one of the most feared complications of therapy with a variety of modern drugs including chloramphenicol, salvarsan, sulfonamides, and anti-inflammatory, anti-rheumatic, anti-epileptic, and anti-diabetic agents (Benestad, 1979). First described by Ehrlich in 1888 as fatty atrophy of the red marrow with cytopenia in the blood, and first so named by Chauffard in 1904, aplastic anemia itself presents a risk of leukemia. Fortunately, this risk appears to be not very high, and to be lower when the anemia is drug-induced than when, as in Fanconi's disease, it is constitutional (Milner and Geary, 1979).

As discussed above, appearance of a second Ph' is one of the Ph'-associated chromosome anomalies in CML. This appearance is usually associated with or heralds the RP. Incidence of the second Ph' in the RP is over 50 per cent but is low in Ph'-positive AML; and this has different survival implications in the two diseases. Thus, Abe and Sandberg (1979) described six cases of AML with the double Ph' anomaly among whom survival varied from under five months to about one year. Also, Hossfeld *et al.* (1971) described a case of erythroleukemia with this anomaly who survived for over two years.

In children, CML is rare, its incidence being less than 3 per cent of all their leukemias; and Ph'-positive CML is an extreme rarity (Smith and Johnson, 1974; see also Section 8.4.3.1). Yet, childhood CML shows all the complexities of the adult counterpart (Chessels *et al.*, 1979; Priest *et al.*, 1980). The Ph'-negative cases show high resistance to therapy while maintaining clinical complications such as skin rash, thrombocytopenia, high fetal hemoglobin, and poor resistance to intercurrent infections. The Ph'-positive cases, as their adult counterparts, can develop sometimes from acute leukemias and can display highly complex therapeutic and other features. Thus, Chessels *et al.* (1979) investigated a series of eight cases of Ph'-positive childhood leukemias diagnosed from 123 consecutive hospital admissions with leukemia. Four of the eight cases presented as acute leukemia; while two of the remaining four cases presenting as typical CML later developed blast crisis. In this total of 6 'acute' cases, the leukemic blasts were lymphoid in three cases, myeloid in one case, and mixed (lymphoid and myeloid) in two cases. Remission was achieved in five of the six acute cases, but it lasted more than one year in only two. In one of these two cases, the blasts at the time of crisis were Ph'-negative. In the other, who presented in myeloid crisis, remission terminated in a lymphoid crisis. Unusual translocations were detected in only two of the eight children.

Thus, on present information, it seems impossible to deduce any consistency in the cytogenetic pattern(s) or in the clinical implications of the pattern(s) in relation to CML. The Ph' anomaly may or may not be present in CML; it may be present in malignancies other than CML; and, when present, it may be associated with variable cytogenetic evolution, hematology, clinical symptomatology, prognosis, and therapeutic response. Perhaps the summation of the situation is exemplified by a recent report of two patients with Ph'-positive AML (Abe and Sandberg, 1979). One patient presented as Ph'-positive, with Ph' being the only detected chromosome anomaly, and the other as karyotypically diploid. In the former, the Ph'-positive clone became *completely* replaced by a newly developed Ph'-negative clone bearing a 21q addition, and the patient died three months later. In the latter, a Ph'-positive clone developed among the karyotypically normal cells, and the patient died one month later.

8.5 Morphological, Biochemical, and Other Features Relative to the Pluripotent Stem Cell

For mainly technical reasons (Chapter Seven, Section 7.3.4; and Section 8.2.2), the cytogenetic and correlated (e.g. biochemical marker) studies of human neoplasms are, up to now, confined largely to the various leukemias, less so to the lymphomas, and least of all to the epithelial cancers. Although this represents a rather unfortunate circumstance in view of the great predominance of the epithelial neoplasms, the studies are beginning to shed some light on the cytogenetic aspects of the development, if not genesis, and the clinical manifestations and behaviour of at least the hematologic neoplasms. These aspects are increasingly being shown to be dependent upon specific differentiational patterns and their aberrations occurring within cell populations containing variable reserve capacities for further differentiation towards final determination. Certain extra-conventional cytogenetic methods, particularly flow cytometry following quantitative DNA fluorochromation (Dosik *et al.*, 1980; Latreille *et al.*, 1980), are also being developed. These are capable of assessing DNA content and ploidy of not only the metaphase cells to which conventional chromosomal analysis is restricted but also the inter-phase cells which can represent up to 90 per cent or more of any given cell population. Although results from use of such methods lack the precise definition of banding studies, they already indicate that aneuploidy may be even commoner in multiple myeloma and other solid malignancies than in either the leukemias or any type of benign neoplasm.

However, a major drawback of these cytogenetic studies, whether conventional or extra-conventional, is that they are measuring gross changes in content or stucture of the DNA of cells which, additionally, are usually from highly advanced neoplasms. It thus seems hardly surprising that the nonrandomness of such changes which is being discovered is superimposed upon an almost overwhelming randomness, and is almost directly proportional to the movement of the measurements towards earlier stages of tumour development and finer structures of DNA. Extrapolation of this trend would predict the ultimate basis of the observed nonrandom chromosomal changes to be genetic rather than chromosomal (cf. Chapter Six, Section 6.5), and that of the ob-served differential prognosis, e.g. in the various leukemias, to be in pluripotent stem-cell differentiation, inclusive of arrested or alternative differentiation involving, perhaps, the blasts at acute stages of the clinical disease. In ALL, for instance, prognosis has been correlated with factors such as blast morphology (Bennett *et al.*, 1976; Keleiti *et al.*, 1978; Van Wering and Vissers-Praalder, 1979) together with the patient's age and WBC count (Vecchi *et al.*, 1980); HLA haplotype (Rogentine *et al.*, 1973; Lawler *et al.*, 1974; Dausset, 1977; Tursz *et al.*, 1978; De Bruyère *et al.*, 1980); and the T-lymphocytic or non-T-lymphocytic character of the dis-ease, with the latter, in comparison with the former, showing a better prognosis and a better response to 'ALL-type' (e.g. VP) therapy (Tsukimoto *et al.*, 1976; Chessels *et al.*, 1977; Sallan *et al.*, 1980; see also Section 8.4.3.4). This last situation may identify that subset of CML patients in lymphoid blast crisis who also share these prognostic and response features, and distinguish them from those CML subsets, perhaps in myeloid or T-lymphoid crisis, who do not.

The Ph' anomaly is a unique example of the above-mentioned proportionality. When it occurs in CML, Ph' can involve all the myeloid cells (e.g. neutrophils, erythroblasts, megakaryocytes, and monocytes) at early stages of the disease such as when the blood leukocyte count is less than 10,000 in prospective studies of individuals at high risk of developing the disease (Kamada and Uchino, 1978). In contrast, as discussed above, with eventual progression of the disease to its refractory phase, factors such as blast morphology and Ph'-associated and other chromosomal changes can become extremely complex and unpatterned.

Despite their undoubted representation of a forward step, none of these features is, by itself, a sufficient diagnostic or prognostic criterion. For instance, as discussed above for the Ph' chromosome itself (Section 8.4.3.1) or blast morphology (Section 8.4.3.4) and diagnosis or prognosis in CML, a persisting and still universal problem is the phenomenon of considerable overlap and non-specificity, i.e. of occurrence of practically any of the features, to variable extents, in some but not all cases of its associated disease, and in other diseases or even in nonpathological conditions. This has led to a state of much confusion, exemplified by the increasing tendency to regard every newly discovered subtype of a neoplastic disease as a separate disease entity. Thus, the conventional acute or chronic forms of lymphoid or myeloid leukemias are increasingly being subclassified on the basis of criteria such as whether an associated cytogenetic anomaly such as Ph' is present or absent, whether the predominant cell-type is B, T, or null, or whether there is or is not a favourable response to a given type of therapy. There is thus no good reason why these same criteria may not be extended also for further diversification of the sub-classification, i.e. on the basis of not only whether or not the features occur but also the extent of their occurrence.

Another related criterion for the subclassification is whether or not a particular biochemical or immunochemical marker is present. Many such markers have been investigated including acid phosphatase, nonspecific esterase, myeloperoxidase, and lysozyme. These are early markers, with the first two occurring earlier than the others (O'Brien *et al.*, 1980), of the cytoplasmic granules whose appearance is one of the first differentiational features of granulocyte and monocyte precursors. Also, acid phosphatase is high in many acute and chronic lymphoproliferative disorders; and α-naphthyl acetate esterase is characteristic of T-lymphocytes and is high in cord blood T-lymphocytes that are apparently masked by sialic acid in their surface receptor structures (Foa *et al.*, 1980). This esterase and β-glucuronidase are high in both T-lymphocytes and T-lymphoid disorders (Basso *et al.*, 1980).

Broadly, certain markers are capable of distinguishing between the three major cell-types of the lymphoreticular system, which is the source of all lymphomas and leukemias. Thus most B cells display surface immunoglobulins (SIg), Ia-like antigens, and receptors for complement and the Fc fragment of IgG. Receptors for Fc of IgG and/or IgM and for sheep erythrocytes, terminal deoxynucleotidyl transferase (TdT) and alloantigens detectable with various T cell specific antisera are found in or on most T cells. The third major cell-type, i.e. null (non-B, non-T) cells, is detectable by specific antisera (Greaves *et al.*, 1975; Roberts *et al.*, 1978). A subset of these null cells bears complement receptors and can be detected by appropriate B cell antisera (Kirov *et al.*, 1980).

Use of such markers to subclassify the leukemias and lymphomas is showing the classes (and even subclasses) to be remarkably heterogeneous. Thus, most non-Hodgkin lymphomas are demonstrable as B-lymphocytic, T-lymphocytic, and/or mononuclear-phagocytic (Cossman and Berard, 1980), and acute leukemias as null ALL, thymic ALL, B cell ALL, and/or AML (Janossy *et al.*, 1980). As recently reviewed by Cossman and Berard (1980), the B-lymphocytic malignancies include chronic lymphocytic leukemia (most cases), 'hairy cell' leukemia (most cases), Waldenstrom's macroglobulinemia, heavy chain diseases, and various lymphomas including well-differentiated lymphocytic, nodular (follicular) and Burkitt's lymphomas. Among the T-lymphocytic malignancies are acute and chronic lymphocytic leukemias (some cases), Sezary's syndrome, and lymphoblastic lymphoma. The so-called 'histiocytic' or large-cell lymphomas are B-lymphocytic (about 60 per cent of cases), T-lymphocytic (5–15 per cent), and histiocytic (about 5 per cent). Further subclassification depends upon other criteria. The T-lymphoblastic lymphomas, for example, have been further subclassified according to their reactivity with a T-cell subset specific (or TH_2) heteroantiserum (Nadler *et al.*, 1980), reflecting the heterogeneity of the normal T-cell population itself.

The nature of the efficacy of these markers is well illustrated by recent findings including those in a multiparametric analysis, using some of the more efficient markers, of 300 cases of various Ph'-negative leukemias (Janossy *et al.*, 1980). The markers included TdT, and immunochemically determined null cell-type ALL-associated antigens, B cell-associated Ia-like antigens, and T lymphocyte-thymocyte antigens termed HuTLA. Tdt, a marker of certain types of immature lymphocyte, is elevated in the neoplastic cells of most patients with acute lymphoblastic leukemia of T or null cell-type. However, it is also elevated in most cases of lymphoblastic lymphoma (Kung *et al.*, 1978), in some cases of acute myeloblastic leukemia (Gordon *et al.*, 1978) and in the refractory but not chronic phase of CML (Marks *et al.*, 1978). Janossy *et al.* found high TdT levels in most cases of adult null cell-type leukemias but not of the childhood counterparts in which the ALL-associated antigens were prominent. In contrast, some of the TdT-positive blasts from both the children and adults were ALL-negative. Blasts in thymic ALL expressed the ALL-associated antigens weakly, TdT and HuTLA strongly, and the Ia-like antigens negatively. The combination of markers was least useful for classification of undifferentiated leukemia.

Perhaps the conceptually most rewarding upshot of these developments is that all human neoplasms of the lymphoreticular system may, fundamentally, represent stage and/or phase related disorders of a single cell-type. This is the apparently pluripotential hematopoietic stem-cell equivalent of the CFU-s described by many workers in mice (Till and McCulloch, 1961; Dexter *et al.*, 1978; Williams *et al.*, 1978; Sharkis *et al.*, 1980) which is capable of self-renewal and of repopulating the myelocytic, monocytic, erythrocytic, platelet, lymphocytic, and other compartments. Basophilia with hyperhistaminemia has recently been associated with CML (Denburg *et al.*, 1980). Various 'stem' cells capable of restricted ranges of hemopoiesis, but often with no or limited self-renewal capacity have been described in cultures of human bone marrow (Martin *et al.*, 1980; Spitzer *et al.*, 1980). Results from a related study (Moore *et al.*, 1980) suggest that the human CFU-s equivalent can replicate for some weeks in culture, and can generate committed precursors such as CFU-c and BFU-e of the myeloid and erythroid compartments, respectively. This pluripotent stem cell seems to lack the Ia-like antigen which, however, is rapidly gained as commitment to the various progenitor cell-types occurs, and is subsequently lost as the latter undergo differentiation within the marrow.

Presumably, the various morphological, biochemical, immunochemical, and/or clinical features of the neoplasm which is being examined are dependent largely upon the stage of differentiation of the CFU-s at which transformation initially occurs. An analogous suggestion, made by Janossy *et al.* (1976,

1980), is that the morphological features of Ph'-positive leukemia will reflect the cell stage at which Ph' induction occurred. A less differentiated cell stage will produce a disease resembling acute undifferentiated, lymphoblastic, or myeloblastic leukemia; but typical chronic phase CML will result from a more differentiated cell stage at Ph' induction.

It may well be that the current distinctions between the leukemias and lymphomas are no more exact than those between the various subclasses of these disorders. Thus, studies of glucose-6-phosphate dehydrogenase mosaicism in cases of Ph'-positive and Ph'-negative CML have shown the two types of disorder to be similar relative to their stem cell and possibly clonal origins but to develop differences only during later, e.g. blast transformation, stages (cf. Fialkow *et al.*, 1980). Blasts in either CML or ALL can be Ph'-positive or Ph'-negative (Section 8.4.3.4); and, in childhood ALL, the Ph'-positive disease tends to present at a later median age (about nine years) than the overall disease (Priest *et al.*, 1980). In general, the two distinctions may have their fundamental basis in the specific (e.g. individual and/or species related) DNA ultrastructures, and in the extragenomic factors such as lactoferrin (Broxmeyer *et al.*, 1980), heme (Hoffman and Ross, 1980), erythropoietin, thymopoietin, and other hormonal and nonhormonal agents (cf. Lacombe *et al.*, 1980) which control CFU-s and their stage-and-phase-specific differentiation. Erythropoiesis alone, for instance, involved at least three major stages: commitment of the stem cell to the erythroid pathway, development of immature 'burst-forming' and 'colony-forming' erythroid precursors to proerythroblasts, and end-stage development involving hemoglobinization and nuclear inactivation (in birds) or elimination (in mammals).

On this basis may be superimposed certain other factors. The latter would include factors responsible for myelofibrosis and aberrant differentiation. Myelofibrosis, including its idiopathic type, occurs quite widely in hematological and other disorders associated with urinary hydroxyproline hyperexcretion (Wang *et al.*, 1980) but the bone-marrow fibroblast involved in appropriate instances appears to be a radiation-resistant mesenchymal cell that is unrelated to hematopoietic stem cells (Golde *et al.*, 1980). Aberrant differentiation may result from superimposition of novel differentiational modes, with gain or loss of one or more of the normal differentiational features of the phenotype or cell stage that becomes frozen (Metcalf and Moore, 1971; Salmon and Seligmann, 1974; Greaves and Janossy, 1978; Sachs, 1978) during the initial neoplastic transformation. Aberrant differentiation, which is presumably behind the widespread neoplastic feature of ectopic synthesis, may be reflected in the capacity of some myeloid leukemias (Srivastava *et al.*, 1976; Catovsky *et al.*, 1979; Janossy *et al.*, 1980), but not normal non-leukemic myeloblasts (Janossy *et al.*, 1979), to express TdT.

Certain recent trends are suggesting that proper understanding of hemopoiesis and its control may pay high dividends in hematological as well as general neoplasia. These are documenting (cf. Donati and Poggi, 1980) a fundamental influence of various components of the hemostatic system, such as endothelial cells, platelets, vascularization, coagulation, and fibrinolysis, in practically all of the basic steps leading to the establishment, growth, and dissemination of neoplasms. These steps include local growth, invasion, and penetration; detachment of neoplastic cells (or emboli) from the primary neoplasm; and subsequent transport of these cells in blood or lymph, their re-entry in extravascular spaces, and their lodgement in metastatic sites.

8.6 Summary and Outlook

Eukaryotic chromosomes are particularly prone to undergo re-combinations and other structural changes such as those occurring at meiosis as a naturally evolved means for establishment of the genetic individuality of germ cells and heterozygotes (Chapter Seven). Although this is almost certainly under strict genetic control, certain features of the currently poorly understood control mechanism(s) can sometimes fail, as indicated by the chromosome anomalies which are not uncommon in spontaneous abortuses (Polani *et al.*, 1979; Chapter Seven, Section 7.3.5.1). It is hence not inconceivable that some of these failures occurring in certain cells may lead to specific chromosome anomalies capable of causing transformation of those cells.

Chromosome anomalies of practically every description have been investigated in cancer cells for almost a century and, in recent decades, by increasingly advanced techniques applied, in particular, to the metaphase cells of clinical neoplasms (Chapter Seven, Section 7.3.4). The major outcome of these investigations is that the anomalies are widespread in such cells but that their occurrences are largely random. Even in those instances marked by a degree of nonrandomness, the occurrences are usually against a background of greater randomness (Section 8.3). The two most important of such instances are the Ph' chromosome that predominates in chronic myelogenous leukemia and the t(8;14) translocation in B-cell neoplasms. The Ph' anomaly is hardly specific since its translocated segment, which is itself structurally variable (Verma and Dosik, 1980), can be found in practically any of the normal chromosomes and in any of the at least 108 different translocations with which the anomaly is involved (Section 8.4.2; also Yunis *et al.*, 1981). In comparison with Ph', the t(8;14) anomaly is structurally less heterogeneous, but it too occurs in only some of the type-specific neoplasms with which it is associated (Section 8.3.2). For instance, t(8;14) has been found in 87 per cent of endemic Burkitt lymphomas and in about 47 per cent of the non-endemic disease; and it also occurs in some cases of other diseases including acute and chronic lymphocytic leukemias, and malignant lymphomas (Mitelman, 1981).

Since the anomalies, when they occur, are seen in some but not other tumour cells of even the same tumour, they may simply reflect the cellular heterogeneity of the tumour(s) (Section 8.2.1) and the high fragility of the tumour cell's chromosomes. In variable extents, this fragility may represent exaggerations of the natural instability of normal chromosomes. The latter are known to contain at least 17 highly fragile sites (LeBeau and Rowley, 1984). In any event, the tumour-associated anomalies have been detected almost exclusively in clinical neoplasms, i.e. at late stages of tumour development; and both the extent and variety of the anomalies tend to increase with tumour progression through stages of increasing malignancy (Section 8.3.3). Hence, any given anomaly may have been absent at an early stage, particularly at tumour initiation. In such a circumstance, the anomaly would have been irrelevant to the molecular mechanism(s) of transformation. This conclusion is amply supported by a variety of major oncologic features such as the capacity of some tumour cells to regress to normal phenotypes (Chapter Nine, Section 9.10.3), and of certain tumour cell genomes to direct normal development (Chapter Nine, Section 9.10.2). Another supporting feature is the absence of any known chromosome anomaly in even some highly advanced clinical neoplasms, such as some 50 per cent of all acute lymphocytic and non-lymphocytic leukemias (Yunis *et al.*, 1981).

The mechanistic significance, if any, of chromosome anomalies in human neoplasia is thus unclear. At best, certain selected anomalies may play some role in one or more of the late stages of development of some tumours. Even this seems a weak possibility, since many tumours develop to fatality in the absence of chromosome anomalies.

Available data on chromosome anomalies in human neoplasia thus give little or no support to the basic tenet of Boveri's hypothesis, i.e. that such anomalies initiate the tumorigenic process.

9 INTERPRETATIONS: FACTS, FANCIES, AND THE FUTURE IN ONCOLOGY

9.1 The Rise and Fall of Oncologic Theories

Among the biological disciplines oncology has proved unsurpassed as a historical graveyard of many and varied once-fashionable theories which have attracted much investigative effort but which, proportionately, have yielded little return in the form of real understanding of the discipline (cf. Chapter Two). Indeed, in terms of cost-effectiveness, cancer research, if viewed as a commercial enterprise, would have been declared bankrupt long ago. Yet, as a long-term investment, this obligatory human endeavour is arguably capable of paying high dividends, hopefully in the not too distant future.

Of all known theories of oncogenesis, the atrabilism of the Greeks and Islam, particularly of Galen and Avicenna, held the longest sway, dominating medical thinking for well over a millennium. Despite this, atrabilism, in retrospect, numbers among the least credible of all such theories, mainly because of its lack of any firm basis in anatomy, or physiology. Thus, popularity and influence, even when highly time-honoured, are not necessarily arguments in favour of an oncologic theory.

It was inevitable that atrabilism should have been most meticulously weighed and found wanting from the time of the Renaissance, marked as this period was by a vigorous upsurge in pathological anatomy which began at the Vesalian school at Padua. The many post-atrabilistic theories then became centred around iatrochemicals, or formless body elements such as lymph, both solidistic and fluidistic, and blastema. Of these, the blastema theory was destined, in terms of survival and popularity, to don the mantle shed by atrabilism, until it too was finally displaced, albeit slowly and reluctantly during the middle decades of the nineteenth century, by Virchow's cellular theory. The latter has remained the only currently known oncologic theory that is beyond dispute and hence, in this sense, as near to perfection as a theory can be. In other ways, however, it was seriously limited. As it stood, it failed to address such important problems as the identity

319

or nature of the cell undergoing neoplastic transformation, or the mechanism or sequelae of the transformation process.

In all fairness, however, these problems have remained, down to this day, extremely difficult. As discussed by Foulds (1969, 1975), the cellular origins of frank neoplasms, mainly because of the latter's long latencies, are usually surmised rather than ascertained. For instance, the cellular origin of retinoblastoma, which is the most common intra-ocular neoplasm of childhood, has variously been suggested to be a neuronal cell, a glial cell, a primitive retinal stem cell, or a primitive neuro-ectodermal cell (Kyritsis *et al.*, 1984).

Such limitations of Virchow's cellular theory became well-recognized during the late nineteenth century. The leading embryologists of the day, notably Waldeyer, Bard, Remak, Conheim, and Zahn, added a dynamic force to the theory by generally proposing maldifferentiation as the mechanism of neoplastic transformation and development. In particular, Conheim, in 1875, advanced his 'cell rest' theory of tumour genesis from errant embryonic cells failing to mature normally. Two years later, Zahn reached the then precocious conclusion that neoplasms more closely resemble embryonic than adult tissues. He thus foreshadowed the modern oncologic doctrine of arrested cellular differentiation of stem cells, this favouring both cellular proliferation and embryofetal expression. Such exploits, inclusive of Weismann's postulate of the inviolate germ line, reflected the contemporary growth not only of embryology, which was founded in Europe by the nineteenth-century Russian biologist Karl Ernst von Baer (but see also Chapter Two, Section 2.7), but also of recognition of the central role of this discipline in oncology. The theory of neoplasia as a developmental disease was thus truly launched.

The late nineteenth century also witnessed a phenomenal growth in light microscopy for the visualization of stained subcellular structures. During the 1870s and 1880s, Miescher's 'nuclein' became Waldeyer's 'chromatin', which corresponded to the 'idioplasm' of Naegeli. Such structures were capable of underpinning a common molecular basis for biological phenomena as diverse as cell function, embryonic development, and hereditary transmission. Then, also, Arnold described chromosomes in human cancer cells.

The stage was thus well set for more detailed study of the chromosomes of cancer cells. Accordingly, during the 1890s, von Hansemann reported 'asymmetrical karyokinesis' (chromosome anomalies) in carcinomas, but Stroebe and others soon showed that such anomalies also occur in other including some normal cells. Despite this, in 1914, Boveri advanced what has since come down as the ever-controversial 'somatic mutation' theory (cf. Chapter Seven, Section 7.2).

Astute clinicians and others from the time of Paracelsus in the sixteenth century have been elucidating a role for an ever-growing roster of environmental factors in cancer genesis (Chapter Three). In modern times there has been an increasing tendency to equate this role with the effects of the factors upon the primary structure or functioning of inherited cellular DNA. The essentials of the modern theories are thus extensions of the older theories based upon differentiation or somatic mutation.

From this brief résumé of the known history of oncologic philosophy it seems unlikely that this ancient saga of chopping and changing fortunes will not continue to make at least some of our currently most cherished theories the atrabilism of tomorrow. None the less each of the major theories of the past was, in its own time, fashionable and hard-won; it epitomized contemporary knowledge; and it represented a development from antecedents and a source of its successors. Even the mystical atrabilism, with its reliance upon diet and melancholy respectively representing environmental and intrinsic factors, had elements of modern theories based upon ecogenetics.

In this final chapter, the essentials of oncology as they are currently understood are critically examined in relation to the major theories in vogue, and with an eye to the probable future of the discipline.

9.2 Basic Facts About Cancer Which Any Acceptable Theory of Oncogenesis Must Accommodate

9.2.1 Antiquity and Ubiquity

It is probable that cancer is as old and as ubiquitous as are the species of *Metazoa* and *Metaphyta* (Chapter Two, Section 2.3.2; Chapter Three, Section 3.2).

This feature suggests that cancer has at least some of its roots in biological evolution. Among other supporting evidence (see below, Section 9.9) is the cellular autonomy which is the prime characteristic of the primitive unicellular organisms generally believed to have been the evolutionary ancestors of the multicellular species. The relative autonomy of cancer cells (cf. Chapter One, Section 1.2.1.5) may hence represent a self-serving resort of these cells to their ancient birthright capacity that is suppressed during normal development but has not been discarded during evolution. Analogously, normally developing cells resort to some of their phylogenetic experiences. The principle involved was generalized over 150 years ago by J.F. Meckel (1781–1833) in his now somewhat tarnished 'ontogeny recapitulates phylogeny' that was later elaborated by E.H. Haekel (1834–1919).

9.2.2 The Continuing Intransigence of the Cancer Problem

Despite the millennia-old and the modern worldwide efforts in the fight against cancer, progress in oncology has remained slow, and the problems posed by neoplasia have remained almost as intransigent as ever they were. For instance, in the treatment of clinical cancer, the modest successes achieved largely through the cytotoxic therapies introduced after the Second World War began to peak soon afterwards. Since the 1950s there has been little significant advance in the treatment of the common adult cancers (Doll and Peto, 1981). For the common childhood cancers, there has been some therapeutic improvement in acute lymphocytic leukemia, Hodgkin's disease, non-Hodgkin's lymphoma, Wilm's tumour, medulloblastoma, and retinoblastoma, but little or none in the others including neuroblastoma, anaplastic astrocytoma, and brain stem glioma (McWhirter and Siskind, 1984). Even for the cancers showing some improvement, the treatment itself may give rise to second primary cancers that prove fatal, e.g. for Hodgkin's disease (Bolvin *et al.*, 1984). This situation recalls the 'tumour of the god Xensu' of ancient Egypt where the medical advice was 'do thou nothing there against'; and also the 'occult' and the 'nolimetangere' (do not touch me) tumours of the later Greeks and medievals (cf. Chapter Three, Section 3.5.1).

9.2.3 Epidemiology, Civilization, and Life Expectancy

At least since the 1930s when, in Denmark and the United States, reliable national cancer registries first began to be established, the overall rates of cancer incidence and mortality have been increasing, to the point where cancer now accounts for about 20 per cent of all deaths in most developed countries.

A popular interpretation of this phenomenon is that cancer is a disease of modern civilization. However, as detailed below (Section 9.3), at least three aspects of the accumulated epidemiological data suggest that this interpretation is an over- simplification of a complex problem. First, the time trends have been non-uniform. They have been rising for some cancers, mainly those of the lung and skin (Doll and Peto, 1981; Urbach, 1983); falling for others such as those of the stomach (Oshima and Fujimoto, 1983) and uterine cervix (Hakama, 1983); and static or mixed for yet others. For instance, in the United States, the mortality rates for prostatic cancer from around 1945 have remained essentially static in Caucasians but have been increasing in others (Mettlin, 1983). For breast cancer, these rates have been increasing in some countries but have remained almost constant in others including the United States, Canada, Australia, the Netherlands, Great Britain, and Japan (Herity, 1983). For colorectal cancer, the rates have been showing all possible time trends: increasing in Japan, Italy, and West Germany; static in the United States (Whites); and decreasing in Great Britain (Miller, 1983).

Second, the true pre-twentieth-century rates, particularly for the internal cancers, are not available for strict comparisons to be made. This is due to factors such as past inadequacies of recording, reporting, and diagnosis. Reliable diagnostic techniques such as sputum cytology, bronchoscopy, chest X-rays, and intrathoracic surgery for lung cancer are introductions of the present century (Doll and Peto, 1981); and others such as double contrast radiology, endoscopy, and X-ray television for stomach cancer are recent innovations (Oshima and Fujimoto, 1983). Before 1900, most cases of lung cancer would not have been correctly diagnosed; and they might even have been recorded on death certificates as 'consumption' or the like. Even today, most cases of non-melanoma skin cancer are not reported (Chapter Six, Section 6.4.1).

Finally, cancer is essentially a disease of older ages, but even this fact needs qualification. In adulthood, but not before, the incidence of many types of cancer increases with age in log-linear fashion (Devesa and Silverman, 1978). For other types, however, the rate of increase is non-uniform. For instance, Hodgkin's disease shows a peak incidence in young adulthood and another in late life (Vianna and Strauss, 1983). Also, the incidence of cervical cancer shows a sharp increase premenopausally but a levelling off thereafter (Hakama, 1983). There is also the 'Clemmeson's Hook' in the incidence of breast cancer (Chapter Six, Section 6.4.4). In addition to such age-related vagaries of various types of cancer incidence, most human populations, at least from around the turn of the present century, have been becoming progressively older (Chapter One, Section 1.2.5). In the United States, for instance, the at-birth life expectancy was 47.3 years in 1900 but 69.7 years in 1959 and it is now over 75 years. As essentially a disease of older ages, cancer would be increasingly common in the increasingly older populations, irrespective of any other change with the progress of civilization.

9.2.4 Natural Specificities in Cancer

Even with an environmental factor which is as strongly associated with a specific cancer as smoking is, many of the even highly exposed individuals fail to develop the cancer within their lifetime; and, moreover, that cancer is not unknown among the unexposed individuals belonging to a susceptible species. This highlights the general principle of natural specificities in oncology: whether between (Chapter Five) or within (Chapter Six) species, the propensity to develop type-specific neoplasms spontaneously or inducibly varies enormously. For instance, the spontaneous neoplasms of laboratory and other nonhuman animals are predominantly mesenchymal (i.e. sarcomas, inclusive of leukemias and lymphomas), and many have a demonstrable species-endogenous viral etiology, e.g. a feline leukemia viral etiology in cats. In man, in contrast, epithelial neoplasms (carcinomas) predominate; and, despite the presence of some suggestive evidence to the contrary (see Zur Hausen, 1980, for a review), not even the sarcomas have such an etiology.

An apt illustration of the inductive specificities is provided by the known relationships between tobacco smoke and neoplasia of the lung and other organs. In man, this factor is the major environmental associate of bronchogenic carcinoma, and it potentiates the broncho-neoplastic propensities of other environmental factors such as asbestos and certain types of metallic and/or mining dust. Yet, appropriate experimental models of this human situation are unknown. In hamsters, for instance, cigarette smoke failed to produce bronchial cancer, even when the smoke was chronically administered in combination with particles of asbestos or of various inorganic oxides (Dontenwill et al., 1973; Wehner et al., 1976), or with coal dust or acrolein. This does not mean that laboratory rodents cannot develop bronchogenic carcinoma. This neoplasm has been induced in hamsters by benzo(a)pyrene in combination with particles of ferric oxide (Sellakumar *et al.*, 1973) or magnesia (Stenbäck *et al.*, 1975), and in rats by point-source irradiation (Gracey *et al.*, 1979). Somewhat analogously to the reported negative association between smoking and colon cancer in man (Williams *et al.*, 1981), smoking has also been associated with reduced body weight but increased lifespan in hamsters (Wehner *et al.*, 1976), and, in F344 rats, with reduced incidence of spontaneous neoplasms of the hematopoietic-lymphoid system, pituitary, uterus, and ovary (Dalbey *et al.*, 1980).

In F344 rats, the spontaneous incidence of many types of neoplasm is high, but that of neoplasms of the upper respiratory tract is low (Sass *et al.*, 1975). In such rats, Dalbey *et al.* reported the induction of some of the latter neoplasms, through lifetime exposure of the animals to 'a maximum tolerated dose of cigarette smoke', i.e. to smoke from 7 cigarettes/day for 2.5 years. In comparative terms of average lifespan and body weight, this exposure is equivalent to that of a single human individual smoking over 2,000 cigarettes/day, every day for about three score and ten years, i.e. over 51 million cigarettes!

Overall, cigarette smoke, the most notorious of known human environmental carcinogens, can, in different species of organism or different organs in the same species, exhibit neoplastic, anti-neoplastic, or even life-prolonging non-neoplastic effects.

The great range of differential cancer susceptibility in humans may be exemplified by the almost legendary cancer-free heavy-smoking octogenarian and the four-year-old child with a malignant lung cancer (Seo *et al.*, 1984). The basis of such differences has been ascribed by Doll and Peto (1981) to 'luck'. They pointed to the well-established fact that the carcinogenic response, whether spontaneous or induced, often varies even among animals of the same inbred strain. However, due to natural factors such as meiotic recombinations it seems highly unlikely that such animals, except for identical twins, can ever be genetically identical, even after hundreds of generations of inbreeding (Chapter Seven, Section 7.3.2).

9.2.5 Physiological Mimicries

All of the known basic properties of neoplasia are, in the words of Rudolph Virchow written over twelve decades ago, 'either a *Heterotopia*, an aberratio loci, or an aberratio temporis, a *Heterochromia*, or lastly, a mere variation in quantity' (Chapter Two, Section 2.6.12). The ensuing decades have documented no necessary modification of this statement.

The modern feverish search for some *qualitative* abnormality in human neoplasia is understandable in terms of the specificity in pathogenesis and/or treatment which has been the common basis of the heady successes in medicine over the past one hundred years. Briefly, this has been the basis of the germ theory of disease as formulated by Virchow and Pasteur (1822–1895); of Pasteur's successes with silkworm disease and anthrax, and also with hydrophobia against which he introduced a specific vaccine; and of the famous postulates of Robert Koch (1843–1910). In the same category belong Koch's discovery of the tubercle bacillus in 1882, to clarify for all times the erstwhile historically enigmatic etiology of the associated disease which had foxed even the great Virchow during most of his professional career. Specificity was also behind the efficacy of antisepsis in the deadly puerperal fever, as was discovered in 1843 in the United States by Oliver Wendell Holmes, and was then extended to obstetrics by the Hungarian, Ignaz Philipp Semmelweiss (1818–1865). In Russia, Elie Mechnikov (1845–1916) demonstrated the specificity of natural immunity, i.e. the capacity of leukocytes to fight against germs and infectious diseases. In 1905, Schaudinn discovered *Spirochaeta pallida* as the cause of the syphilis known to Europe since the time of Columbus; and, in 1910, Ehrlich introduced the arsenic compound Salvarsan as a specific remedy. Analogously, during 1889–93, Joseph von Mering established the symptomatic cause of diabetes mellitus; and, in 1922, Banting and Best introduced insulin as a remedy. Succeeding years saw the introduction of the sulfonamides, the antibiotics, the tetracyclines, the anticholinergics, the anti-histamines, the hormones and hormonoids, and a host of other 'wonder' drugs displaying diverse specificities against a variety of infectious and other diseases.

Against such a background, it can be neither surprising nor unexpected that the search for specificity in human neoplasia has already encompassed features as diverse as genetic mutations (Section 9.6) or environmental factors (Section 9.3) as specific causes, and chromosome anomalies (Chapter Eight) or tumour products as specific diagnostic aids in clinical cancer. However, as discussed in the Sections and Chapter indicated, none of the sought objects has been found to have the desired specificity. This principle of non-specificity also applies equally to the other major features of clinical cancer, i.e. its treatment (Section 9.2.2) and prevention (Chapter Six, Section 6.5) and also to preclinical cancer detection and management (reviewed by Koss and Greenebaum, 1983; see also Chapter Six, Section 6.4.4).

Among the tumour products which have been found, perhaps the most important are the hormones because of their powerful universal effects which are often exerted independently of normal host homeostasis (Chapter Four). In the amine-precursor-uptake-and-decarboxylation (APUD) series, for instance, which includes oat-cell carcinomas and carcinoid tumours of the lung as well as small-cell nonkeratinizing carcinomas of the uterine cervix, multiple immunoreactive polypeptide hormones are produced. These include adrenocorticotropic hormone (ACTH), the historical prototype of the ectopic hormones described by Liddle *et al.* in 1965 as part of the 'ACTH syndrome' (cf. Liddle *et al.*, 1969; also Chapter Four, Section 4.5), as well as somatostatin, pancreatic polypeptide, calcitonin, vasoactive intestinal polypeptide, glucagon, and melanocyte stimulating hormone (Odell *et al.*, 1977; Odell and Saito, 1983; Inoue *et al.*, 1984). It is almost certain that the worst effects of cancer, particularly the wasting away (cachexia) that is often almost mercifully relieved by death, are secondary ('paraneoplastic') effects of such hormones produced uncontrollably rather than primary effects of the cancerous growths themselves.

Structurally normal representatives of practically all of the major types of physiological substances have been found as tumour products. Indeed, this is so general that any rare report of a structurally abnormal tumour product may well be regarded as the exception that proves the rule. Other than hormones, the tumour products of note include alpha-fetoprotein (AFP) and various 'antigens' such as the carcino-embryonic antigen (CEA) (cf. Chapter One, Section 1.2.1) and various lymphocyte differentiation antigens (Olsson *et al.* 1984). Monoclonal antibodies to the latter antigens are proving useful as aids in the classification of certain leukemias and in the gaining of insights into normal lymphocyte differentiation (Linch *et al.*, 1984). The tumour products also include immunoglobulins; enzymes such as aldolase, hexokinase, thymidine and pyruvate kinases, and acid and alkaline phosphatases (Balinsky *et al.*, 1984; Hagberg *et al.*, 1984); prostaglandins (PGs) such as PGE_2 and PGE_{2x} (Rolland *et al.*, 1980; Watson *et al.*, 1984); and intracellular, cell surface-bound, and extracellular glycolipids, glycoproteins, and other glyco-conjugates (Yogeeswaran, 1983; Blaszczyk *et al.*, 1984).

(For detailed discussions of fetal phenotypic expressions in neoplasia, see Coggin and Anderson, 1974; Mintz and Fleischman, 1981.)

9.2.6 Cancer and Genetic Susceptibility

Despite its traditional unpopularity, the concept of neoplasia as a disease with a firm basis in variable inherited susceptibility has, in recent years, been becoming increasingly well-documented (Chapter Six).

The validity of this concept has already been supported by practically all of the well-established major features of neoplasia. These include the antiquity and ubiquity of the disease (Section 9.2.1); its nonrandom occurrences interspecifically, and also intraspecifically among animals (Chapter Five) and humans (Chapter Six); and its physiological mimicries (Section 9.2.5). With the recent upsurge of molecular genetics, certain inherited genes capable of stimulating (Bishop, 1982; Weinberg, 1983) or suppressing (Lilly, 1972; Bubbers, 1984) oncogenesis are increasingly being discovered. Among the former are the so-called 'oncogenes', which were discovered initially by use of transforming retroviruses rather than by gene transfer of cellular DNA. However, the evolutionary origin of the oncogenes is cellular, not viral. Moreover, they are of widespread if not universal distribution within the biosphere. The oncogene associated with human bladder cancer, for instance, has homologues in the DNA of all vertebrates examined, and also in that of the fruit fly, *Drosophila melanogaster*.

The oncogenes are therefore of very ancient lineage, they having been conserved in evolution from at least as far back as the primitive common metazoan ancestors of the arthropods and chordates. Such a high degree of conservation, analogous to that of the genes for the core histones and other vital proteins (Wilson *et al.*, 1977), points to indispensable roles for the oncogenes in cellular and organismic physiology (cf. Müller *et al.*, 1982). Their association with oncogenesis may hence represent only a minor departure from their normal functions. Their designation as oncogenes, rather like the term 'HLA' (cf. Chapter Six, Section 6.3), is hence unfortunate.

The already known oncogenes may represent but a small sampling of the developmentally vital normal genes which are secondarily associated with the stimulation or suppression of oncogenesis. Bentvelzen (1984), for instance, demonstrated the transforming capability of certain fragments of normal cellular DNA from several strains of mouse and rat. In *Drosophila melanogaster*, at least 25 of the some 5,000 normal genes present in the genome are causally associated with neoplastic development. In her recent review of this situation, Gateff (1982) stressed her 'strong conviction' that in all instances 'cancer has a genetic base . . . and is a problem of cell differentiation and the maintenance of this state'.

9.3 Cancer and the Environment

9.3.1 A Plethora of Experimental Carcinogens and Some Extrapolative Difficulties

The human environment, or 'nurture', has been described as 'what people do or have done to them' (Doll and Peto, 1981), or as 'the totality of the effects of that which we eat, breathe or are otherwise exposed to' (Nicholson, 1984). That this environment plays an important role in establishment of the frequency of many types of clinical cancer has become well-documented through two distinct approaches (Chapter Three, Section 3.4): the direct approach involving the anecdotal and epidemiological observations in humans, and the indirect approach involving laboratory testing.

Jointly, these two approaches have implicated practically every aspect of the environment as determinants of human cancer. Among the implicated physical factors is cosmic radiation, which has antedated the origin of biological life. Among the biological factors are certain types of intestinal and fecal flora; liver flukes such as *Opisthorchis felineus* and *Chlonorchis sinensis*; and viruses such as the Epstein-Barr virus, the herpes simplex viruses types 1 and 2, the hepatitis B virus, and even the mouse mammary tumour virus (cf. Caldwell, 1983). Some of the other implicated factors are not readily classifiable as physical, biological, or chemical, e.g. psychosomatic stress, and practices related to industry, occupation, and sex and reproduction. (For some reviews, see IARC Working Group, 1980; Doll and Peto, 1981; Kodama and Kodama, 1983; and Bourke, 1983).

As determined mainly by the indirect approach, the implicated chemical factors are especially numerous, simply because defined chemical substances are readily available and are more amenable than the other factors to laboratory testing under controlled conditions. Literally hundreds of such substances, from both natural and artificial sources, have been reported to produce cancer of one type or another in at least one of the few test systems in common use (Chapter Three, Sections 3.6 and 3.7). Among the natural substances are cellular products such as hormones and cholesterol metabolites; fungal and microbial metabolites such as aflatoxins, mitomycin C, and griseofulvin; dietary factors such as animal fat and protein, as well as certain secondary amines capable of forming nitrosamines in the stomach or intestines; inorganic substances such as asbestos and compounds of chromium, beryllium, nickel, and arsenic; and a variety of plant products. The latter comprise a growing list (Bull *et al.*, 1968; McLean, 1970; Mattocks, 1972; Culvenor and Jago, 1979) which already includes carrageenan, coumarin, cycasin, parasorbic acid, pyrrolizidine alkaloids, safrole and related compounds, shikimic acid, tannins, and certain polycyclic arylhydrocarbons (PAHs). Some of the PAHs, including their historical prototype 3,4-benzo(a)pyrene (Chapter Three, Section 3.6.3.2), have been known for some time to occur naturally in vegetables and perhaps all green plants (Graf and Diehl, 1966). Also, among the some 200 known pyrrolizidine alkaloids isolated from over 300 species in 12 plant families, about 85 are esters of unsaturated pyrrolizidine amino-alcohols, i.e. the common structural feature of the known hepatotoxic and/or carcinogenic analogues. There are also the alkaloids from major carcinogenic sources such as nicotine, nornicotine, and cotinine from tobacco, and arecoline and arecaidine from betel (*Areca catechu L.*).

The implicated artificial substances outnumber even the natural ones. They include useful substances such as the pesticides DDT and dieldrin, and medicinals such as cyclophosphamide, synthetic hormone analogues (Chapter Four, Section 4.2.5), melphalan, ethylene oxide, mustard gas, thiotepa, reserpine, phenobarbitone, phenacetin, and even aspirin. Interestingly, most of these medicinals are used in clinical cancer chemotherapy, underlining the old adage that like destroys like. Also implicated are the ubiquitous PAHs (see above) which are partial combustion products of tobacco, fossil fuels, and also of many foodstuffs during cooking. During cooking also, heterocyclic amines capable of forming nitrosamines (e.g. through interaction with nitrite present in saliva and preserved foods) are produced from free or protein-bound tryptophan and certain other amino acids. One of the major implicated factors, tobacco smoke, is a mixture of at least 2,000 different chemicals, of which at least 30 are associated with carcinogenesis (Wynder and Hoffmann, 1967, 1976).

Some four million synthetic chemicals have been recorded up to around 1979. Of these, the first million took almost 150 years to produce, i.e. from the birth of modern organic chemistry in the early nineteenth century to around 1947; but the second, third, and fourth took just about 14, 9, and 9 years (Miller, 1979). To this list, over 6,000 new entries are recorded weekly, so that the fifth or even the sixth million would already have been reached. In view of the high rate (about 25 per cent) of activity found in random testing experiments (Chapter Three, Section 3.7), at least one million of these synthetic chemicals should be experimental carcinogens. Moreover, a substance found inactive in one or more of the few tests in common use may well prove active in another. For instance, phenacetin is carcinogenic in the hamster but not in the rat, and 2-naphthylamine in several species but not in the rat and rabbit. Consequently, it cannot be certain that a substance found inactive in all of the usual tests will not be active in a new test, or even in man. For instance, neither arsenic nor benzene has thus far produced experimental tumours; but, in man, the former is associated with cancers of the skin and lung, and the latter with acute nonlymphocytic and other leukemias. Finally, a given carcinogen may act upon different tissues in different species of organism. For instance, beryllium is associated with lung cancer in humans, but with bone cancer in rabbits. Analogously benzidine is associated with liver cancer in rats and hamsters, chlornaphazine with lung cancer in mice and sarcomas in rats, and 2-naphthylamine with hepatomas in mice. In man, however, all three of these substances are associated with bladder cancer. (For references, see IARC Working Group, 1980, 1982.)

The experimentally painted picture of environmental carcinogenesis is thus too complex to see the wood for the trees. It yields no reliable information on features such as the identity of an experimental noncarcinogen, of a human carcinogen or noncarcinogen, or of the human tissue at risk from exposure to an experimental carcinogen.

9.3.2 The Role of Human Cancer Epidemiology in the Simplification and Grading of Environmental Cancer-risk Factors

In recent years, the epidemiological data accumulated over the past 14 decades, i.e. since the times of Tanchou and Rigoni-Stern (Chapter Three, Section 3.4.6), have been widely reviewed and evaluated (e.g. Wynder and Gori, 1977; Higginson and Muir, 1979; IARC Working

Group, 1980, 1982; Doll and Peto, 1981; Byers and Graham, 1984). As summarized in table 9.1, the overall results of this enterprise represent a considerable simplification and a reasonably clear-cut grading of the environmental cancer-risk factors to humans. However, the actual percentages given in the table are rough estimates due to factors such as the great complexity of both cancer etiology and human exposures. Even rougher are the figures given for the role of geophysical factors since most cases of sunlight-associated cancers, i.e. of the non-melanoma variety, are not recorded (Chapter Six, Section 6.4.1). Also, as used by Higginson and Muir, lifestyle refers to factors such as 'dietary fiber, excess fat and calorie intake, and possibly hormone carcinogenesis'.

Five features of the data summarized in Table 9.1 are noteworthy. First, the figures given are purely statistical, referring only to 'excess' cancer incidences or mortality (Section 9.4). Sec-

Table 9.1: Proportions of Human Cancer Incidence or Mortality Attributed to Various Different Factors according to Three Independent Estimates

Factor or class of factors	Percentage of all cancers in:				
	Birmingham (England)[a]		The United States		
			b		c
	M	F	M	F	M + F
Diet	—	—	40	57	35
Tobacco	30	7	28	8	30
Tobacco/alcohol	5	3	4	1	—
Alcohol	—	—	—	—	3
Lifestyle	30	63	—	—	—
Sunlight	10	10 }	8	8	3
Ionizing radiation	1	1 }			
Occupation	6	2	4	2	4
Iatrogenic	1	1	—	—	1
Sexual/reproduction	—	—	—	—	7
Exogenous hormones	—	—	—	4	—
Pollution	—	—	—	—	2
Industrial products	—	—	—	—	‹1
Congenital	2	2 }	16	20	—
Unknown	15	11 }			

Notes: Data from *a*, Higginson and Muir (1979), *b*, Wynder and Gori (1977), *c*, Doll and Peto (1981); *a* and *b* based on incidence data, *c* on mortality data. *M*, males; *F*, females; —, figure not given. See text for further details and explanations.

ond, the major risk factors are few, i.e. dietary, smoking, cosmic, and sexual and reproductive factors. Third, these factors are all highly complex. Fourth, with the exception of smoking (but see Chapter Three, introductory section) they have probably always involved all of mankind. As associates of cancer, diet has been suspected at least since the time of Galen (Chapter Two, Section 2.4.2); sex and reproduction since 1700 (Chapter Three, Section 3.4.2.2); and tobacco since 1761 (Chapter Three, Section 3.4.2.6.2). Finally, contrary to the results from laboratory testing (Section 9.3.1) and to the notion popularized largely by Epstein (1978) and Epstein and Schwartz (1981), factors such as occupational exposure and pollutants in air, water, food, and soil do not pose any substantial risk of human cancer. This is not to deny the vital importance of exposure, e.g. to asbestos, to the small populations involved. However, according to the IARC Working Group (1980), only 18 defined chemicals or industrial processes are associated with sufficient evidence for a substantial risk of human cancer (Table 9.2).

9.4 Epidemiology and Cancer Causation: Interpretative Difficulties and a Re-interpretation

A popular interpretation of the epidemiological data summarized in Table 9.1 is that over 90 per cent of human cancers are directly caused by the environment (cf. Chapter Five, Section 5.1). This interpretation is based upon the largest observed geographical differences in the frequencies of specific types of cancer. Supporting evidence, also suggestive of an environmental role, has come from studies of time trends, of alteration of risks in migrants and other populations (e.g. ex-smokers), and from the case-control and cohort analyses which attempt to identify specific risk factors.

Some major features of the data, however, suggest that the grounds for the interpretation are not always firm. Certainly, the geographical differences are large for some specific cancers. For instance, breast cancer is four to five times commoner in the British Isles and the Netherlands than in Costa Rica, Mexico, and Japan (Herity, 1983); and stomach cancer is over 25 times commoner in Japan and Chile than in Thailand and Nicaragua (Oshima and Fujimoto, 1983). However, as indicated by the

Table 9.2:   A Complete List of Chemicals or Industrial Processes for Which There Is Sufficient Evidence for Their Association with Risk of Human Cancers at Specific Body Sites

Chemical or process	Site(s) of cancer
4-Aminobiphenyl	Urinary bladder
Arsenic and certain arsenic compounds	Skin, lung, liver
Asbestos	Lung (pleural and peritoneal mesotheliomas)
Auramine manufacture	Urinary bladder
Benzene	Hematopoietic tissues (leukemias)
Benzidine	Urinary bladder
Chlornaphazine	Lung
Chloromethyl ethers	Lung
Chromium and certain chromium compounds	Lung
Diethylstilbestrol	Vagina
Hematite mining (underground)	Lung
Isopropyl alcohol manufacture (strong acid process)	Nasal sinuses
Melphalan	Lung
Mustard gas	Lung
2–Naphthylamine	Urinary bladder
Nickel refining	Lung; nasal sinuses
Soots, tars, mineral oils	Skin, lung, scrotum
Vinyl chloride	Liver (angiosarcoma)

Source: As reviewed by the IARC Working Group (1980, 1982).

Japanese experience with cancers of the breast and stomach, in practically all populations, low incidences for some types of cancer are offset by high incidences for others. Nigerians, for instance, have low incidences for several cancers including cancers of the colon, rectum, lung, larynx, corpus uteri, pancreas, and kidney; but they have high incidences for others including childhood lymphosarcoma and adult cancers of the liver, prostate, breast, and cervix uteri. In overall terms, the geographical differences are threefold or less (Doll and Peto, 1981). This suggests that, in any human population which is sufficiently large to give statistically significant results, only a small and approximately fixed proportion of people will develop cancer of one type or another, regardless of environmental vagaries. Another difficulty concerns proper apportionment of the associated environmental factors in accordance with the rate variations for different cancers in that population.

A further difficulty concerns proper identification of the implicated environmental cancer-risk factors. Broadly, some strong associations have been found for certain epithelial neoplasms of adults, mainly of the skin but excluding most cases of malignant melanoma (Chapter Six, Section 6.4.1), and also of the respiratory organs and the upper digestive tract. For certain other neoplasms such as Burkitt's lymphoma in children and adult neoplasms of the gastrointestinal and genital tracts, the associations are weak and/or nonspecific (Muir and Parkin, 1983). No environmental association is known for the remaining neoplasms, particularly those of childhood such as neuroblastoma, retinoblastoma, and Wilm's tumour, and most adult neoplasms having a well-recognized genetic basis (Chapter Six).

Even the well-established environmental associations present interpretative difficulties. As shown in Table 9.1, for instance, diet is held responsible for some 40 per cent of all cancers in males and 57 per cent in females in the United States (Wynder and Gori, 1977). Many reports have implicated animal fat and protein, particularly for cancers of the breast, colon, rectum, and endometrium. However, in the United States, the frequency of these cancers is similarly low among the ovo-lacto-vegetarian Seventh Day Adventists of California (Phillips *et al.*, 1980) and the high meat-eating Mormons of Utah (Lyon *et al.*, 1980). In a recent review of reviews, the latter numbering over 60 within the past decade alone, Byers and Graham (1984) concluded that the entire epidemiological effort conducted over the past fifty years and in many parts of the world 'has not led to a single unequivocal conclusion regarding the relationship between dietary factors and cancer risk'.

Equivocation similarly surrounds the other complex risk factors. Examples are tobacco smoke, betel, and sexual and reproductive factors (Sections 9.2.3 and 9.2.4), as well as industrial factors such as those associated with high risk of cancers of the nose, stomach, lung, bladder, and other organs in woodworkers (Stellman and Garfinkel, 1984). A related example is provided by farmers, who have elevated risk of multiple myeloma, leukemia, lymphoma, and certain other neoplasms (Cantor and Blair, 1984). Conversely, elevated risk of pancreatic cancer has been associated with some

Table 9.3: Some Epidemiologically Derived Risk Factors for Various Human Cancers

Cancer site	Risk factors
Mouth[a]	Sunlight (for lip cancer in the fair-skinned); betel chewing, smoking of 'bidi' (a tobacco-and-dried-leaf cigarette) (mainly in India); alcohol; smoking and/or chewing of tobacco; tobacco snuff (mainly among women in southern USA); chronic deficiency of iron and vitamin A (e.g. in the Plummer-Vinson syndrome); defective dentition and poor oral hygiene
Nasopharynx[a]	Genetic factors (e.g. HLA-A2 and B-sin2 in southern Chinese); EBV infection; (Cantonese-type) diets high in salted and fried fish and croton oil; cigarette smoking; bacterial fatty acids
Esophagus[a]	Cigarette smoking and/or alcohol; nutritional deficiency of zinc, magnesium, riboflavin, nicotinic acid; low socioeconomic status; natural and mycotoxins in food
Stomach[b]	Genetic factors (e.g. blood group A and pernicious anemia); (Japanese-type) diets high in salted, fried, and starchy foods and low in fresh fruit, vegetable, and vitamin C
Pancreas[c]	Genetic factors; radiation; cigarette smoking, but not alcohol; coffee; (Western-type) diets high in animal fat and protein and low in fresh vegetable (fibre); certain associated diseases or disturbances such as diabetes mellitus, hyperglycemia, uterine myoma, spontaneous abortion, oophorectomy, ovarian hyperplasia, and neoplasms of breast, uterus, and ovary; some 50 distinct occupations (cf. Mack, 1982)
Colon[d]	Gentic factors (e.g. Peutz-Jehger's syndrome and familial polyposis coli); inflammatory bowel conditions such as ulcerative colitis and Crohn's disease; high socioeconomic status; Western-type diets (as above); low dietary but high drinking-water selenium; intestinal flora; bile salts; beer; low serum cholesterol; nulliparity
Lung[e]	Cigarette smoking; asbestos; arsenic; benzo(a)pyrene; chloromethyl ethers; chromium; radon; genetic factors (e.g. arylhydrocarbon hydroxylase inducibility)
Breast[f]	Genetic factors, e.g. some strong familial aspects, possibly associated with endogenous hormones and with the glutamate-pyruvate-transaminase locus (King *et al.*, 1980); sex (female predominance); high socioeconomic status; nulliparity; late first parity; early menarche; late menopause; high dietary fat; diagnostic, therapeutic, and other radiation, e.g. in X-ray, mammography, and A-bomb exposure; oral contraceptives; alcohol; body height and weight
Skin[g]	Genetic factors, e.g. xeroderma pigmentosum and, especially for malignant melanoma (MM) of the non-lentigo maligna variety, unknown constitutional factors; UV-B radiation for non-MM types; arsenic; X-ray; soot; tars; mineral oils

Sources: Data called from the following (mainly reviews): a. Henderson and Louie (1978), Hirayama and Ito (1981), McMichael (1983); b. Oshima and Fujimoto (1983); c. Macdonald *et al.* (1982), Mabuchi (1983); d. Bruce *et al.* (1981), Miller (1983); e. Doll and Peto (1981), Smith and Troop (1983); f. Haagensen *et al.*(1981), Herity (1983); g. Uhrbach (1983).

fifty different industries or occupations, but the identity of any particular risk factor remains obscure (Mabuchi, 1983).

Yet another interpretative difficulty concerns the multiplicity of the implicated risk factors for even a single type of neoplasm (Table 9.3). For breast cancer, for instance, such factors include dietary fat, endogenous and exogenous hormones, cold climate, benign breast disease, hypercorticoidism, radiation, reserpine, ethnic or familial background, early menarche, late menopause, late first parity, low parity, nulliparity, increased frequency of ovulation failure, mammographic features including breast parenchymal pattern, and body height and weight (Herity, 1983; Kodama and Kodama, 1983; Brisson *et al.*, 1984; see also Chapter Six, Section 6.4.4). A related example is esophageal cancer, which has been associated with alcohol, particularly when combined with smoking. However, this association is significant in some high-risk areas such as most Western countries but not in others such as Iran and Central Asia (McMichael, 1983). It has been suggested by van Rensberg (1981) that the risk factors are those which will increase the predisposition of the esophageal epithelium to neoplastic transformation and promote tumour growth, i.e. factors such as chronic deficiencies of zinc, magnesium, riboflavin, and nicotinic acid, together with an adequate energy and protein intake.

A final interpretative difficulty is that the same risk factor(s) may be associated positively with one type of cancer but negatively with another. For instance, cold climate, dietary fat, and delay of or abstention from sexual experience reportedly increase the risk of breast cancer but decrease that of cervical cancer (Kodama and Kodama, 1983). Analogously, among other dietary factors, milk has been reported to increase the risk of pancreatic cancer (Mabuchi, 1983) but to decrease that of stomach cancer (Oshima and Fujimoto, 1983). Risk of breast cancer is also increased by oral contraceptives, though somewhat controversially except perhaps in older women (Hennekens *et al.*, 1984); but these agents protect against fibrocystic and other benign breast disease (Hiasa *et al.*, 1984). Even smoking, the most well-established of the environmental cancer risk factors, has been associated with reduced risk of colon cancer (Williams *et al.*, 1981). Its association with pulmonary fibrosis is controversial (Weiss, 1984; Kilburn, 1984).

Conceptually, the major reason for such difficulties is the assumption by the medical paradigm that all humans are genetically equal or that such genetic differences as do exist become insignificant when sufficiently large human populations are studied epidemiologically (cf. Chapter Five, Section 5.1). However, like the undoubtedly strong association between birds and the air or between fish and water, that between a cancer and an environmental factor does not, by itself, establish a cause and effect relationship. As compared with the medical paradigm-based interpretation given at the beginning of this section a more logical interpretation of the epidemiological data is that the established associations are, at best, causes of the increased incidence or mortality rates for the cancers involved, but that they are not the causes of the cancers themselves (Chapter Six, Section 6.5). The interindividual differential (positive, negative, or neutral) responses to even the same environmental factor(s) would then be due to the appropriate interindividual differences in inherited cancer susceptibility. The currently widespread and almost unquestioned notion of the environment as the prime cause of human cancer, in the words of Mulvihill (1980), 'ignores the facts that the cause of cancer in most patients is unknown and that gene frequencies, as well as environment, can differ worldwide' (Chapter Six, Section 6.1).

Human cancer epidemiology, as at present constituted and executed, has as its prime mandate the establishment of significant specific associations between cancer and environment, to serve as pointers to appropriate preventive measures. In this mandate, it may well have already reached the limits of its capabilities. Its future seems to lie in biochemical and especially genetic epidemiology, mandated to address problems such as the nature of the interindividual cancer-susceptibility variations and of the latter's interactions with even the same environment to produce widely different oncologic responses. A related problem, that of the molecular mechanism(s) of oncogenesis, has remained almost exclusively the domain of the experimental method.

9.5 Carcinogenic Mechanisms: Clues From Experimental Chemical Carcinogenesis

9.5.1 The Two-stage Hypothesis

Molecular mechanisms of chemical carcinogenesis based upon a need for interactions, mainly covalent, between the chemical and one or more cellular macromolecules have been widely proposed or reviewed (e.g. Heidelberger, 1973; Irving, 1979; Weinstein *et al.*, 1979; Miller and Miller, 1974, 1981). This major contribution of experimental chemical carcinogenesis has resulted from a concerted international effort signposted by four pioneer findings. First, in 1915 in Japan, Yamagiwa and Ichikawa demonstrated the practicability of experimental chemical carcinogenesis (Chapter Three, Section 3.6.3.1). Second, in the 1930s in England, Kennaway and his colleagues demonstrated experimental carcinogenesis by single well-defined chemicals (Chapter Three, Section 3.6.3.2). Third, in the 1940s and 1950s in Israel, Berenblum and others demonstrated that chemical carcinogenesis in mouse skin proceeds in two distinct stages: an irreversible 'initiation' stage and a subsequent reversible 'promotion' stage (reviewed by Berenblum, 1954). Finally, in 1960 in the United States, Miller and his colleagues (Cramer *et al.*) showed that, contrary to the older notion that xenochemical metabolism is perhaps exclusively detoxification (cf. Williams, 1959), the chemically inert experimental carcinogen 2-acetylaminofluorene (AAF) is metabolized into a chemically reactive and potentially more carcinogenic derivative (Chapter Three, Section 3.6.3.6). This finding implied that initiation involved irreversible structural modification(s) of a 'critical cellular target' such as DNA, and that this was followed by reversible stimulation of 'uncontrolled' division or promotion of the initiated or 'transformed' cell.

9.5.2 Initiation, Metabolic Activation, and the Concept of Procarcinogens, Proximate Carcinogens, and Ultimate Carcinogens

Viewed with hindsight, the finding by Cramer *et al.* (1960) of N-hydroxyglucuronyl-AAF in the urine of AAF-treated rats carried some major implications to the molecular mechanisms of tumour initiation in experimental chemical carcinogenesis. First, some chemically inert carcinogens ('procarcinogens') can become metabolically activated by oxidation and subsequent conjugation, through derivatives of intermediate reactivity ('proximate carcinogens'), into those of high reactivity ('ultimate carcinogens'). Second, the ultimate carcinogens may then combine covalently and hence irreversibly with suitable cellular macromolecules that thereby become structurally and perhaps also functionally modified. Finally, unless correctly repaired, such a structural modification of cellular DNA could, during subsequent rounds of DNA replication, lead to a heritable permanent mutation such as a base substitution (point mutation) or, through deletion of the modified base, a frameshift mutation.

Numerous subsequent studies have tended to confirm and extend these implications. The metabolic activation of several types of procarcinogen (mainly aromatic amines and amides, carbamates, polycyclic arylhydrocarbons, and nitrosamines) has been shown to generate proximate carcinogens containing one or more highly polarized bonds capable of undergoing ready heterolysis or homolysis and thus of producing strong electrophilic cations or free radicals (cf. Miller and Miller, 1974; Nery, 1976). Benzo(a)pyrene, for instance, is metabolized variously into free or conjugated arene oxides, phenols, dihydrodiols, dihydrodiol epoxides, and quinones (Nebert *et al.*, 1979; Phillips and Sims, 1979), as well as into the 6-oxo-benzo(a)pyrene (Nagata *et al.*, 1974) and other types of free radical or radical cation (Sullivan *et al.*, 1978). Consequently, the subsequent interactions of the ultimate carcinogens with cellular macromolecules are substitutions, bimolecular (S_N2) rather than unimolecular (S_N1), occurring at suitable electron-dense centres such as the N–7, C–8, and, in particular, the 0–6 of guanyl residues in nucleic acids. In DNA, guanyl 0–6 methylation can cause mispairing of guanine, i.e. with thymine instead of, as normally, with cytosine (Eadie *et al.*, 1984).

In general, the ultimate carcinogens react as strong electrophiles to alkylate, arylate, arylaminate, or, more rarely, acylate suitable sites in cellular macromolecules. They fall into two distinct categories: those which are metabolically generated from the chemically inert species, i.e. the procarcinogens; and those which, being inherently reactive, require no metabolic activation. The latter include the nitrogen and sulfur mustards used in cancer chemotherapy, and the nitrosamides. The inorganic carcinogens such as compounds of nickel, chromium, and beryllium are also not known to require metabolic activation. Their mode of action is unknown, but this may involve inhibitory and other co-factor effects upon vital enzymatic functions.

9.5.3 Metabolic Activation and Its Implications for Cancer Prevention

An implication of the above-mentioned generalization is that agents capable of inhibiting the formation or subsequent interactions of the ultimate carcinogens should also inhibit tumorigenesis in appropriate instances. Among such agents for which there is some supporting, though mainly experimental, evidence are ascorbic acid and certain other antioxidants, largely phenols such as butylated hydroxyanisole and ethoxyquin; selenium; vitamin E; and, in particular, vitamin A and other retinoids (Wattenberg, 1980). Selenium seems to have a vitamin E-like action. It activates the glutathione peroxidase-catalase system responsible for the breakdown of hydrogen peroxide and lipid and other hydroperoxides, as well as some of the enzymes catalyzing carcinogen detoxification (Griffin, 1979). The retinoids, which are of widespread natural distribution particularly in certain vegetables, can, like the natural body hormones (Chapter Four, Section 4.4), control epithelial cell differentiation and induce terminal differentiation in leukemia, teratocarcinoma, and other types of neoplastic cell (Section 9.10.3, below; also Sporn, 1983). Their antineoplastic action may thus occur at the level of promotion during oncogenesis (Section 9.5.6, below). However, although they have been reported to inhibit experimental tumorigenesis of various types (e.g. of breast, skin, lung, and urinary bladder), they tend to become sequestered in the liver. This can cause serious liver injury and, moreover, prevent the administered retinoid from reaching, via the blood stream, nonhepatic targets in sufficient threshold concentrations to produce the desired therapeutic effect. This would encourage higher retinoid dosage, thereby exacerbating the hepatotoxicity.

9.5.4 *Limitations of the Metabolic Concept*

The metabolic concept as outlined above has a degree of simplicity and neatness that, against the background of the complex problem which it addresses, seems to border upon naiveté. Its central theme is that chemical carcinogenesis is initiated by strong electrophiles producing irreversible and heritable structural alterations, explicitly or implicitly gene mutations in cellular DNA (cf. Miller and Miller, 1974, 1981).

Unsurprisingly, the concept suffers from a number of serious limitations. First, oxidative metabolism is not restricted to procarcinogens, neither as a process nor in terms of the responsible enzymes. The latter constitute a complex natural system of perhaps a dozen CO-binding hemoproteins, the cytochrome P450-dependent monooxygenases. Like the arylhydrocarbon hydroxylases, these enzymes appear to be highly inducible, under genetic control, to varying extents among tissues, individuals, and species of organisms. They occur in the endoplasmic reticulum mainly but also in other (e.g. nuclear) cellular membranes of the liver predominantly and of other organs (mainly skin, lung, bladder, and intestines) in smaller amounts. In addition to procarcinogens, their substrates include noncarcinogenic xenochemicals such as methyl and butyl carbamates and drugs such as meprobamate and pentobarbital. Such xenochemical-oriented metabolizing activities of the monooxygenases, and also of the linked conjugating (e.g. with sulfate, phosphate, and glucuronate) enzymes, are secondary to the main function of the enzymes. This function is to render water-soluble (hydrophilic) those of the body's unwanted cellular products (e.g. steroid hormones, fatty acids, and other lipids) which are too hydrophobic for ready renal and other excretions. (For reviews or extensive discussions, see Chapter Five, Section 5.3.2; Gorrod, 1978; Arnott *et al.*, 1979; Irving, 1979).

Second, the major site (the liver) of metabolic activation of a procarcinogen and that of the latter's tumorigenic activity are rarely identical. For instance, the bladder is the major site of tumorigenesis by benzidine in dogs and by 2-naphthylamine in dogs, hamsters, and non-human primates (for references and other examples, see Chapter Five; this chapter, Section 9.2.4; IARC Working Group, 1980, 1982). Indeed, practically any tissue or organ has been implicated as the major site of tumorigenesis by one procarcinogen or another.

Third, the correlation between procarcinogen activation and tumorigenesis is poor. For instance, the guinea pig is refractory to the carcinogenic influences of 2-acetylaminofluorene (AAF). Yet, this animal metabolically activates the O-glucuronide of N-hydroxy-AAF by deacetylation, and also AAF by N-hydroxylation (Gutmann and Bell, 1977). In fact, regardless of its oncogenicity or otherwise, AAF is uniformly activated metabolically in the livers of all mammals tested (Weisburger and Weisburger, 1973; Irving, 1979).

Fourth, the marked interspecies and intraspecies differences in innate susceptibility to oncogenesis by a given procarcinogen (Chapter Five, Sections 5.2 and 5.3) are not necessarily due to corresponding differences in innate capacity to metabolically activate the agent. For instance, in different strains of rats and mice selected for their differential subsceptibility to colon carcinogenesis by 1, 2-dimethylhydrazine (DMH), the same differential susceptibility is expressed in response to administered DMH (the procarcinogen) as to administered methylazoxymethanol, the proximate carcinogen of DMH (Deschner *et al.*, 1984).

Finally, for a considerable number of experimental and/or human carcinogens, neither metabolic activation nor the mediation of electrophiles, strong or weak, is known to be involved or necessary. These include certain natural or synthetic hormones (Chapter Four, Section 4.2), mineral oils, strongly anionic (nucleophilic) carcinogens (discussed below, Section 9.5.5), and foreign bodies (FBs) such as asbestos, plastic films, and glass fibre. The FBs are usually complex mixtures that may, like tobacco smoke and fossil fuels that are associated with lung and other cancers in man, contain trace amounts of various carcinogens. However, the oncologic activity of the FBs depend upon their physical rather than chemical properties (Brand *et al.*, 1975; Stanton *et al.*, 1977; Wagner *et al.*, 1984). This activity may be augmented by natural body substances such as histones and polyamines (Lavelle and MacIomhair, 1984).

9.5.5 *The Elusive Critical Cellular Target in Tumour Initiation*

In the initiation of experimental chemical carcinogenesis, practically all of the major cellular substructures or macromolecular classes, as well as the intercellular matrix, have been variously implicated as the major site of interaction with the ultimate carcinogens. This can be hardly surprising since, by definition (Section 9.5.2), these agents are highly reactive so that they would be expected to undergo rapid interactions with any suitable ligand present at their *situ nascendi* or within their reaction radii. Thus, they, though not necessarily their precursors, have short biological half-lives. In comparative studies in rats, for instance, complete metabolism of the procarcinogen dimethylnitrosamine required from three to six hours and that of the diethyl analogue somewhat longer; whereas the half-lives of the proximate carcinogens, the N-methyl and the N-ethyl derivatives of nitrosourea, were two and five minutes respectively (Margison and O'Connor, 1979). Since procarcinogen metabolism is predominantly a cytoplasmic event (Section 9.5.4), the major targets of the metabolically generated ultimate carcinogens would be cytoplasmic nucleophils such as water, proteins, and transfer and messenger RNAs. In contrast, the major targets of the intrinsically reactive carcinogens such as the nitrosamides and biological alkylating agents would be extracellular nucleophils. The latter would include collagen, fibronectin, laminin, and other matrix proteins, as well as the glycoproteins and other glycoconjugates of the plasma membrane. Many experimental studies have consistently demonstrated the covalent binding of chemical carcinogens preferentially to functional groups such as methionyl-S, ε-lysyl-NH_2, histidyl-N, seryl-OH, and threonyl-OH in proteins (Barry and Gutman, 1973; Kriek and Westra, 1979; Allfrey et al., 1979). The binding sites have also included various hydroxyl, ethylenic, and other nucleophilic centres in lipids, glycolipids, and other glycoconjugates (Yogeeswaran, 1983); and N–7, C–8, and 0–6 of guanine in DNA and RNA, as well as 0–4 of thymine in DNA (Lawley, 1979). Some chemical carcinogens such as mitomycin C and benzo(a)pyrene, like the natural polyamines spermine and spermidine, bind non-covalently (intercalate) in the groove of double-helical DNA, causing conformational changes (Irving, 1979). However, such physicochemical binding is not correlatable with tumorigenicity (Ts'o et al., 1974). Many chemical as well as physical carcinogens interact preferentially with the transcriptionally inactive (heterochromatic) rather than active (euchromatic) regions of DNA (Tomura and van Lancker, 1980). Finally, among the various sites considered as the targets of the ultimate carcinogens are the nucleus (Lawley, 1979), the mitochondrion (Anghilieri, 1978; Backer and Weinstein, 1980), the plasma membrane (Yogeeswaran, 1983), and the intercellular matrix (Alitalo and Vaheri, 1982).

Other than its great variety, this binding concept in the initiation of tumorigenesis has several interpretative difficulties. For instance, as demonstrated with a homologous series of alkyl carbamates and their N-hydroxy derivatives (Nery, 1968), the binding is neither restricted to carcinogens nor correlatable with tumorigenicity. Further, at least one type of binding, methylation, which is effected by a large group of experimental carcinogens (e.g. certain methyl derivatives of nitrosamines, nitrosamides, nitrosoureas, hydrazines, sulfates, and sulfonates), is also a vital physiological process. The latter is effected by S-adenosyl-L-methionine in the presence of appropriate cytosolic and/or nuclear methyltransferases. Physiological methylation of histone lysyl, arginyl, and carboxyl residues potentiates histone function, including the higher organization of chromatin which is itself associated with eukaryotic gene expression and tumorigenesis (Lipetz et al., 1982). Indeed, physiological methylation of cellular macromolecules such as histones and DNA is an essential part of eukaryotic gene control (Bird, 1984). Perhaps other types of alkylating carcinogens such as ethionine, which is a rodent hepatocarcinogen and a biological ethylating agent (Miller and Miller, 1974), interfere with physiological methylation by blockage of the methylation sites or by transferase inactivation (Cox and Tuck, 1981). This rationalization is not feasible for the carcinogen-mediated methylation which, however, may be un-physiological and may thus induce aberrations of the associated normal gene control mechanisms.

There is clearly no convincing evidence for the identity of the presumed critical cellular target in chemical carcinogenesis or, indeed, for the necessity for such a target. There are, for instance, the neoplastic transformations and related changes which are undergone spontaneously by cells through the latter's serial sub-culturing or through alterations in the nutrients or other culture conditions, i.e. without the mediation of any known carcinogen (Chapter Three, Section 3.6.2.3). Among the features involved in such changes are morphology, chromosome and biochemical analysis, growth characteristics, and tumorigenicity (Aubert *et al.*, 1984) as well as increasing heterogeneity due apparently to induced adaptation rather than to mutation or selection of pre-existing variants (Rubin, 1984). There is also the above-mentioned (Section 9.5.4) phenomenon of the tumorigenicity of agents such as asbestos and other foreign bodies (FBs).

Like the FBs, certain experimental carcinogens, among them trypan blue, may be engulfed by phagocytes but they are incapable of even entering the cells they transform. They thus can undergo neither metabolic activation nor chemical interaction with any intercellular target in the latter cells. In fact, it is this incapacity that is the basis of the traditional histological use of trypan blue to distinguish dead from living cells. This agent is highly anionic, and hence highly nucleophilic instead of, like the proposed ultimate carcinogens (Section 9.5.2), electrophilic. Among other strongly anionic experimental carcinogens are the carageenans, i.e. a heterogeneous group of sulfated polygalactans obtainable from red seaweed and other sources (Wakabayashi *et al.*, 1978); and dextran sulfate, a potent but non-mutagenic inducer of intestinal neoplasms in rats (Hirono *et al.*, 1981). Such carcinogens also include artificial sweeteners such as the alkali metal salts of cyclamate and saccharin (IARC, 1980), which may also act as promoters of tumorigenesis (Hicks *et al.*, 1975).

9.5.6 Promotion and Cellular Differentiation

Reversibility or potential reversibility of the neoplastic state to normal or near-normal phenotypes is not an unknown feature of established neoplasms (Section 9.10.3). Consequently, with its essential feature of reversibility, promotion is apparently more relevant to carcinogenesis in humans than is initiation with its corresponding irreversibility (Section 9.5.1). Curiously, however, an inordinately greater investigative effort has been made to define a molecular basis for initiation than for promotion during the past four decades since the birth of the two-stage hypothesis (Section 9.5.1).

Currently, fundamental information on the nature of promotion is sparse but significant, pointing increasingly to a basis in cellular differentiation. The active agents in croton oil, the traditional promoter, are phorbol esters, particularly 12-tetradecanoylphorbol 13-acetate (TPA). Some other agents have also been found to be active as promoters in the mouse skin and few other (e.g. thyroid, renal, hepatic, bladder, and intestinal) experimental systems. Examples are 4, 4'-diaminodiphenylmethane in thyroid carcinogenesis (Hiasa, *et al.*, 1984) and nephrotoxic compounds such as folic acid and basic lead acetate in renal carcinogenesis (Shirai *et al.*, 1984). In various nondifferentiating untransformed cell lines in culture, TPA and other promoters can, without the aid of an initiator, reversibly elicit some of the growth, cell surface, and other features usually associated with transformed cell lines (Rovera *et al.*, 1980). As further reviewed by Rovera *et al.*, these agents can also *induce* differentiation in some cell lines, e.g. lines of mouse erythroleukemia, mouse myeloid leukemia, and human leukemias, but *inhibit* differentiation in others. Among the latter are Friend erythroleukemia and some lines of meyloid leukemia in the mouse, and of embryo myoblasts and chondroblasts in the chick.

Such effects of the promoters are probably associated with cellular products acting as differentiation factors. Polypeptides with differentiation inducing activity have been produced through mitogen-stimulation of both normal and neoplastic cells, e.g. human mononuclear blood cells and cells of the T-lymphocytic leukemic cell line HUT-102 (Olsson *et al.*, 1984; see also Diamond *et al.*, 1980).

9.6 The Somatic Mutation Hypothesis

9.6.1 Carcinogenicity and Bacterial Mutagenicity

As discussed above (Sections 9.5.4 and 9.5.5) uncertainty still surrounds the nature or even the reality of initiation and critical cellular targets in carcinogenesis. Despite this, the somatic mutation hypothesis, particularly since its recent revival (Ames *et al.*, 1973) after a long period in the doldrums (Chapter Seven, Section 7.2), has proclaimed the initiating event to be a mutation in nuclear DNA as the target. Ames *et al.*, showed that many chemical carcinogens, presumably as their ultimate forms (Section 9.5.2), are mutagens in selected strains of *Salmonella typhimurium* in the presence of rodent hepatic microsomes. In recent years, this bacterial system (the 'Ames test') has been gaining in popularity as a rapid and cheap means of screening the increasingly complex human chemical environment (Section 9.3.1) for mutagens as potential human carcinogens (for reviews see Ames, 1979; Epstein and Swartz, 1981; Miller and Miller, 1981).

9.6.2 Problems of Definition

Much confusion currently surrounds the precise definition of a mutation that is relevant to the somatic mutation hypothesis. As usually defined, a mutation is any 'permanent heritable change in genetic information carried by deoxyribonucleic acid (DNA) in the cell nucleus' (cf. Coulter, 1983).

However, there are many known examples of such a change which occur naturally in biological evolution and development, but for which there is little or no evidence for their causal connection with oncogenesis. The most important of these are the germ-line meiotic recombinations which, if regarded as mutations, would make all humans and other heterozygotes except identical twins mutants in interindividual comparisons. This principle would apply equally to the nondisjunctions with their resulting monosomies and trisomies, the translocations, the ring chromosomes such as those described by Schmid *et al.* (1983), and the other heritable anomalies which sometimes accompany the normal meiotic process (Chapter Seven, Section 7.3.5). There are also somatic mutations .such as those associated with normal ageing (Burnet, 1974; Bertell, 1977) and possibly with ageing-related features such as interference with normal hematopoiesis (Lipschitz *et al.*, 1984); mutations associated with severe malnourishment in children (Murthy and Rahiman,

1983); and the various gene amplifications which accompany processes such as development of drug resistance and, in rabbits, of attenuation in myxomatosis (Doolittle *et al.*, 1984). Even a definition restricting the DNA structural change to the cell undergoing neoplastic transformation would have to exclude a prezygotic 'mutation' such as that presumed to be associated with retinoblastoma (cf. Vogel, 1979) or one of the cancer-predisposing conditions such as xeroderma pigmentosum or polyposis coli (Chapter Seven, Section 7.5). Such a prezygotically inherited mutation would occur equally in all of the nucleated cells of the affected individual.

In the context of the hypothesis a mutation may be redefined as a permanent and heritable structural change which occurs in the nuclear DNA of a somatic cell *and which is the primary cause of the transformation and a distinguishing feature of that cell.* The accurate identification of such a change must be at least as difficult as that of the originating cell of a frank neoplasm (Section 9.1).

9.6.3 Somatic Mutation, Oncogenes, and Cancer

A so-far unique example of a known cancer-associated genetic mutation in somatic cells is that of a recently discovered oncogene of human bladder cancer (Section 9.2.6; for a review, see Weinberg, 1983). This oncogene carries a single point mutation, a guanine-thymine transversion, that results in a glycine-valine substitution in the twelfth amino acid residue of the oncogene-encoded 21,000-dalton protein.

This oncogene has sometimes been regarded as evidence for a human cancer having been initiated by a somatic mutation (e.g. Coulter, 1983). However, such a conclusion would appear premature. It would depend upon still unresolved questions such as whether or not the point mutation is absent from the normal bladder cells of the patient bearing the cancer, and whether or not the oncogene but not its unmutated counterpart can and in fact did transform one or more of these cells that developed into the cancer. Most important would be the question as to how such a simple mutation could have produced such devastating effects as those produced by the cancer. A great variety of non-pathogenic point and other mutations, such as the over 100 normal genetic variants of just one type of adult hemoglobin (Chapter Five, Section 5.1), occurs in the general human population.

These are complex questions. For instance, by itself, the bladder cancer oncogene transformed NIH3T3 mouse fibroblasts; but it required the co-operation of another oncogene in order to transform primary embryo mouse fibroblasts (Weinberg, 1983). In contrast with the latter, normal cells, the former are highly abnormal, they having been immortalized by extensive serial passaging and apparently been thus already primed for transformation.

Such an indication of transformation being an effect of cooperating factors, a major one of which is the intrinsic nature of the target cell itself, is amply supported by related findings. The avian leukosis virus (ALV), for instance, produces a fatal lymphoma in chickens, but it has no oncogene and it is not transforming. Sometimes, ALV integrates its DNA copy close to the cellular oncogene *c-myc* in an immunoglobulin (Ig) heavy chain locus (Bishop, 1982). In both man and mouse, ALV may thus, via its transcriptional promoter or enhancer element, stimulate *c-myc* transcription and oncogenicity (Hayday *et al.*, 1984). In man, *c-myc* is located 5' to the Ig genes (Hollis *et al.*, 1984), on that part of chromosome 8 that is involved in the t(8;14) translocation found in many Burkitt's lymphomas (Neel *et al.*, 1982). However, any role for *c-myc* activation in production of the translocation is problematical. For instance, the translocation is far from being a universal feature of the lymphomas, although it does predominate in B-lymphocytic neoplasms (Chapter Eight, Section 8.3; see also Mitelman, 1981). Other associated problems, as pointed out by Bishop (1982), are that ALV does not always integrate close to *c-myc*, and that its tumorigenic effect is not restricted to B lymphocytes. For instance, ALV sometimes produces renal tumours. Also, the activation of *c-myc* is sometimes also effected by agents other than ALV, e.g. chicken syncytial virus. Moreover, *v-myc*, the viral analogue of *c-myc*, is not known to produce lymphomas. Finally, some oncogenic viruses contain more than one oncogene. The avian retrovirus Mill Hill no.2, for instance, contains two unrelated and independently expressed cell-derived oncogenes, *v-mil* and *v-myc* (Jansen *et al.*, 1984). In contrast, only about 20 per cent of human tumours thus far investigated have yielded oncogenes upon transfection (Weinberg,1983).

9.6.4 Limitations of the Hypothesis: Some Unrealized Great Expectations

Consideration of the basic tenets of the somatic mutation hypothesis leads to certain testable expectations which, in actual practice, have remained unfilfilled. First, the primary cause of the requisite informational change is DNA damage (e.g. base modification and/or chain breakage) effected by the carcinogenic mutagen in the cell undergoing transformation. This damage must be sufficiently slight for it to be effectively repaired, so as to maintain the viability of the cell and the continuity and readability of the DNA chain. Cells containing extensive, unrepaired, or irreparable DNA damage are unlikely to survive or replicate. Hence, DNA damage is not synonymous with mutagenesis, and a potent DNA-damaging agent such as UVB radiation would be cytotoxic rather than mutagenic. However, this agent is associated with one of the commonest of human cancers, i.e. non-melanoma skin cancer (Chapter Six, Section 6.4.1).

Second, the DNA damage must be incorrectly repaired, in order to introduce the requisite structural change. Faulty DNA repair is thus an integral part of mutagenesis. Consequently, in the presence of a mutagen, an inhibitor of DNA repair such as caffeine (Timson, 1977) would increase cytotoxicity but inhibit both mutagenesis and carcinogenesis. However, coffee-drinking, particularly with cigarette-smoking, has been associated with cancers of the human bladder and pancreas (MacMahon *et al.*, 1981; Mabuchi, 1983). Caffeine and other xanthines have been reported to be mutagenic (Kuhlmann *et al.*, 1968); but, in a case-control study, caffeine-free but not regular coffee was significantly associated with pancreatic cancer (Lin and Kessler, 1981).

Third, the twin need for the introduced mutation to be permanent and heritable requires the mutation to be faithfully replicated with DNA and passed on to all of the progenies of the initially transformed cell. According to the hypothesis, all tumours are of monoclonal origin; and, in fact, this has been repeatedly claimed by its proponents from the time of Boveri himself (Chapter Seven, Section 7.2). However, most if not all single neoplasms are heterogeneous in features such as morphology, drug resistance, antigen expression, metastatic potential, degree and kind of cellular differentiation, and other features (Poste and Fidler, 1980; Heppner and Miller, 1983; Talmadge, 1983; Layton and Franks, 1984) including transforming *ras* (rat sarcoma-associated) oncogenes (Albino *et al.*, 1984). However, like the ultimate cellular origins of neoplasms (Section 9.1), the points of origin of these various types of heterogeneity during oncogenesis are not known with certainty.

Fourth, the initiating mutation is more likely to be intragenic than chromosomal, although the founding basis of the hypothesis was chromosomal abnormalities or asymmetrical karyokinesis (Chapter Seven, Section 7.2). In recent times, most carcinogenic mutagens have been described to modify specific DNA bases (Section 9.5.2). Consequently, in appropriate circumstances, mainly change of one or more of the triplet codons in the protein encoding region of the affected gene, the mutation would lead to the corresponding mutated gene products (RNA and protein), analogous to the mutated protein encoded by the human bladder cancer oncogene described above (Section 9.6.3). Such products of the mutated gene, as well as the gene itself (cf. the third feature described above), would be specific diagnostic features capable of un-equivocally distinguishing the tumour or any of its component neoplastic cells from the normal counterparts. However, despite the inordinate expenditure of research effort in this direction, such a specificity has remained unknown in the annals of human oncology (Section 9.2.5).

Finally, the frequency of the oncogenesis-initiating mutation should show a one-to-one correlation with that of transformation or carcinogenesis. However, this expectation has also not been realized. As incisively reviewed by Rubin (1980), in comparative *in vitro* studies, the frequency of transformation can be up to 540 times (Barrett and T'so, 1978) or even 1,000 times (Parodi and Brambilla, 1977) that of mutation. Moreover, the *in vitro* systems, in their use of isolated and dispersed cells, drastically alter the cell density, cell matrix, junctional communication, and related features which are so vital for the regulation of cell behaviour *in vivo*. *In vitro*, transformation can be induced by the culture conditions alone, such as low population density or alteration of the plasma membrane (e.g. by proteases) or the cell matrix (Parshad and Sanford, 1968; Alitalo and Vaheri, 1982; Aubert *et al.*, 1984). The frequency of induced transformation in the *in vitro* systems at low cell density has been estimated to be some ten thousand million times that in intact animals (Parodi and Brambilla, 1977).

Neither is mutagenicity in the bacterial tests correlatable with carcinogenicity in the animal tests. As further reviewed by Rubin (1980) some potent animal carcinogens are nonmutagenic; and many noncarcinogens, including even the indispensable oxygen, are mutagenic. Further, in view of well-established oncologic features such as the natural specificities in neoplasia (Section 9.2.4), there can be no certainty that a factor found active or inactive in one of the mutagenicity tests will not show the opposite effect in another; and, analogously, that it will not show variable carcinogenic or noncarcinogenic activities among animals or humans. Consequently, for certainty, any risk of human cancer that may be associated with an untested factor might be indicated roughly by animal testing. However, in the final analysis, it will have to be determined by human cancer epidemiology (cf. Section 9.3).

In view of such limitations of the somatic mutation hypothesis, it seems difficult to justify, in theoretical or practical terms, the currently widespread and growing use of the bacterial and other mutagenicity tests, avowedly as rapid and cheap means for screening the increasingly complex human chemical environment for cancer-risk factors. That the limitations may stem from a misconceived foundation of the hypothesis itself is further substantiated by an appropriate consideration of the fundamental differences which exist between bacteria and humans, or between prokaryotes and eukaryotes.

9.7 Bacterial and Other Non-human Systems as Inappropriate Models for the Study of Human Cancer

Despite the likelihood that bacteria and humans represent two different lines of biological evolution (Gilbert, 1978), the many unifying features of the biosphere might suggest that any one of the latter's organisms is a suitable model for the study of cancer in any other. Among such features are a cellular basis, the same six predominant elements (C, H, O, N, P, S), the same five nucleic acid bases, a largely identical genetic code (cf. Section 9.8.5), the same 21 amino acids, many similar types of cellular components and products, and a reliance for survival upon reproduction, nutrition, and ecogenetic relationships.

However, the diversifying features seem sufficiently fundamental to suggest that the only proper (though often impracticable) model for the study of human cancer is man. For instance, many bacterial features have little or no counterparts in humans and other higher species. These include independent cellularity, propagation by binary fission, cell wall (for an extensive discussion, see Hammond *et al.*, 1984), operons, a 'streamlined' genome lacking nonfunctional DNA (Gilbert, 1978), and a practically simultaneous occurrence of transcription and translation. Conversely, bacteria have no need for a eukaryotic feature such as the nuclear membrane. Except in some mitotic stages marked by spindle movements and a virtual absence of macromolecular biosynthesis, this membrane separates nuclear phenomena such as DNA, DNA repair, replication, and transcription, and RNA processing from related cytoplasmic phenomena. Among the latter are the polyribosomes, mRNA translation, postsynthetic modifications of the translated products, and metabolic activation or detoxification of carcinogenic and other potentially hazardous substances of either intrinsic or extrinsic origin.

It is perhaps the subtle differences in such nuclear and cytoplasmic phenomena that underpin the natural specificities in neoplasia which make even the common laboratory animals unreliable as models for the proper study of human cancer (Section 9.2.4). This is despite the fact that all higher animals share other unifying features not found in bacteria. These include certain basic morphological and anatomical features, sexual reproduction involving meiosis and heterogametic fertilization, and, above all, multicellular development involving an integrated interdependent stage-and-phase specific differentiation of a constant genome (Britten and Davidson, 1969; Davidson and Britten, 1979). As a rough measure of the complexity of this development, some ten million million cells in man, i.e. about 200 times the number in the rat, participate in the phenomenon at any one time; and almost a thousand times as many (10^{16}) cell divisions are undergone by the human zygote and its progenies in the average human individual (Enesco and Leblond, 1962; Cairns, 1978). The normal gene controls in such a complexity, and the possibilities of their operational errors in carcinogenesis, are far beyond current comprehension.

9.8 Some Unique Features of the Eukaryotic Cell

9.8.1 Nucleosomes and Chromatin Superstructure

Eukaryotic chromatin is a complex mixture of DNA, RNA, and protein that, in man, respectively constitute about 15, 10, and 75 per cent of its total weight. Its basic building block, the nucleosome, consists of an octameric core of a pair each of the four 'core' histones (H2A, H2B, H3, and H4) and a supercoil of double-helical DNA wrapped around the core. The nucleosomes are arranged like beads on a string of DNA, with the fifth histone (H1) occurring as a stabilizing feature within the internucleosomal linker regions. The nucleosomal beads are coiled and supercoiled into cylinders made up of concentric layers of rows of nucleosomes. This nucleosomal structure, with its arcs and helices, is dynamic, showing large variability in conformation, folding, and unfolding, particularly in euchromation, the transcriptionally active regions of DNA (Dubochet and Noll, 1978). At least four subchromosomal levels of organization are present, and there are indications that gene expression and tumorigenesis are modulated by this complex superstructure and its dynamicity (Lipetz *et al.*, 1982).

9.8.2 Heterochromatin and 'Useless' DNA

Unlike the fully functional prokaryotic chromatin, eukaryotic chromatin contains variable amounts of 'nonfunctional','excess' or 'useless' mainly repetitive DNA sequences found largely in heterochromatin. Such sequences are virtually absent in some primitive eukaryotes such as *Aspergillus*, are minimal in others such as *E. coli* and *Saccharomyces*, but are abundant in higher organisms (Doolittle and Sapienza, 1980). They thus seem to have been progressively accumulated during eukaryotic evolution, as evolutionary hitch-hikers claimed to serve no useful purpose in the cell's economy (Orgel and Crick, 1980). However, they may serve as a buffer against some types of cellular injury, e.g. as the preferential binding sites of physical and chemical carcinogens (Tomura and van Lancker, 1980). They may also play a role in eukaryotic gene control (Davidson and Britten, 1979).

9.8.3 Gene Rearrangement and RNA Splicing: the Generation of Diversity

A particularly important feature of the eukaryotic cell is the pronounced capacity of its chromatin to generate a great diversity of genetic structure or of gene products from identical sets of inherited genes or gene segments. The highly controlled gene rearrangements occurring at meiosis generate the genetic individuality of eggs, sperms, and heterozygotes. Those occurring during lymphocyte ontogeny are behind the previously perplexing features such as the remarkable diversity and specificity of lymphocyte clones and immunoglobulins (Igs) (Sakano *et al.*, 1979;

Schilling *et al.*, 1980; Kurosawa *et al.*, 1981; Tonegawa, 1983); and the sequence switch, during antibody production, from IgM to IgD to IgG, IgA, or IgE (Liu *et al.*, 1980; Robertson and Hobart, 1981).

Splicing of primary RNA transcripts of structural genes containing transcribable but untranslatable intervening sequences ('introns') was postulated by Gilbert in 1978 as a eukaryote-specific means for generating variants of a single protein. Since then, this postulate has been amply verified and extended, to dispel for ever the once tenacious doctrine of 'one gene, one protein'. The phenomenon of more than one mRNA or polypeptide from single genes has been described for, among others, cancer-associated genes such as those of SV40, adenoviruses, immunoglobulins, calcitonin, growth hormone, and prolactin (Gubbins *et al.*, 1980; Chien and Thompson, 1980; Malcolm, 1981). In some instances, the diversification can result from a combination of events, such as the two myosin light chains produced from the same myosin gene through two modes of splicing combined with transcription from two different initiation sites (Nabeshima *et al.*, 1984).

Differential splicing of primary transcripts is also a contributory factor to the tissue-specific expressions of the same structural genes, such those for α-amylase (Schibler *et al.*, 1980; Young *et al.*, 1981; Hagenbüchle *et al.*, 1981; Flavell, 1981). This enzyme occurs physiologically at significantly higher levels in some glands such as the pancreas and salivary glands than in liver. Other contributory factors may be the tissue-specific differences in promoters or other diffusible factors affecting expression of the relevant structural genes rather than differences in the genes themselves or in *cis*-acting regulatory sites (Ziff, 1980).

9.8.4 *Selective Gene Amplification: Transformation as a Dosage Effect*

The eukaryote cell exhibits a marked capacity for selective gene amplification. This process involves discrete genetic elements which are sometimes regarded as molecular parasites. They replicate independently of the chromosomes in which they are embedded, and the copies then become transposed to new genomic positions without loss of the originals. Apparently, the selected gene is co-amplified with variable lengths of flanking DNA, at a frequency that is influenced by the chromosomal position of the gene (Wahl *et al.*, 1984). Also, the co-amplified DNA itself may have undergone various recombinational events (Fox, 1984a).

The identity of the amplified gene is rarely known. In spontaneous neoplasms it may be an oncogene. Several oncogene-derived transforming proteins, some with tyrosine-phosphorylating activity are present in normal cells, but at greatly increased concentrations in transformed cells (Bishop, 1982). This led Bishop to suggest that transformation is a dosage effect. It is definable as aberrant gene control causing amplification and translocation with or without enhanced expression of selected normal gene(s). A supporting finding is that of an oncogene which occurs normally as a single copy but which is greatly amplified in human neuroblastoma cells (Schwab *et al.*, 1984).

9.8.5 *The Mitochondrion: the Enigmatic Symbiont of the Eukaryotic Cell*

The endosymbiotic relationship that exists between the eukaryotic cell and the mitochondrion, the ATP-dependent powerhouse of the cell, is of ancient ancestry. It may well have existed at least 1.5 thousand million years ago, to provide the vast energy requirements of the primitive chlorophyll-containing plants responsible for the initial conversion of the prebiotic reducing atmosphere into its present oxygenated form. In modern plants, the organelle has become especially well-developed, as indicated by its DNA being very large and multiformed (Fox, 1984b). In man and other higher animals, a mitochondrial function is the burning up of excess fat, apparently through the mediation of brown adipose tissue. In exchange for such services, the cell affords protection to the mitochondrion, through the latter's safe intracellular localization. It also provides mitochondrial proteins, most of which are nuclear-coded, suggesting the existence of extensive unidirectional gene transfer, i.e. from nucleus to mitochondrion, but not the reverse.

As an organelle, the mitochondrion is remarkable in that it displays a unique mixture of prokaryotic, eukaryotic, and independent properties. For instance, its inner membrane resembles the bacterial cell wall in a richness of cardiolipin. In contrast, its outer membrane, like that of the eukaryotic cell, is rich in cholesterol and phosphatidylinositol. Its eukaryotic features also include a genome with AT-rich unique and repetitive sequences, in fact one of the AT-richest known; and also with introns, e.g. in its cytochrome genes. Among its unique properties is its incomplete complement of the 31 tRNA species, e.g. in HeLa cells it has 23 species (Barrell *et al.*, 1980) and 24 in yeast (Bonitz *et al.*, 1980). Also, some of its codon-anticodon arrangements, particularly in their third or 'wobble' positions, differ significantly from the cellular counterparts. For instance, in the mitochondria of mammals (Barrell *et al.*, 1980), yeast (Bonitz *et al.*, 1980), and *Neurospora crassa* (Heckman *et al.*, 1980), UGA codes for tryptophan instead of termination, as does UGG in the UG family. In the AU family, the code is unconventional only in mammalian mitochondria. In general, the mitochondrial code is deviant in such respects as UGA coding for tryptophan, CUA for threonine instead of leucine, and AUA for methionine instead of isoleucine. Mitochondria appear to represent the unique deviants from an otherwise universal genetic code. Consideration of such properties has led to different theories of mitochondrial origin and evolution, e.g. the conventional endosymbiosis theory and theories based upon prokaryote-independent evolution or special creation (for a review, see Harington and Thornley, 1980).

The mitochondrion has been suggested to play an important role in oncogenesis (Section 9.5.5). Anghilieri (1978), for instance, has reviewed evidence to suggest that neoplastic transformation is a consequence of changes in the permeability of cellular membranes to calcium ions. This leads to unphysiological concentrations of the ions in mitochondria, to mitochondrial damage, and to disruptions of oxidative phosphorylation that enforce cellular shift towards glycolysis for energy production. The damage includes DNA fragmentation, resulting in incorporation of some of the fragments in cellular DNA, i.e. in reversal of the normal unidirectional gene flow. It also includes disturbance of mitochondrial role in membrane specification, resulting in cellular loss of growth inhibition and intercellular communication.

9.9 Conservatism in Biological Evolution and Development

The unifying principle underlying the above-discussed features of the eukaryotic cell is that of natural conservatism. Rather than upon unusual structures such as novel or mutated genes, this cell relies for its adaptations and diversifications upon existing features such as the dynamicity of its chromatin superstructure, the recombination and amplification of its inherited genes, the splicing of its primary RNA transcripts, and changes in its membrane and cytoplasmic properties.

The general applicability of this principle suggests that Nature does not lightly discard or change those of its past triumphs which have been useful in the past. Thus fixation of a single mutation in vital genes such as those for the core histones can require millions of years of evolutionary time (Wilson *et al.*, 1977). Also, rearrangement with or without amplification, rather than mutation, of inherited genes is the essential basis of features such as antigenic variation in trypanosomes, translocatable elements in maize, antibody diversity, yeast mating types, and transposons and insertion elements in bacteria (Williams *et al.*, 1979; Hoeijmakers *et al.*, 1980; Turner, 1980). In mutant salamanders, abnormal heart development has been corrected under the influence of normal endoderm (Lemanski *et al.*, 1979). Interspecifically, undifferentiated corneal epithelium of the chick has been induced by mouse embryonic dermis to produce feathers (Coulombre and Coulombre, 1971). More strikingly, chick embryonic epithelium has been induced by mouse molar mesenchyme to produce a variety of mammalian dental structures. The latter included perfectly formed crowns with differentiated ameloblasts depositing enamel matrix (Koller and Fisher, 1980). Homology between the genes for rat α-lactalbumin and chick lysozyme is extensive (Quasba and Safaya, 1984). Anaerobic glycolysis for energy production, i.e. the 'Warburg effect' that was almost traditionally regarded as a distinguishing feature of cancer cells, is an adaptation of the goldfish to anoxic conditions (Shoubridge and Hochachka, 1980). The newly discovered 'oncogenes' are turning out to be highly conserved normal genes of apparently vital importance in evolution and development (Sections 9.2.6, 9.6.3, and 9.8.4).

Clearly, the metazoan genome inherits adaptive and developmental capabilities which exceed those that are expressed during the normal development of the species to which it belongs. According to the DNA constancy rule, all of these capabilities are transmitted intact to all of the normal nucleated cells of the individual organism. It is thus possible that one or more of these cells, when faced with an appropriate microenvironmental threat, may, in the interest of self-survival and perhaps fortuitously in abrogation of the normal controls of the host organism, resort to some of these capabilities to generate cancer.

9.10 The Developmental Hypothesis

9.10.1 Tumorigenic Capabilities of the Normal Genome

It is now just around the centenary of the old controversy as to whether the essential basis of the body's phenotypic differences established during ontogeny is structural or functional (Chapter Two, Section 2.6.16). Weismann's fourth postulate, i.e. that the heredity-specifying particles (nuclear DNA) are intact in germ cells but are differently doled out to somatic cells, has long ago yielded to Naegeli's principle of differential expression of a structurally intact genome in both types of cells. However, the analogous controversy, that concerning the essential basis of normoneoplastic differences, still rages. In contrast with the mutational hypothesis, the developmental hypothesis specifies that Naegeli's principle applies equally to both sets of differences. In modern terms, the latter hypothesis envisages oncogenesis as natural or induced aberrations of fundamental ontogenic principles, i.e. of the still poorly understood differentiational controls of structurally intact inherited genes. This places oncogenetic mechanisms in the mainstream of the molecular biology of life itself.

Despite this poor understanding of what may well be the most crucial of all outstanding biological problems, there has been a growing appreciation that the mammalian and other metazoan genomes have evolved and retained all the information necessary for neoplastic expression (for some reviews see Markert, 1968; Nery, 1976; Pierce *et al.*, 1978; Braun, 1977; Mintz and Fleischman, 1981; Gateff, 1982). Among the prominent features of this expression, for instance, is the aberrant synthesis of normal embryofetal products such as AFP, CEA, isoenzymes, and hormones (Section 9.2.5).

The other prominent features of malignant expression are the pronounced propensities of cancer cells to proliferate at the expense of normal differentiation, to invade and metastasize, and eventually to effectively abrogate the normal controls, needs, and economy of the host organism. These features, like the embryofetal expressions, are also close mimicries of events in normal ontogeny. Thus, soon after fertilization, the mammalian zygote proliferates at the expense of differentiation until a considerable pool of stem cells has been produced. Ontogeny then proceeds apparently through a series of stem cell constellations with increasingly restricted developmental options. Embryofetal growth is one of the most rapid known to developmental biology. Moreover, it receives preferential treatment, as exemplified by the many annuals which bear seed once and then die or by the species of fish such as the Pacific salmon which stop feeding during spawning and then also die. In the developing mammalian embryo, melanoblasts migrate actively through many tissues before finally becoming localized at specific sites and differentiating into non-migrating melanocytes. Neural crest cells migrate from the primordial neural tube and then invade tissues with a degree of freedom comparable to that enjoyed throughout life by macrophages, leukocytes, lymphocytes, and other circulating cells. During pregnancy, pieces of placental tissue may metastasize to the maternal lung only to disappear after term.

Such a behaviour of placental tissue is a mimicry of the 'conditional' neoplasms, i.e. tumorous growths that are dependent for their existence upon the continued presence of the inciting agent(s). A related example is the mammalian corpus luteum that is formed from granulosa and theca cells in the ruptured Graffian follicles, and which regularly undergoes hormone-dependent cyclical growth and disappearance. Analogously, conditional neoplasms such as those of *Drosophila melanogaster* (Gateff, 1982) are also formed in rabbits under the influence of the dye Scarlet Red placed in contact with the epithelial cells of the ear (cf. Chapter Three, Section 3.6.3.5.). Continued presence of the dye causes the cells to multiply rapidly, invade underlying tissues deeply, and even enter the blood and lymphatic systems. As reviewed by Braun (1978) similar effects have also been produced in many other systems including overgrowth stimulating factor, trypsin, or pronase on cultured chick embryo fibroblasts, and plant hormones (auxins, gibberelins, cytokinins) on plant cells. In the latter cells, the effects have included growth stimulation, production of seedless fruits from unfertilized flowers, and abnormal growth leading to cytoxicity and plant death. Further, as already discussed (Section 9.5.6), phorbol esters and other promoters can reversibly elicit many of the growth and differentiational characteristics associated with transformation.

There are many other known indications of the neoplastic propensities of the normal genome. Among these are the capacities of certain normal genes to stimulate or suppress transformation (Sections 9.2.6 and 9.6.3). Also, established neoplasms generally reflect the stage of stem cell differentiation or of ontogeny at which transformation presumably occurs (Pierce *et al.*, 1978; Mintz and Fleischman, 1981). This determines the differentiational characteristics of the neoplasms produced, within the range from the well-differentiated (benign) to the poorly differentiated (malignant) with a preponderance of proliferative (anaplastic) cells. Thus, as reviewed by Gardner (1983), comparisons of features such as the cellular heterogeneity and antigenic properties of teratocarcinoma stem cells from man and mouse suggest that the human neoplasms originate at an earlier stage of ontogeny than the murine counterparts. Analogously, in *Drosophila melanogaster*, the tumours occurring in the embryo are of mixed types; but in the larva they are malignant neuroblastomas, imaginal disc neoplasms, and malignant blood cell neoplasms, and benign gonial neoplasms in the adult. Finally, abrogation of normal host logistics seen in neoplasia has its non-neoplastic counterparts in features such as overhealing during tissue regeneration, and ectopic or super-numerary tissues, organs, and digits. In fact, Pierce *et al.* (1978) have envisaged oncogenesis as various caricatures of normal tissue regeneration.

9.10.2 Normal Developmental Capabilities of the Neoplastic Genome

The phenomenon of widespread cytogenic anomalies, some quite bizarre and even hypodiploid, in neoplastic cells from established tumours (Chapter Eight) would make it unlikely that the genomes of such cells have retained intact the full developmental capabilities of their normal counterparts. However, the well-established fact that some neoplastic genomes do express such capabilities suggests strongly that such anomalies, at least those occurring in develop-mentally vital genetic elements, are not necessary for oncogenesis. Thus, McKinnell and others have repeatedly shown that nuclei containing incorporated herpesviral DNA and derived almost certainly from frog (*Rana pipiens*) renal adenocarcinoma cells, when transplanted into enucleated frog ova and allowed to develop normally, sometimes produced normally appearing larvae and even swimming tadpoles though, as yet, not adult frogs (McKinnell *et al.*, 1969, 1976; King and DiBerardino, 1965). Such nuclear trans-plantation experiments are fraught with technical difficulties that complicate even analogous experiments involving normal nucleus-donor cells, e.g. from *Xenopus laevus* (Gurdon, 1974). Analogously, teratocarcinoma cells or even just one of these cells from mice of the 129 or the LT strain, when microinjected into mouse blastocyst and allowed to develop normally, participated in the development of all of the tissues of the allophenic mice which were produced (Ilmensee and Mintz, 1976). As recently reviewed by Mintz and Fleishman (1981), the murine teratocarcinomas contain neoplastic stem cells called embryonal carcinoma cells, as well as tissue representatives of all three embryonic germ layers including nerve (neurons, ganglion cells, glial cells), bone, cartilage, muscle (striated, smooth, cardiac), adipose tissue, pigmented cells, hair, and a variety of epithelia, e.g. in ducts, tubules, and cysts. However, representatives of liver, kidney, lung, thymus, and certain other organs or tissues are absent. The human teratocarcinomas are sometimes even more heterogeneous than the murine counterparts, as they display some highly organized structures such as teeth, fingers, eyes, and hair (Gardner, 1983). There are other indications of the totipotency of the neoplastic genome. These include the capacity of transformed rodent cells to produce a variety of normal tissues (Rabinowitz and Sachs, 1970). In plants also, neoplastic cells from Kostoff genetic, *Agrobacterium tumefaciens*-induced, and other types of neoplasm (Braun, 1977) including mature root callus of *Panax ginseng* (Chang and Hsing, 1980) can undergo all of the complex events involved in the normal development of embryos, organs, and sometimes even flowering and seed-bearing plants. Analogously to the herpesvirus-containing frog tumour-cell nuclei described above, the bacterial plasmid of *A. tumefaciens* can persist in the plants grown from the crown gall tumour cells of tobacco (Drummond *et al.*, 1977).

9.10.3 Reversibility in Cancer: Immunological versus Differentiational Mechanisms

The central premises of the somatic mutation hypothesis are that the cancer phenotype is permanent and irreversible, and that this phenotype is initiated by somatic mutation with similar properties (Sections 9.6.1 and 9.6.2). However, there are indications that the phenotype is not necessarily any more permanent than are the body's normal phenotypes established during ontogeny without the intervention of somatic mutation. In fact, it has already become one of the basic tenets of oncology that many types of even highly advanced cancer or cancer cells can undergo spontaneous or induced reversions into their normal or near-normal counterparts. In 1966, for instance, Everson and Cole documented 176 cases of spontaneous reversions of established human cancers such as hypernephroma, malignant melanomas, choriocarcinomas, and neuroblastomas. Among other related examples are the 67 cases of spontaneous reversions of human metastatic renal carcinomas reviewed by Fairlamb in 1981.

Neuroblastoma is the classic example of spontaneous reversion of a highly advanced and potentially fatal human cancer. Despite its poor therapeutic response (Section 9.2.2; see also McWhirter and Siskind, 1984), this childhood cancer sometimes reverses spontaneously, usually into benign ganglioneuroma, even in the case of the Stage IV-S disease (Evans *et al.*, 1971). The latter usually afflicts children under three months of age and commonly involves the liver, skin, and bone marrow. Tsuchida *et al.* (1984) recently described a case involving ectopic liver tissue attached to one of the adrenal glands.

The biochemical basis of the reversions in cancer is controversial. The popular view that it is immunological (cf. Bloom, 1973; Pochedly, 1976) seems inconsistent with general features such as the inception and at least early development of perhaps most human cancers in apparently immunologically competent individuals, and the consistent failure of the numerous attempts to diagnose or treat the disease effectively and specifically by immunological means. Further, the conceptual basis of cancer immunity has changed in keeping with conflicting data that have been accumulating ever since it became suspected (cf. Gorer, 1938) that the immune system might recognize and reject allogeneic tumours. Thus, the basis was variably held to be specific in humoral immunity that may be abrogated by 'blocking factors' (Hellstrom and Hellstrom, 1974), in cellular immunity and immune surveillance (Burnett, 1970), or in non-specific immunity effected by macrophages (Eccles and Alexander, 1976; Hibbs *et al.*, 1982) or natural killer cells (Clark and Harmon, 1980). However, other results have shown that the immunological effect may not be anti-tumour at all, but neutral or even essential for tumour development (reviewed by Stutman, 1975). In some instances, either T-lymphocytes or phagocytes may increase cancer risk (Naor, 1979). Some immunologically incompetent individuals experience no unusual cancer-risk. These include congenitally athymic ('nude') mice (Stutman, 1975; Rygaard and Povlsen, 1976), as well as patients with Hansen's disease, who may have generalized depression of cellular immunity (Brinton *et al.*, 1984). In some cases, such individuals may even display increased resistance to cancer development. Such an already confused state of current cancer immunology is further exacerbated by the fact that the awesome destructive power of the immune system is sometimes turned against self (in the autoimmune diseases). Hence, even a demonstrable instance of antitumour immunity may have its basis in some defect of the immune self-recognition apparatus rather than in some non-self expressed feature of the cancer cell.

In recent years, various *in vitro* studies have consistently demonstrated the basis of the reversions to be differentiational. Leukemia and teratocarcinoma cells, for instance, have been induced into terminal differentiation by retinoids through unknown mechanisms that, however, involve cytoplasmic receptors for retinoic acid (Sporn, 1983). Also, changes in nutrients and other culture conditions have induced differentiation of human malignant melanocytes (Aubert *et al.*, 1984). So have a membrane solvent (dimethylsulfoxide) and a sodium transport inhibitor (amiloride) in the case of human promyelocytic leukemia cells, suggesting the differentiation to be a membrane phenomenon (Carlson *et al.*, 1984). Analogously, according to Brugarolas and Gonsalvez (1980), several thioprolines ('norgamems') induce differentiation of a large variety of cancer cells through normalization of the cellular membranes. Differentiation of myeloid leukemia cells into mature granulocytes has also been induced by dimethyl sulfoxide and by other agents including butyrate, hypoxanthine, retinoic acid, and phorbol esters (Rovera *et al.*, 1980). This probably involved specific polypeptides than can be produced through mitogenic stimulation of human mononuclear blood cells or human T-lymphocytic leukemia cells (Olsson *et al.*, 1984). In neuroblastoma, the numerous differentiation-inducing factors which have been described include nerve growth factor which, like the phorbol esters (Rovera *et al.*,), can also induce cell division (Revoltella and Butler, 1980). Among these factors are also mitomycin C (Goldstein and Plurad, 1980) and agents which may or may not act via cyclic AMP (Portier *et al.*, 1980; Sandra *et al.*, 1981), a factor which has been correlated with experimental metastasis of B16 melanoma cells (Sheppard *et al.*, 1984).

Nerve growth factor belongs to the important group of natural regulators of cellular growth and differentiation. The intimate involvement of such regulators in the reversions as well as in oncogenesis is indicated by the close structural homologies between some of the regulators and the transforming proteins of specific oncogenes. For instance, the regulators' epidermal growth factor and platelet-derived growth factor are homologous with the transforming proteins of respectively the *v-erb-B* oncogene of avian erythroblastosis virus and the *sis* oncogene of simian sarcoma virus (Downward *et al.*, 1984).

9.10.4 Molecular Mechanisms: Differentiation and Dedifferentiation

Probably the major spurt to metazoan evolution is the phenomenon of the inherited genome diversifying and propagating its own species through the type of sexual reproduction that has become so well-developed in modern mammals. Accordingly, metazoan evolution has become far more advanced than the bacterial counterpart which has not relied upon this phenomenon. During mammalian ontogeny the somatic line cells produced by the zygote generate a dispensable somatic body, through a predetermined and highly controlled branching series of stem-cell populations with progressively decreasing differentiational options. The prime mandate of this body is to provide the protection, the nutrition, and the other means (e.g. selection of sexual partner and care of the offspring) whereby the germ line cells diversify and propagate the inherited genome. Of the two cell lines, only the somatic line, with its major feature of differentiation, is highly programmed for ageing and inevitable death. In contrast, the germ line, with its major feature of cell division with haploidization and genetic recombination being non-differentiative, is highly programmed for immortality. Against this evolutionary-developmental background, immortality is as unbiological as post-reproductive death is appropriate in any metazoan individual. This is because the latter's genesis as a contribution to the phenomenon of genomic diversification and propagation occurs only once. It may hence be that cancer, as one of the diseases largely of older ages, i.e. of ages past the peak of the capacity to fulfil the above-mentioned mandate, is also, like ageing and somatic death, an evolved means to facilitate the phenomenon. Even the earlier cancers may be a means of selection against early developmental errors. The genetically programmed differentiation of somatic cells thus seems to be the essential basis for their phenotypic heterogeneity, their ageing leading to death, and, as aberrant differentiation, probably also their transformation leading to frank neoplasia.

In oncogenesis, cellular transformation occurring within specific stem-cell constellations (cf. Chapter Eight, Section 8.5; this chapter, Section 9.10.1) appears to inhibit further differentiation along normal pathways but to stimulate cell division. This has several implications, all of which have become well-documented. First, in adults, primary tumours occur more rarely in tissues (e.g. nerves and muscles) with low normal cell turnover rates than in others (e.g. bone marrow and epithelia) with high rates. In young children, in whom many types of tissue are still maturing, correspondingly all types of tumours tend to occur, though with a predominance of hematological, sarcomatous, and neural tumours. This may not be wholly due to any presumably embryonic nature of the cells which become transformed since, in plants with their predominance of embryonic cells (e.g. in roots and growing tips), tumours are not particularly widespread. Second, wherever they occur, tumours generally exhibit higher turnover rates (cf. Hobson and Danecamp, 198) and lower states of differentiation than their normal progenitor tissues. Third, the less differentiated the tumour, the more aggressive, totipotent or multipotent, and potentially immortal it is likely to be, e.g. teratocarcinomas (Section 9.10.2) in contrast with benign neoplasms (Chapter One, Section 1.2.1.3). Finally, effective tumour therapy would depend largely upon selective inhibition of cell division through stimulation of cytodifferentiation (Section 9.10.3).

It seems unlikely that the inhibition of normal differentiation during oncogenesis also inhibits abnormal differentiation. Probably all single neoplasms express maldifferentiational heterogeneity in their component neoplastic cells (Section 9.6.5). This expression, albeit aberrant, is not necessarily haphazard. The APUD series of tumours, for example, expresses variable combinations of specific hormones (Section 9.2.5). The expression may be ectopic, suggesting inappropriate derepression of normally repressed gene(s); or it may be eutopic, suggesting over-activation of normally expressed gene(s), e.g. by amplification (Section 9.8.4). Analogously, alpha-fetoprotein is expressed by several tumours including hepatomas and teratocarcinomas, but not by pure germ-cell tumours such as seminomas and dysgerminomas (Abelev, 1974). In general, the same tumour may aberrantly expresss several differentiated functions, while several tumours may express the same function. Thymidine kinase, for instance, is elevated in acute myelogenous leukemia, acute lymphocytic leukemia, chronic granulocutic leukemia, non-Hodgkin lymphoma, and small cell carcinoma of the lung, among other tumours (Hagberg *et al.*, 1984). In contrast, breast cancer is associated with elevations of carcinoembryonic antigen, several hormones, and enzymes such as lactate dehydrogenase, malate dehydrogenase, hexokinase, and pyruvate kinase (Balinsky *et al.*, 1984). Breast cancers also variably express hormone receptors such as those for estrogens and progesterone. This feature is partly prognostic of the variable responses of these tumours to endocrine therapy (Sledge and McGuire, 1983). Overall, such vaguely patterned expressions and variable hormone-responsiveness of highly advanced (i.e. clinical) neoplasms suggest that the escape from normal host controls during oncogenesis is a slow, variable, and rarely complete process.

The phenomenon of maldifferentiation in neoplasia raises the question as to whether the progression from a normal cell to neoplastic cells at various states of aberrant differentiation is basically a differentiational (cf. Mintz and Fleischman, 1981) or dedifferentiational (cf. Uriel, 1979) process. At present, however, this question cannot be satisfactorily answered. This is primarily because of the lack of proper understanding of the molecular mechanisms of normal differentiation. There are also the difficulties associated with proper identification of the normal progenitor cell of a given neoplasm (Section 9.1). Without such basic background understanding, it would seem nothing more than mere lashing out in the dark in any serious attempt to address questions such as the molecular mechanisms of neoplastic differentiation, the differentiational characteristics of the initially transformed cell, or the similar characteristics of this cell's progenies at various 'preneoplastic' stages of tumour development. That 'nothing could be further from the truth' than the notion that the study of 'precancerous lesions in man is an exact science' (Koss and Greenebaum, 1983) thus comes as no surprise.

9.11 The Long Road Ahead

It is already reasonably certain that the on-off gene-switching network relationships which exist between a normal cell and its descendant neoplastic cells at various stages and phases of tumour development are extremely complex, are closely related to ontogeny, and are fundamental to oncology. Whether differentiational, dedifferentiational, or a mixture of the two, these relationships fall within a range that is sufficiently broad to accommodate all tumours, from the most differentiated to the least, and all shades in between. At the far extremes of this range may be placed cellular proliferation occurring without cytodifferentiation, representing the ultimate state of tumour development, and the exact reverse, representing the ultimate state of tumour regression.

It is unlikely that either of these extremes is ever reached naturally *in vivo*. However, the above-mentioned network relationships may bear some resemblance to a series of chemical equilibria, in the restricted sense that in both of these situations it is possible to direct a shift towards one extreme or the other (cf. Section 9.10). In this view, renewed efficacy in the biochemical prevention of preclinical neoplastic development or in the treatment of clinical neoplasia would depend upon ways and means to direct the cellular shift towards terminal differentiation at the expense of proliferation. Like birth itself relative to the metazoan individual, such a direction would lead to the eventual death of the neoplastic cell.

The finding of such ways and means, however, represents an extremely daunting though perhaps not impossible task. Were this not so daunting, cancer would hardly have remained the historic and persisting enigma it is.

The main difficulty in this task centres around the high probability of cancer being a disease of stem cells (Section 9.10; Chapter Eight, Section 8.5). In both normal and neoplastic tissues, particularly in those that are still developing or have remained embryonic, these cells are characterized by their dual capacities for self-renewal and for generation of progeny cells that differentiate either normally towards termination along preprogrammed lines or aberrantly in the interest of self-survival. Consequently, any manipulated or other depletion or destruction of these progeny cells would tend to stimulate the stem cells to re-establish the *status quo*. This is a common occurrence, e.g. in all types of wound healing, and after specific events such as loss or donation of blood, desquamation of damaged or effete epithelial cells of skin or digestive tract, or liver damage or partial hepatectomy. The same principle also applies to the many plants and lower animals which, after appropriate loss or damage, regenerate tissues, organs, or even entire organisms. More significantly, after cytotoxic cancer therapy that presumably fails to obliterate the neoplastic stem cell population, the cancer tends to recur after a period of remission and then to prove fatal. In contrast, prolonged remission in leukemia may be attained after successful transplant of bone marrow, the seat of the tumour's stem cell population. The upshot is that the above-mentioned efficacy in preclinical cancer prevention and clinical cancer treatment would also depend upon inhibition of the self-renewal capacity of the neoplastic stem cells while potentiating their differentiational capacity. Moreover, this, or complete destruction of these stem cells, would have to be achieved tumour-specifically, i.e. without similarly affecting any of the normal stem-cell populations of the body.

The task thus set by neoplasia is that for man first to understand and then to sensibly exploit the relevant features of the intrinsic molecular biology of his own development. However, a further difficulty associated with this task is the inordinately greater capacity of the human mind to unravel and exploit the natural mysteries outside than inside his being or, more succinctly, to conquer the stars than himself. The stark contrast between the striding manhood of his nucleonic, electronic, space, warfare, and other technology and the toddling infancy of his developmental biology speaks for itself. In the former situation, one day's science fiction soon becomes the next day's reality and the third day's history. In the latter, even the periphery of the nature and interrelationships pertaining to gene control in normal and neoplastic developments still constitutes largely uncharted territory.

The continuing outward orientation of cancer research is understandable in terms of the historical impetus this discipline has received from a similar orientation behind the heady successes achieved by medicine over the past one hundred years (Section 9.2.5). However, the successes thus far achieved through the study of cancer as an environmental disease are few. These are mainly to the effect that certain sensible precautions relating to smoking, drinking, dietary, sexual, and reproductive practices can reduce the risk of some cancers (Section 9.3.2). Such precautions recall the basic teachings (the 'eightfold path') of the Lord Buddha about 26 centuries ago. However, as in China and Japan, devout adherence to these teachings, or to the similar ones by the Seventh Day Adventists in California (Section 9.4), is associated with reduced incidence of certain types of cancer, but it is no guarantee against the occurrence of the disease itself. Moreover, the environmental approach has yielded little or no clearly helpful information about vital questions such as those concerning the true cause(s) of cancer (Section 9.4) or the molecular mechanisms of carcinogenesis (Sections 9.5 and 9.6).

In this mechanistic context, the worst weaknesses of the somatic mutation hypothesis, over and above those already discussed (Section 9.6.4), are in its capacity to act as a red herring. Thus, it diverts research attention and resources from man (in the words of the poet, 'the proper study of mankind'), i.e. from the central theme of the developmental hypothesis (Section 9.10). It also effectively ignores even its own experimental controls, in using them as mere baseline passive parameters, rather as does the medical paradigm with the bulk of the human population (Chapter Five, Section 5.1). The developmental hypothesis, in contrast, regards these controls, whether human or experimental, as the real repositories of the basic natural secrets which cancer research is endeavouring to fathom. It stresses that since the abnormal is an aberration of the normal, proper understanding of the former can hardly be independent of that of the latter. This red herring situation vividly recalls the dictum of Peyton Rous (1959), the Nobel laureate, that the introduction of the somatic mutation hypothesis into oncologic thinking resulted in 'no good thing but much that is bad' and in 'fatalism to blast many a hope and effort'.

From the mists of recorded human history to the present day, the problem of cancer has remained stubbornly intractable. It has represented a fertile field, a veritable free-for-all, for all kinds of mechanistic and other speculations, most unfounded in established facts (cf. Chapter Two). In this field, the current favourites are the two hypotheses under discussion. Were the somatic mutation hypothesis eventually proven to be entirely erroneous, the expended research effort would have been wasted. Were this also the eventual fate of the developmental hypothesis, the effort could not but still be rewarding, e.g. in terms of the many genetic diseases and the worst ravages of the later ageing process which so increasingly afflict mankind. Of these two hypotheses, only the latter distributes its eggs in many baskets and promises a gem-strewn road ahead. It is necessarily a long-term promise, but one which the developmental hypothesis cannot but honour in one way or another.

In its broad sense, the developmental hypothesis depicts man as an entity made up of parts which, through their interactions, make the entity greater than the sum of the parts. This entity is, in turn, an integral part of an interacting cosmic whole. To the extent that this hypothesis recalls the holistic approaches of the ancients, the historical wheel has turned full circle. However, for the first time, a firm scientific basis for such approaches seems possible, particularly in terms of the influence of environmental cancer-risk factors upon the on-off gene-switching network relationships which exist between normal and neoplastic developments.

BIBLIOGRAPHY

Abe, S. and Sandberg, A. A. (1979). Chromosomes and causation of human cancer and leukemia: XXXII. Unusual features of Ph-positive acute myeloblastic leukemia (AML), including a review of the literature. *Cancer, 43*: 2352–64

Abe, S. and Sandberg, A. A. (1980). Sister chromatid exchange and growth kinetics of marrow cells in aneuploid acute nonlymphocytic leukemias. *Cancer Research, 40*: 1292–9.

Abelev, G. I. (1974). α-Fetoprotein as a marker of embryo specific differentiation in normal and tumor tissues. *Transplantation Reviews, 20*: 3–37.

Adair, F. E., Pack, G. T. and Farrior, J. H. (1932). Lipomas. *American Journal of Cancer, 16*: 1104–20

Adam, A. and Hochholzer, L. (1981). Ganglioneuroblastoma of the posterior mediastinum: a clinopathologic review of 80 cases. *Cancer, 47*: 373–81.

Adami, H. O., Rimsten, A., Stenkvist, B. and Vegelius, J. (1977). Influence of height, weight and obesity on risk of breast cancer in an unselected Swedish population. *British Journal of Cancer, 36*: 787–92

Adamson, R. H. and Sieber, S. M. (1972). Antineoplastic agents as potential carcinogens. In: H. H. Hiatt, J. D. Watson and J. A. Winstein (eds.), *Origins of Human Cancer*, Cold Spring Harbor Laboratory, Cold Spring Harbor, New York, pp. 429–43

Agricola, G. (1556). *De Re Metallica, 1556*. Translated by H. C. Hoover and L. H. Hoover, *Mining Magazine*, London, 1912

Albino, L. P., Le Strange, R., Oliff, A. I., Furth, M. E. and Old, L. J. (1984). Transforming *ras* genes from human melanoma: a manifestation of tumour heterogeneity? *Nature, 308*: 69–72

Albright, S. G. and Hook, E. B. (1980). Estimates of the likelihood that a Down's syndrome child of unknown genotype is a consequence of an inherited translocation. *Journal of Medical Genetics, 17*: 273–6

Alitalo, K. and Vaheri, A. (1982). Pericellular matrix in malignant transformation. *Advances in Cancer Research, 37*: 111

Al-Khouri, H. and Greenstein, B.D. (1980). Role of corticosteroid binding globulin in interaction of corticosterone with uterine and brain progesterone receptors. *Nature, 287*: 58–60

Allfrey, V. G., Boffa, L. C. and Vidali, G. (1979). Effects of carcinogens on nuclear protein composition and metabolism. A. C. Griffin and C. R. Shaw (eds.), *Carcinogenesis: Identification and Mechanisms of Action*, Raven Press, New York, pp. 419–37

Altenburger, W., Steinmetz, M. and Zachau, M. G. (1980). Functional and non-functional joining in immunoglobulin light chain genes of a mouse myeloma. *Nature, 287*: 603–7

Ames, B. N. (1979). Identifying environmental carcinogens causing mutations and cancer. *Science, 204*: 587

Ames, B. N., Durston, W. E., Yamasaki, E. and Lee, F. D. (1973). Carcinogens are mutagens: a simple test system combining liver homogenates for activation and bacteria for detection. *Proceedings of the National Academy of Sciences (USA), 70*: 2281–5

Anders, A. and Anders, F. (1978). Etiology of cancer as studied in the platyfish-swordtail system. *Biochemica et Biophysica Acta, 516*: 61–95

Anderson, D. E. (1978). Familial cancer and cancer families. *Seminars on Oncology*, 5: 11–6

Anderson, D. E. (1980). Muir's syndrome. *Cancer*, 45: 1103–7

Andrewes, C. H. (1932). The transmission of fowl tumours to pheasants. *Journal of Pathology and Bacteriology*, 35: 407–13

Anghilieri, L. J. (1978). Cell membrane ionic permeability, calcium ion, mitochondria, and carcinogenesis. *Archiv für Geschwulstforschung*, 48: 497–503

Arcos, J. C. (1972). In memory of Nguyen Phuc Buu-Hoi, 1915–1972. *Cancer Research*, 32: 2856A–56

Ardashnikov, S. N. (1937). Genetics of leukemia in man. *Journal of Hygiene*, 37: 286–302

Arlett, C. F. and Harcourt, S. A. (1980). Survey of radiosensitivity in a variety of human cell strains. *Cancer Research*, 40: 926–32

Armstrong, B. and Doll, R. (1975). Environmental factors and cancer incidence and mortality in different countries, with special reference to dietary practices. *International Journal of Cancer*, 15: 617–31

Armstrong, R. W., Kutty, M. K., Dharmalingham, S. K. and Ponnudurai, J. R. (1979). Incidence of nasopharyngeal carcinoma in Malaysia. *British Journal of Cancer*, 40: 557–67

Arnold, J. (1879a). Uber feinere struktur der Zellen unter normalen und pathologischen Bedringungen. *Virchow's Archiv für Pathologische Anatomie und Physiologie und für Klinische Medizin*, 77: 181–206

Arnold, J. (1879b). Beobachtungen über Kernteilungen in der Zellen der Geschwülste. *Virchow's Archiv für Pathologische Anatomie und Physiologie und für Klinische Medizin*, 78: 279–301

Arnott, M. S., Yamauchi, T. and Johnston, D. A. (1979). Aryl hydrocarbon hydroxylase in normal and cancer populations. In: A. C. Griffin and C. R. Shaw (eds.), *Carcinogens: Identification and Mechanisms of Action*, Raven Press, New York, pp. 145–56

Arya, S. K. (1980). Phorbol ester-mediated stimulation of the synthesis of mouse mammary tumour virus. *Nature*, 284: 71–2

Atkin, N. B. (1976). Prognostic significance of ploidy levels in human tumours. 11 extra-uterine cancers and summary of data on 1171 tumours. *Cytobios*, 15: 233–7

Atkin, N. B. and Baker, M. C. (1977a). Chromosome 1 in cervical carcinoma. *Lancet*, 2: 984

Atkin, N. B. and Baker, M. C. (1977b). Pericentric inversion of chromosome 1: frequency and possible association with cancer. *Cytogenetics and Cell Genetics*, 19: 180–4

Atkin, N. B. and Baker, M. C. (1977c). Abnormal chromosomes and number 1 heterochromatin variants revealed in C-banded preparations from 13. *Cytobios*, 18: 101–9

Atkin, N. B. and Baker, M. C. (1978). Duplication of the long arm of chromosome 1 in a malignant vaginal tumour. *British Journal of Cancer*, 38: 468–71

Atkin, N. B. and Baker, M. C. (1979). Chromosome 1 in 26 carcinomas of the cervix uteri. *Cancer*, 44: 604–13

Atkin, N. B. and Piokthall, V. J. (1977). Chromosomes 1 in 14 ovarian cancers. Heterochromatin variants and structural changes. *Human Genetics*, 38: 25–33

Atkins, H., Bulbrook, R. D., Falconer, M. A., Hayward, J. L., MacLean, K. S. and Schurr, P. H. (1968). Ten years' experience of steroid assays in the management of breast cancer. *Lancet*, 2: 1255–60

Atkinson, K., Kay, H. E. M., Lawler, S. D., Wells, D. G. and McElwain, T. J. (1975). Meningeal leukemia after blast transformation of chronic myeloid leukemia. *Cancer*, 35: 529–33

Aubert, C., Rouge, F. and Galindo, J.-R. (1984). Differentiation and tumorigenicity of human malignant melanocytes in relation to their culture conditions. *Journal of the National Cancer Institute*, 72: 3–12

Azzopardi, J. G. and Evans, D. J. (1971). Argentaffin cells in prostatic carcinoma: differentiation from lipofuscin and melanin in prostatic epithelium. *Journal of Pathology*, 104: 247–51

Backer, J. M., and Weinstein, I. B. (1980). Mitochondrial DNA is a major cellular target for a dihydrodiol-epoxide derivative of benzo[a]pyrene. *Science*, 209: 297–9

Baikie, A. G., Court-Brown, W. M., Buckton, K. E., Harnden, D. G., Jacobs, P. A. and Tough, I. M. (1960). A possible specific chromosome abnormality in human chronic myeloid leukemia. *Nature*, 188: 1165–6

Balakrishnan, V. and Gangadharan, P. (1982). Cancer of the nasopharynx in man: younger age peak and related aspects. In: G. Reznik (ed.), *Comparative Nasal Cavity Tumors in Animals and Man*, CRC Press, Boca Raton, Louisiana

Baldwin, R. W. (1973). Immunological aspects of chemical carcinogenesis. *Advances in Cancer Research*, 18: 1–75

Balinsky, D., Platz, C. E. and Lewis, J. W. (1984). Enzyme activities in normal, dysplastic and cancerous human breast tissue. *Journal of the National Cancer Institute*, 72: 217–24

Baltimore, D. (1970). RNA-dependent DNA polymerase in virions of RNA tumor viruses. *Nature*, 226: 1209–11

Bang, F. B. (1978). Genetics of resistance of animals to viruses: 1. Introduction and studies in mice. *Advances in Virus Research*, 23: 269–348

Bank, A., Mears, J. G., Ramirez, F., Burns, A. L., Feldenzer, J. and Spence, S. (1980). Detection and gene defects in the thalassemias and related disorders. *Annals of the New York Academy of Sciences*, 344: 1–11

Bara, J., Nardelli, J., Gadenna, C., Prade, M. and Burtin, P. (1984). Differences in the expression of mucus-related antigens between proximal and distal human colon adenocarcinomas. *British Journal of Cancer*, 49: 495–502

Bardin, C. W. and Catterall, J. F. (1981). Testosterone: a major determinant of extragenital sexual dimorphism. *Science*, 211: 1285–94

Barnekow, A., Schartl, M., Anders, F. and Bauer, H. (1982). Identification of a fish protein associated with a kinase activity and related to the Rous sarcoma virus transforming protein. *Cancer Research*, 42: 2429–33

Barnes, H. E. (ed.) (1965). *An Intellectual and Cultural History of the Western World*. Dover Publications, London. 3 volumes

Barr, M. L. and Bertram, E. G. (1949). A morphological distinction between neuroses of the male and female, and the behaviour of the nuclear satellite during accelerated nucleoprotein synthesis. *Nature*, 163: 676–7

Barrell, B. G., Anderson, S., Bankier, A. T., Debruijn, M. H. L., Chen, E., Coulson, A. R., Smith, A. J. H., Staden, R. and Young, I. G. (1980). Different pattern of codon recognition by mammalian mitochondrial tRNAs. *Proceedings of the National Academy of Sciences, USA*, 77: 3164–6

Barrett, J. and Ts'o, P. (1978). Relationship between somatic mutation and neoplastic transformation. *Proceedings of the National Academy of Sciences, USA*, 75: 3297–301

Barry, E. J. and Gutmann, H. R. (1973) Protein modifications by activated carcinogens. *Journal of Biological Chemistry*, 248: 2730–7

Bass, H. N. and Sparkes, R. S. (1979). Two balanced translocations in three generations of a pedigree: t(7;10)(q11;q22) and +(14;21)(14qter cen 21qter). *Journal of Medical Genetics*, 16: 215–18

Basso, G., Cocito, M. G., Semenzato, G., Pezzutto, A. and Zanesco, L. (1980). Cytochemical study of thymocytes and T-lymphocytes. *British Journal of Haematology*, 44: 577–82

374   *Bibliography*

Baum, J. K., Holtz, F, Bookstein, J. J. and Klein, E. W. (1973). Possible association between benign hepatomas and oral contraceptives. *Lancet*, *2*: 926–9

Baxter, P. J., Langlands, A. O., Anthony, P. P. Macsween, R. N. M. and Schever, P. J. (1980). Angiosarcoma of the liver: a marker tumor for the late effects of thorotrast in Great Britain. *British Journal of Cancer*, *41*: 446–53

Baylin, S. B. and Mendelsohn (1980). Ectopic (inappropriate) hormone production by tumors: mechanisms involved and the biological and clinical implications. *Endocrinological Reviews*, *1*: 45–77

Bayon, H. P. (1927). Parasites and malignant proliferations. *Journal of Tropical Medicine and Hygiene*, *39*: 73–80

Beard, M. E. J., Durrant, J., Catovsky, D., Wiltshaw, E., Amess, J. L., Brearley, R. L., Greaves, M. F. and Galton, D. A. G. (1976). Blast crisis of chronic myeloid leukemia (CML). *British Journal of Haematology*, *34*: 167–8

Beatson, G. T. (1896). On the treatment of inoperable cases of carcinoma of the mamma: suggestions for a new method of treatment with illustrative cases. *Lancet*, *2*: 104–7 and 162–5

Becher, R., Schmidt, C. G., Theis, G. and Hossfeld, D. K. (1979a). Sister chromatid exchange in Phl-positive chronic myelocytic leukemia. *International Journal of Cancer*, *24*: 713–16

Becher, R., Schmidt, C. G., Theis, G. and Hossfeld, D. K. (1979b). The rate of sister chromatid exchange in normal human bone marrow cells. *Human Genetics*, *50*: 213–16.

Becker, F. F. (1979). Keynote address: evolution, chemical carcinogenesis, and mortality: the cycle of life. In: A. C. Griffin and R. K. Shaw (eds.), *Carcinogens: Identification and Mechanisms of Action*. Raven Press, New York, pp. 5–17

Becker, F. F., Fox, R. A., Klein, K. M. and Wolman, S. R. (1971). Chromosome patterns in rat hepatocytes during N-2-fluorenylacetamide carcinogenesis. *Journal of the National Cancer Institute*, *46*: 1261–9

Becker, F. F., Klein, K. M., Wolman, S. R., Asofsky, R. and Sell, S. (1973). Characterisation of primary hepatocellular carcinomas and initial transplant generations. *Cancer Research*, *33*: 3330–8

Bell, P. A., Borthwick, N. M. and Dembinski, T. C. (1980). The regulation of transcription in lymphocytes by glucocorticoids. In: S. Iacobelli, R. J. B. King, H. R. Lindner and M. E. Lippman (eds.), *Hormones and Cancer*, Raven Press, New York, pp. 99–112

Bellevue, R., Dosik, H. and Rieder, R. F. (1979). Alpha thalassemia in American blacks: a study of a family with five cases of haemoglobin H disease. *British Journal of Haematology*, *41*: 193–202

Bence-Jones, H. (1848). On a new substance occurring in the urine of a patient with 'mollities ossium'. *Philosophical Transactions of the Royal Society*, *138*: 55–62

Bender, M. A., Griggs, H. G. and Bedford, J. S. (1974). Mechanisms of chromosomal aberration production III. Chemical and ionising radiation. *Mutation Research*, *23*: 197–212

Bender, R. A. (1980). Vinca alkaloids and epipodophyllotoxins. In: H. M. Pinedo (ed.), *Cancer Chemotherapy 1980*, Excerpta Medica, Amsterdam and Oxford, pp. 95–106

Benestad, H. B. (1979). Drug mechanisms in marrow aplasia. In: C. G. Geary (ed.), *Aplastic Anaemia*, Baillière Tindall, London, pp. 26–42

Ben-Galim, E., Gross-Kieselstein, E., and Abrahamov, A. (1977). Beckwith-Weidemann syndrome in a mother and her son. *American Journal of Diseases of Childhood*, *131*: 801–3

Benjannet, S., Seidah, N. G., Routhier, R. and Chrétien, M. (1980). A novel human pituitary peptide containing the α-MSH sequence. *Nature*, *285*: 415–16

Bennett, J. M., Catovsky, D., Daniel, M. T., Flandrin, G., Galton, D. A. G.,

Gralnik, H. R. and Sultan, C. (1976). Proposals for the classification of the acute leukaemias. *British Journal of Haematology, 33*: 451–8.

Bentvelzen, P. (1984). Presence of fibroblast-transforming genes in normal DNA of several mouse and rat strains. *European Journal of Cancer and Clinical Oncology, 20*: 567–71

Berenblum, I. (1941). The mechanism of carcinogenesis. A study of the significance of carcinogenic action and related phenomena. *Cancer Research, 1*: 807–14

Berenblum, I. (1954). Carcinogenesis and tumor pathogenesis. *Advances in Cancer Research, 2*: 129–75

Berenblum, I. (1979). Theoretical and practical aspects of the two-stage mechanism of carcinogenesis. In: A. C. Griffin and C. R. Shaw (eds.), *Carcinogens: Identification and Mechanisms of Action*, Raven Press, New York, pp. 25–36

Berenblum, I. and Shubik, P. (1947). A new qualitative approach to the study of the stages of chemical carcinogens in the mouse's skin. *British Journal of Cancer, 1*: 383–91

Berg, J. M., Gardner, H. A., Gardner, R. J. M., Goh, E. G., Markovic, V. D., Simpson, N. E. and Worton, R. G. (1980). Dic (21, 21) in a Down's syndrome child with an unusual chromosome 9 variant in the mother. *Journal of Medical Genetics, 17*: 144–8

Berger, R. (1971). Anomalies chromosomiques constitutionnelles et neoplasies. *Presse Médicale, 79*: 1107–9

Berger, R., Bernheim, A., Brouet, J. C., Daniel, M. T. and Flandrin, G. (1979). t(8;14) Translocation in a Burkitt's type of lymphoblastic leukemia (L3). *British Journal of Haematology, 43*: 87–90

Berger, R., Bernheim, A., Weh, H. F., Daniel, M. T., and Flandrin, G. (1980). Cytogenetic studies on acute monocytic leukemia. *Leukemia Research, 4*: 119–27

Bernal, J. D. (1965). *Science in History*, 3rd edn, 4 vols. MIT Press, Cambridge, Massachusetts

Bernstein, R., Jenkins, T., Dawson, B., Wagner, J., Dewald, G., Koo, G.C. and Wachtel, S. S. (1980). Female phenotype and multiple abnormalities in sibs with a Y chromosome and partial X chromosome duplication: H-Y antigen and Xg blood group findings. *Journal of Medical Genetics, 17*: 291–300

Berry, A. C., Belton, E. M. and Chantler, C. (1980). Monozygotic twins discordant for Weidemann-Beckwith syndrome and the implications for genetic counselling. *Journal of Medical Genetics, 17*: 136–8

Berry, A. C., Honeycombe, J. and Macoun, S. J. (1979). Two children with partial trisomy for 7p. *Journal of Medical Genetics, 16*: 320–1

Bertell, R. (1977). X-ray exposure and premature ageing. *Journal of Surgery and Oncology, 9*: 379

Bichat, X. (1801). *Anatomie Générale Appliquée à la Physiologie et à la Médecine*, 2 vols, Brosson, Gabon et Cie, Paris

Bigozzi, U., Simoni, G., Montali, E., Dalpra, L., Rossella, F., Piazzini, M. and Borghi, A. (1980). 47.XXX chromosome constitution in a male. *Journal of Medical Genetics, 17*: 62–6

Bird, A. P. (1984). DNA methylation — how important in gene control? *Nature, 307*: 503–4

Bishop, J. M. (1982). Retroviruses and cancer genes. *Advances in Cancer Research, 37*: 1–32

Biskind, G. R., Bernstein, D. E. and Gospe, S. M. (1953). The effect of exogenous gonadotropins on the development of experimental ovarian tumors in rats. *Cancer Research, 13*: 216–20

Biskind, M. S. and Biskind, G. R. (1944). Development of tumors in the rat ovary after transplantation into the spleen. *Proceedings of the Society of Experimental Biology and Medicine,5*: 176–9

Bitman, J. and Cecil, H. C. (1970). Estrogenic activity of DDT analogs and polychlorinated biphenyls. *Journal of Agricultural and Food Chemistry, 18*: 1108–12

Bittner, J. J. (1935). Some possible effects of nursing on the mammary gland tumor incidence in mice. *Science, 84*: 162

Black, H. S. and Douglas, D. R. (1972). A model system for the evaluation of the role of cholesterol α-oxide in ultraviolet carcinogenesis. *Cancer Research, 32*: 2630–2

Blackett, N. M. and Gordon, M. Y. (1978). Observations on the distribution of granulocytic progenitor cells (CFU-C) in human bone marrow: the importance of the manner in which the results of *in vitro* cultures are reported. *British Journal of Haematology, 40*: 355–6

Blacklock, J. E. and Stanton, J. D. (1980). Common pathways of interferon and hormonal action. *Nature, 283*: 406–8

Blaszczyk, M., Ross, A. H., Ernst, C. S., Marchisio, M., Atkinson, B. F., Pak, K. Y., Steplewski, Z. and Koprowski, H. (1984). A fetal glycolipid expressed on adenocarcinomas of the colon. *International Journal of Cancer, 33*: 313

Bloom, H. J. G. (1973). Adjuvant therapy for adenocarcinoma of the kidney: present position and prospects. *British Journal of Urology, 45*: 237–57

Blundell, T., Dodson, G., Hodgkin, D. and Mercola, D. (1972). Insulin: the structure in the crystal and its reflection in chemistry and biology. *Advances in Protein Chemistry, 26*: 279–402

Blundell, T. and Humbel, R. E. (1980). Hormone families: pancreatic hormones and homologous growth factors. *Nature, 287*: 781–7

Bodmer, W. F. (ed.) (1978). The HLA system. *British Medical Bulletin, 34*: 213–316

Bodmer, W. F. and Bodmer, J. G. (1978). Evolution and function of the HLA system. *British Medical Bulletin, 34*: 309–16

Bolvin, J.-F., Hutchinson, G. B., Lyden, M., Godbold, J., Chorosh, J. and Schottenfeld, D. (1984). Second primary cancers following treatment for Hodgkin's disease. *Journal of the National Cancer Institute, 72*: 233–41

Bonitz, S. G., Berlani, R., Corlizzi, G. W. M., Macino, G., Nobrega, F.C., Nobrega, M. P., Thalenfeld, B. E. and Tzagoloff, A. (1980). Codon recognition rules in yeast mitochondria. *Proceedings of the National Academy of Sciences (USA), 77*: 3167–70

Bostock, C. J. and Sumner, A. T. (1978). *The Eukaryotic Chromosome*. North-Holland Publishing Co., Amsterdam

Boston Collaborative Drug Surveillance Program (1974). Reserpine and breast cancer. *Lancet, 2*: 669–71

Bourke, G. J. (ed.) (1983). *The Epidemiology of Cancer*, Croom Helm, London

Boveri, T. (1914). *Zur Frage der Einstehung maligner Tumoren*, Gustav Fischer, Jena. English version: *The Origin of Malignant Tumors*, Baillière, Tindall, and Cox, London, 1929

Boyd, W. (1977). *The Spontaneous Regression of Cancer*, C. C. Thomas, Springfield, Illinois

Boyland, E. (1969). The correlation of experimental carcinogenesis and cancer in man. *Progress in Experimental Tumor Research, 11*: 222–34

Bramwell, M. E. and Harris, H. (1978). Some further information about the abnormal membrane glycoprotein associated with malignancy. *Proceedings of the Royal Society [Biology], 203*: 93–9

Brand, K. G., Bouen, L. C., Johnson, K. H. and Brand, I. (1975). Etiological factors, stages and the role of the foreign body in foreign body tumorigenesis. *Cancer Research, 35*: 279–86

Braun, A. C. (1977). *The Story of Cancer. On its Nature, Causes, and Control*, Addison-Wesley Publishing Company, Reading, Massachusetts

Breasted, J. H. (1930). *The Edwin Smith Surgical Papyrus*, University of Chicago Press, Chicago

Breasted, J. H. (1933). *The Dawn of Conscience*, Scribner, New York

Brennan, B. G. and Carr, D. H. (1979). Parental origin of triploidy and D and G trisomy in spontaneous abortions. *Journal of Medical Genetics, 16*: 285–7

Brinton, L. A., Hoover, R., Jacobson, R. R. and Fraumeni, J. F. (1984). Cancer mortality among patients with Hansen's disease. *Journal of the National Cancer Institute, 72*: 109–14

Brisson, J., Morrison, A. S., Kopans, D. B., Sandowsky, N. L. Kalisher, L., Twaddle, J. A., Meyer, J. E., Henske, C. I. and Cole, P. (1984). Height and weight, mammographic features of breast tissue and breast cancer risk. *American Journal of Epidemiology, 119*: 371–8

Britten, R. J. and Davidson, E. H. (1969). Gene regulation for higher cells: a theory. *Science, 165*: 349–57

Bodeur, G. M., Sekhon, G. S. and Goldstein, M. N. (1977). Chromosomal aberrations in human neuroblastomas. *Cancer, 40*: 2256–63

Brooks, D. E. (1983). Epididymal functions and their hormonal regulation. *Australian Journal of Biological Science, 36*: 205

Brothwell, D. (1967). The evidence for neoplasms. In: D. Brothwell and A. T. Sandison (eds.), *Diseases of Antiquity*, C. C. Thomas, Springfield, Illinois, pp. 320–45

Brown, D. E., Mulrow, Y. H. and Stoudemire, G. A. (1984). The anxiety disorders. *Annals of Internal Medicine, 100*: 558–64

Brownlie, S. A., Campbell, J. G., Head, K. W., Imlah, P., McTaggart, H. S. and McVie, J. C. (1978). Prednisolone treatment of hereditary pig lymphoma. *European Journal of Cancer, 14*: 983–94

Broxmeyer, H. E., Desouse, M., Smithyman, A., Ralph, P., Hamilton, J., Kurland, J. I. and Bognacki, J. (1980). Specificity and modulation of the action of lactoferrin, a negative feedback regulator of myelopoiesis. *Blood, 55*: 3324–33

Broxmeyer, H. E., Grossbard, E., Jacobsen, N. and Moore, M. A. S. (1978). Evidence for a proliferative advantage of human leukemia colony-forming cells in vitro. *Journal of the National Cancer Institute, 60*: 513–21

Bruce, W. R., Correa, P., Lipkin, M., Tannenbaum, S. R. and Wilkins, T. D. (eds.) (1981). *Gastrointestinal Cancer: Endogenous Factors*, Banbury report 7, Cold Spring Harbor Laboratory, Cold Spring Harbor, New York

Brugarolas, A. and Gonsalvez, M. (1980). Treatment of cancer by an inducer of reverse transformation. *Lancet, 1*: 68–70

Brynes, R. K., Golomb, H. M., Desser, R. K., Recant, W., Reese, C. and Rowley, J. (1976). Acute monocytic leukemia. *American Journal of Chemical Pathology, 65*: 471–82

Bubbers, J. E. (1984). Identification and linkage analysis of a gene, Rcs-1, suppressing spontaneous SJL/J lymphoma expression. *Journal of the National Cancer Institute, 72*: 441–6

Buell, P. (1973). Changing incidence of breast cancer in Japanese-American women. *Journal of the National Cancer Institute, 51*: 1479–83

Buick, R. N., Till, J. E. and McCulloch, E. A. (1977). Colony assay for proliferative blast cells circulating in myeloblastic leukemia. *Lancet, 1*: 862–3

Bull, L. B., Culvenor, C. C. and Dick, A. T. (1968). *The Pyrolizidine Alkaloids. Their Chemistry, Pathogenicity, and Other Biological Properties*, North-Holland Publishing Company, Amsterdam

Bulow, H., Wullstein, H. K., Bottger, G. and Schroder, F. H. (1973). Mammacarcinom bei oestrogenbehandeltern Prostata-carcinom. *Urologe, A12*: 249–53

Burgoyne, P. S. (1979). Evidence for an association between univalent Y chromosomes and spermatocyte loss in XYY mice and men. *Cytogenetics Cell Genetics, 23*: 84–9

Burke, P. J., Karp, J. E., Braine, H. G. and Vaughan, W. P. (1977). Timed sequential therapy of human leukemia based upon the response of leukemic cells to humoral growth factors. *Cancer Research, 37*: 2138–46

Burkitt, D. and Wright, D. H. (1970). *Burkitt's Lymphoma*. Churchill Livingstone, Edinburgh

Burnet, F. M. (1970). The concept of immunological surveillance. *Progress in Experimental Tumor Research, 13*: 1–27

Burnett, M. (1974). *Intrinsic Mutagenesis: A Genetic Approach to Ageing*, Medical and Technical Publishing Co., Lancaster

Buschke, F. (ed.) (1958). *Progress in Radiation Therapy*, Grune and Stratton, New York

Bustad, L. K., Goldman, M. and Rosenblatt, L. (1976). Inferences on radiation carcinogenesis revealed by selective studies in animals. In: J. M. Yuhas, R. W. Tennant and J. D. Regan (eds.), *Biology of Radiation Carcinogenesis*, Raven Press, New York, pp. 13–29

Butenandt, A. (1929). Über 'Progynon'. Ein krystallisiertes weibliches Sexualhormon. *Naturwissenschaften, 17*: 879

Byers, T. and Graham, S. (1984). The epidemiology of diet and cancer. *Advances in Cancer Research, 41*: 1–71

Cairns, J. (1978). *Science and Society*, W. H. Freeman and Co., San Francisco

Caldwell, G. G. (1983). Infections, infestations, and cancer. In: G. J. Bourke (ed.), *The Epidemiology of Cancer*, Croom Helm, London, pp. 292–326

Campbell, P. N. and Craig, R. K. (1979). Hormonal regulation of specific gene expression. *FEBS Letters*, 99:223–37

Canellos, G. P. (1979). Chronic granulocytic leukemia. *Medical Clinic, 60*: 1001–18

Cantor, K. P. and Blair, A. (1984). Farming and mortality from multiple myeloma: a case-control study with the use of death certificates. *Journal of the National Cancer Institute, 72*: 251–5

Cardona, R. A. and King, C. H. (1976). Activation of the O-glucuronide of the carcinogen N-hydroxy-N-2-fluorenylacetamide by enzymatic deactylation in vitro: formation of fluorenylamine-tRNA adducts. *Biochemical Pharmacology, 25*: 1051–6

Cardy, R. H. and Lijinsky, W. (1980). Comparison of the carcinogenic effects of five nitrosamines in guinea pigs. *Cancer Research, 40*: 1879

Carlson, J., Dorey, F., Cragoe, E. and Koeffler, E. P. (1984). Amiloride potentiation of differentiation of human promyelocytic cell line HL-60. *Journal of the National Cancer Institute, 72*: 13–17

Carpenter, N. J., Say, B. and Browning, D. (1980). Gonadal dysgenesis in a patient with an X;3 translocation: case report and review. *Journal of Medical Genetics, 17*: 216–21

Carrel, A. and Burrows, M. T. (1911). Cultivation of tissues *in vitro* and its technique. *Journal of Experimental Medicine, 13*: 387–96

Carter, L. J. (1974). Cancer and the environment (1): a creaky system grinds on. *Science, 86*: 239–42

Case, R. A. M. (1956). Cohort analysis of cancer mortality in England and Wales, 1911–1954, by site and sex. *British Journal of Preventive and Social Medicine, 10*: 172–99

Casey, H. W., Giles, R. C., and Kwapien, R. P. (1979). Mammary neoplasia in animals: pathologic aspects and the effects of contraceptive steroids. *Recent Results in Cancer Research, 66*: 129–60

Caspersson, T., Gahrton, G., Lindsten, J. and Zech, L. (1970). Identification of the Philadelphia chromosome as a number 22 by quinacrine mustard fluorescence analysis. *Experimental Cell Research, 63*: 238–40

Caspersson, T., Zech, L., Modest, E. J., Foley, G. E., Wagh, U. and Simonsson,

E. (1969). DNA-binding fluorochromes for the study of the organisation of the metaphase nucleus. *Experimental Cell Research*, 58: 141–52

Castiglioni, A. (1958). *A History of Medicine*, 2nd edn. Trans. E. B. Krumbhaar, A. A. Knopff, New York

Catovsky, D. and Galton, D. A. G. (1977). Cell markers and the classification of acute leukemia. *Haematology and Blood Transfusion*, 20: 25–31

Catovsky, D., Pittman, S., O'Brien, M., Cherchi, M., Costello, C., Foa, R., Pearce, E., Hoffbrand, A. V., Janossy, G., Ganeshaguru, K. and Greaves, M. F. (1979). Multiparameter studies in lymphoid leukemias. *American Journal of Clinical Pathology*, 72: 736–45

Chaganti, R. S. K., Schoberg, S. and German, J. (1974). A manyfold increase in sister chromatid exchanges in Bloom's syndrome lymphocytes. *Proceedings of the National Academy of Sciences (USA)*, 71: 4508–12

Chambers, A. F., Hill, R. P. and Ling, V. (1981). Tumor heterogeneity and stability of the metastatic phenotype of mouse KHT sarcoma cells. *Cancer Research*, 41: 1368–72

Chan, P. C. and Dao, T. L. (1981). Enhancement of mammary carcinogenesis by a high fat diet in Fischer, Long-Evans and Sprague-Dawley rats. *Cancer Research*, 41: 164–7

Chan, P. C., Didato, F. and Cohen, L. A. (1975). High dietary fat elevation of rat serum prolactin and mammary cancer. *Proceedings of the Society for Experimental Biology and Medicine*, 149: 133–5

Chandley, A. C. (1979). The chromosomal basis of human infertility. *British Medical Bulletin*, 35: 181–6

Chang, R. S. and Le, C. T. (1984). Failure to acquire Epstein-Barr virus infection after intimate exposure to the virus. *American Journal of Epidemiology*, 119: 392–5

Chang, T. D., Biedler, J. L., Stockert, E. and Old, L. J. (1977). Trisomy of chromosome 15 in X-ray-induced mouse leukemia. *Proceedings of the American Association for Cancer Research*, 18: 225

Chang, W. and Hsing, Y. (1980). In vitro flowering of embryoids derived from mature root callus of ginseng (*Phanax ginseng*). *Nature*, 284: 341–2

Cheng, W. S., Mulvihill, J. J., Greene, M. H., Pickle, W., Tsai, S. and Whang-Peng, J. (1979). Sister chromatid exchanges and chromosomes in chronic myelogenous leukemia and cancer families. *International Journal of Cancer*, 23: 8–13

Chessels, J. M., Hardisty, R. M., Rapson, N. T. and Greaves, M. F. (1977). Acute lymphoblastic leukemia in children: classification and prognosis. *Lancet*, 2: 1307–9

Chessels, J. M., Janossy, G., Lawler, S. D. and Walker, L. M. S. (1979). The Ph' chromosome in childhood leukemia. *British Journal of Haematology*, 41: 25–41

Chien, Y. H. and Thompson, E. B. (1980). Genomic organization of rat prolactin and growth hormone genes. *Proceedings of the National Academy of Sciences (USA)*, 77: 4583–7

Childs, G., Maxson, R., Cohn, R. H. and Kedes, L. (1981). Orphons: dispersed genetic elements derived from tandem repetitive genes of eucaryotes. *Cell*, 23: 651–63

Choi, E., Ruehl, M. and Wall, R. (1980). RNA splicing generates a variant light chain from an aberrantly rearranged κ gene. *Nature*, 286: 776–9

Cimino, M. C., Rowley, J. D., Kinnealey, A., Variakojis, D. and Golomb, H. M. (1979). Banding studies of chromosomal abnormalities in patients with acute lymphocytic leukemia. *Cancer Research*, 39: 227–38

Claesson, M. H., Rodger, M. B., Johnson, G. R., Whittingham, S. and Metcalf, D. (1977). Colony formation by human T lymphocytes in agar medium. *Clinical and Experimental Immunology*, 28: 526–34

Clark, E. A. and Harmon, R. C. (1980). Genetic control of natural cytotoxicity and hybrid resistance. *Advances in Cancer Research, 31*: 227–83

Clarkson, B. D. (1969). Review of recent studies of cellular proliferation in acute leukemia. *National Cancer Institute Monographs, 30*: 81–120

Clarren, S. K. and Smith, D. W. (1978). The fetal alcohol syndrome. *New England Journal of Medicine, 298*: 1063–7

Cleaver, J. E. (1974). Repair processes for photochemical damage in mammalian cells. *Advances in Radiation Biology, 4*: 1–75

Clemmeson, J. (1965). *Statistical Studies in the Aetiology of Malignant Neoplasms*, 4 vols, Munksgaard, Copenhagen

Cleveland, L. R. (1947). The origin and evolution of meiosis. *Science, 195*: 287–9

Clunet, J. (1910). *Recherches Experimentales sur les Tumeurs Malignes*. Steinheil, Paris

Coggin, J. H. and Anderson, N. G. (1974). Cancer differentiation and embryonic antigens: some central problems. *Advances in Cancer Research, 19*: 105–65

Cohen, A. J. (1979). Critical reviews of the toxicology of coumarin with special reference to interspecies differences in metabolism and hepatotoxic response and their significance to man. *Food and Cosmetics Toxicology, 17*: 277–89

Cohen, B. H. (1978) Common familial component in lung cancer and chronic obstructive pulmonary disease. *Lancet, 1*: 95–6

Cohen, B. H., Diamond, E. L., Graves, C. G., Kreiss, P., Levy, D. A., Menkes, H. A., Permutt, S., Quaskey, S. and Tockman, M. S. (1977). A common familial component in lung cancer and chronic obstructive pulmonary disease. *Lancet, 2*: 523–6

Cohen, L. A., Chan, P. C. and Wynder, E. L. (1981). The role of a high-fat diet in enhancing the development of mammary tumors in ovariectomised rats. *Cancer, 47*: 66–71

Cohen, P. and Dix, D. (1981). Lactation and breast cancer. Are they unrelated? *European Journal of Cancer, 17*: 259–60

Cohle, S. D., Tschen, J. A., Smith, F. E., Lane, M. and McGavran, M. H. (1979). ACTH-secreting carcinoma of the breast. *Cancer, 43*: 2370–6

Cohnheim, J. (1889). *Lectures on General Pathology*, 3 vols, New Sydenham Society, London

Coiffier, B., Sicard, B., Bryon, P. A. and Germain, D. (1980). Observations on human bone marrow granulocytic progenitor cell culture: a comparison of two ways to express results. *British Journal of Haematology, 44*: 335–7

Coldman, A. J., Fryer, C. J. H., Elwood, J. M. and Sonley, M. J. (1980). Neuroblastoma: influence of age at diagnosis stage, tumor site, and sex on prognosis. *Cancer, 46*: 1896–1901

Cole, M. P., Jones, C. T. A. and Todd, I. D. H. (1971). A new anti-oestrogenic agent in late breast cancer. An early clinical appraisal of ICI46474. *British Journal of Cancer, 25*: 270–9

Cole, P. and Merletti, F. (1983). Occupational cancer. In: G. J. Bourke (ed.), *The Epidemiology of Cancer*, Croom Helm, London, pp. 260–91

Coleman, M., Silver, R. T., Pajak, T. F., Cavalli, F., Rai, K. R., Kostinas, J. E., Glidewell, O. and Holland, J. F. (1980). Combination chemotherapy for terminal-phase chronic granulocytic leukemia: cancer and leukemia group B studies. *Blood, 55*: 29–36

Coley, W. B. (1898). The treatment of inoperable sarcoma with the mixed toxins of erysipelas and *Bacillus prodigiosus*: immediate and final results in 140 cases. *Journal of the American Medical Association, 31*: 389–95 and 456–65

Conley, G. L., Misiti, J. and Laster, A. J. (1980). Genetic factors predisposing to chronic lymphocytic leukemia and to autoimmune disease. *Medicine, 59*: 323–34

Connors, T. A. (1980). Alkylating drugs, dinitrosourea and dimethyltriazenes. In:

H. M. Pinedo (ed.), *Cancer Chemotherapy 1980*, Excerpta Medica, Amsterdam and Oxford, pp. 27–65

Cook, J. W., Hieger, I., Kennaway, E. L. and Mayneord, W. V. (1932). The production of cancer by pure hydrocarbons. *Proceedings of the Royal Society B.*, *3*: 455–84

Cook, J. W. and Kennaway, E. L. (1940). Chemical compounds as carcinogenic agents. *American Journal of Cancer*, *39*: 381–428

Cooke, I. D. (1976). Oestrogens as a cause of endometrial carcinoma. *British Medical Journal*, *1*: 1209–10

Cossman, J. and Berard, C. W. (1980). Malignant lymphomas: the role of immunologic markers in diagnosis, subclassification and management. *Human Pathology*, *11*: 309–11

Coulombre, J. L. and Coulombre, A. J. (1971). Metaplastic induction of scales and feathers in the corneal anterior epithelium of the chick embryo. *Developmental Biology*, *25*: 464–78

Coulter, J. R. (1983). The role of drugs in the production of human cancer. In: G. J. Bourke (ed.), *The Epidemiology of Cancer*, Croom Helm, London, pp. 327–42

Court-Brown, W. M. (1964). Chromosomal abnormality and chronic lymphatic leukemia. *Lancet*, *1*: 986

Cowen, J. M., Walker, S. and Harris, F. (1979). Trisomy 13 and extended survival. *Journal of Medical Genetics*, *16*: 155–7

Cox, R. and Tuck, M. T. (1981). Alteration of methylation patterns in rat liver histones following administration of ethionine, a liver carcinogen. *Cancer Research*, *41*: 1253–6

Cramer, J. W., Miller, J. A. and Miller, E. C. (1960). N-Hydroxylation: a new metabolic reaction observed in the rat with the carcinogen 2-acetylaminofluorene. *Journal of Biological Chemistry*, *235*: 885–8

Creasy, M. R., Crolla, J. A. and Alberman, E. D. (1976). A cytogenetic study of human spontaneous abortions using banding techniques. *Human Genetics*, *31*: 177–96

Crittenden, L. B., Witter, R. L. and Fadly, A. M. (1979). Low incidence of lymphoid tumours in chickens continuously producing endogenous virus. *Avian Diseases*, *23*: 646–53

Crooke, S. T. (1980). Antitumor antibiotics II: actinomycin D, bleomycin, mitomycin and other antibiotics. In: H. M. Pinedo (ed.), *Cancer Chemotherapy 1980*, Excerpta Medica, Amsterdam and Oxford, pp. 84–94

Crossen, P. E. (1975). Giemsa banding patterns in chronic lymphocytic leukemia. *Humangenetik*, *27*: 151–6

Cullen, B. R., Lomedico, P. T. and Ju, G. (1984). Transcriptional interference in avian retroviruses — implications for the promoter insertion model of leukaemogenesis. *Nature*, *307*: 241–5

Culvenor, C. C. J. and Jago, M. V. (1979). Carcinogenic plant products and DNA. In: P. L. Grover (ed.), *Chemical Carcinogens and DNA*, CRC Press, Boca Raton, Louisiana. Vol. 1, pp. 161–86

Cunningham, I., Gee, T., Dowling, M., Changanti, R., Bailey, R., Hopfan, S., Bowden, L., Turnbull, A., Knapper, W. and Clarkson, B. (1979). Results of treatment of Ph′+ chronic myelogenous leukemia with an intensive treatment regimen. *Blood*, *53*: 375–95

Cutler, B. S., Forbes, A. P., Ingersoll, F. M. and Scully, R. E. (1972). Endometrial carcinoma after stilbestrol therapy in gonadal dysgenesis. *New England Journal of Medicine*, *287*: 628–31

Daar, A. S., Merrill, C. R., Moolla, S. M. and Clarke, T. N. S. (1981). Rectal examination and acid phosphatase: evidence for persistence of a myth. *British Medical Journal*, *282*: 1378–9

Dalbey, W. E., Nettesheim, P., Griesemer, R., Caton, J. E. and Guerin, M. R. (1980). Chronic inhalation of cigarette smoke by F344 rats. *Journal of the National Cancer Institute, 64*: 383–90

Dallapiccola, B., Lungarotti, M. S., Falorni, A., Magnani, M. and Dacha, M. (1980a). Evidence for the assignment of GuKl gene locus to 1q32-q43 segment from gene dosage effect. *Annals of Genetics, 23*: 83–5

Dallapiccola, B., Bruni, L., Boscherini, B., Pasquino, A. M., Chessa, L. and Vignetti, P. (1980b). Segregation of an x ring chromosome in two generations. *Journal of Medical Genetics, 17*: 306–8

Damjanov, I., Solter, D. and Skreb, N. (1979). Teratomas. In: V. S. Turusov (ed.), *Pathology of Tumours in Laboratory Animals. Volume 2 — Tumours of the Mouse*, World Health Organization/International Agency for Research on Cancer, Lyon, p. 655

Danes, B. S. (1979). In vitro evidence for adenoma-carcinoma sequence in large bowel. *Lancet, 2*: 44–5

Daniel, A., Perel, I. D., Clarke, A. J. and Saville, T. (1979). Familial dicentric translocation t(13;18)(p13;p11.2) ascertained by recurrent miscarriages. *Journal of Medical Genetics, 16*: 73–5

Dannies, P. S. and Rudnick, M. S. (1980). 2-Bromo-ergocryptine causes degradation of prolactin in primary cultures of rat pituitary cells after chronic treatments. *Journal of Biological Chemistry, 255*: 2776–81

Darby, G. (1980). The uninvited guests. *Nature, 285*: 13–15

Das, P. K. (1980). Chromosome change during growth in *Puschkinia libanotica L. (Liliaceae)*. *Experientia, 36*: 315–16

Dausset, J. (1977). HLA and association with malignancy. In: G. P. Murphy (ed.), *HLA and Malignancy*, A. Liss, New York, pp. 131–44

Dausset, J. and Svejgaard, D. A. (eds.) (1977). *HLA and Disease*, Williams and Wilkins, Munksgaard

Davidson, E. H. and Britten, R. J. (1979). Regulation of gene expression: possible role of repetitive sequences. *Science, 204*: 1052–9

Davidson, R. L., Kaufman, E. R., Dougherty, C. P., Ouelette, A. M., Difolco, C. M. and Latt, S. A. (1980). Induction of sister chromatid exchanges by BUdR is largely independent of the BUdR content of DNA. *Nature, 284*: 74–6

De Boer, L. E. M. (1980). Do the chromosomes of the Kiwi provide evidence for a monophyletic origin of the ratites? *Nature, 287*: 84–5

De Bruyère, M., Cornu, G., Heremans-Bracke, T., Malchaire, J. and Sokal, G. (1980). HLA haplotypes and long survival in childhood acute lymphoblastic leukemia treated with transfer factor. *British Journal of Haematology, 44*: 243–51

De Grouchy, J. and Turleau, C. (1977). *Clinical Atlas of Human Chromosomes*, Wiley and Sons, New York

De la Chapelle, A. (1972). Analytic review: nature and origin of males with XX sex chromosomes. *Journal of Human Genetics, 24*: 71–105

De la Chapelle, A., Hortling, H., Sanger, R. and Race, R. R. (1964). Successive non-disjunction at first and second meiotic division of spermatogenesis: evidence of chromosomes and Xg. *Cytogenetics, 3*: 334–41

Del Villano, B. C. Miller, S. I., Schacter, L. P. and Tischfield, J. A. (1980). Elevated superoxide dismutase in black alcoholics. *Science, 207*: 991–3

Denburg, J. A., Wilson, W. E. C., Goodacre, R. and Bienenstock, J. (1980). Chronic myeloid leukemia: evidence for basophil differentiation and histamine synthesis from cultured peripheral blood cells. *British Journal of Haematology, 45*: 13–21

Denef, C., Manet, D. and Dewals, R. (1980). Dopaminergic stimulation of prolactin release. *Nature, 285*: 243–6

Denman, T. (1810). *Observations on the Cure of Cancer*, J. Johnston, London

DeOme, K. B., Nandi, S., Bern, H. A., Blair, P. and Pitelka, D. (1962). The preneoplastic hyperplastic alveolar nodule as the morphological precursor of mammary cancer in mice. In: L. Severs (ed.), *The Morphological Precursors of Cancer*, Division of Cancer Research, Perugia, pp. 349–68

Deschner, E. E., Long, F. C., Hakissian, M. and Cupo, S. H. (1984). Differential susceptibility of inbred mouse strains forecast by acute colonic proliferative response to methylazoxymethanol. *Journal of the National Cancer Institute, 72*: 195–8

De Sombre, E. R. and Jensen, E. V. (1980). Estrophilin assays in breast cancer: quantitative features and application to the mastectomy specimen. *Cancer, 46*: 2783–8

De-Thé, G. and Ito, Y. (eds.) (1978). *Nasopharyngeal Carcinoma: Etiology and Control*, International Agency for Research on Cancer, Lyon

Devesa, S. S. and Diamond, E. L. (1980). Association of breast cancer and cervical cancer incidences with income and education among whites and blacks. *Journal of the National Cancer Institute, 65*: 515–28

Devesa, S. S. and Silverman, D. T. (1978). Cancer incidence and mortality trends in the United States 1935–74. *Journal of the National Cancer Institute, 60*: 545–71

De Waard, F. (1975). Breast cancer incidence and nutritional status with particular reference to body height and weight. *Cancer Research, 35*: 3351–6

De Weerd-Kastelein, E. A., Keijzer, W., Rainaldi, G. and Bootsma, D. (1977). Induction of sister chromatid exchanges in xeroderma pigmentosum cells after exposure to ultraviolet light. *Mutation Research, 45*: 253–61

De Wolf, W. C., Dupoint, B. and Yunis, E. J. (1980). HLA and disease: current concepts. *Human Pathology, 11*: 332–7

Dexter, T. M., Allen, T. D., Lajtha, L.G., Krizsa, F., Testa, N. G. and Moore, M. A. S. (1978). In vitro analysis of self-renewal and commitment of hematopoietic stem cells. In: B. Clarkson, P. Marks and J. Till (eds.), *Differentiation of Normal and Neoplastic Hematopoietic Stem Cells*, Cold Spring Harbor Symposium, Cold Spring Harbor, pp. 63–80

Diamond, L., O'Brien, T. G. and Baird, W. M. (1980). Tumor promoters and the mechanism of tumor promotion. *Advances in Cancer Research, 32*: 1

Dicke, K. A., Spitzer, G. and Ahearn, M. J. (1976). Colony formation in vitro by leukaemic cells in acute myelogenous leukaemia with phytohaemagglutinin as stimulating factor. *Nature, 259*: 129–30

Dicker, P. and Rozengurt, E. (1979). Retinoids enhance mitogenesis by tumour promotor and polypeptide growth factors. *Biochemical and Biophysical Research Communications, 91*: 1203–10

Dicker, P. and Rozengurt, E. (1980). Phorbol esters and vasopressin stimulate DNA synthesis by a common mechanism. *Nature, 287*: 607–12

Dingerkus, G. (1976). Karyotypic analysis and evidence of tetraploidy in the North American paddlefish, *Polyodon spathula*. *Science, 194*: 842–3

Dmochowski, L. (1949). Some data on the distribution of the milk factor. *British Journal of Cancer, 3*: 525–33

Dodds, E. C., Goldberg, L., Lawson, W. and Robinson, R. (1938). Oestrogenic activity of certain synthetic compounds. *Nature, 141*: 247–8

Dofuku, R., Beidler, J. L., Spengler, B. A. and Old, L. J. (1975). Trisomy of chromosome 15 in spontaneous leukemia of AKR mice. *Proceedings of the National Academy of Sciences (USA), 72*: 1515–7

Doll, R. (1977). Introduction. In: H. H. Hiatt, J. D. Watson and J. A. Winstein (eds.), *Origins of Human Cancer*, Cold Spring Harbor Laboratory, Cold Spring Harbor, New York, pp. 1–12

Doll, R. and Peto, R. (1981). Avoidable risks of cancer in the United States. *Journal of the National Cancer Institute, 66*: 1193–1308

Donati, M. B. and Poggi, A. (1980). Malignancy and haemostasis. *British Journal of Haematology, 44*: 173–82

Dontenwill, W., Chevalier, H. J., Harke, H. P., Lafrenz, U., Reckzeh, G. and Schneider, B. (1973). Investigation on the effects of chronic cigarette-smoke inhalation in Syrian golden hamsters. *Journal of the National Cancer Institute, 51*: 1781–1832

Doolittle, W. F., Kirkwood, T. B. L. and Dempster, M. A. H. (1984). Selfish DNAs with self-restraint. *Nature, 307*: 501–2

Doolittle, W. F. and Sapienza, C. (1980). Selfish genes, the phenotype paradigm and genome evolution. *Nature, 284*: 601–3

Dorn, H. F. and Cutler, S. J. (1959). *Morbidity from Cancer in the United States, Public Health Monograph No. 56*, United States Government Printing Office, Washington, DC

Dosik, G. M., Barlogie, B., Göde, W., Johnston, D., Tekell, J. L. and Drewinko, B. (1980). Flow cytometry of DNA content in human bone marrow: a critical reappraisal. *Blood, 55*: 734–40

Douglass, E. C., Magrath, I. T., Lee, E. C. and Whang-Peng, J. (1980). Cytogenetic studies in non-African Burkitt lymphoma. *Blood, 55*: 148–55

Downward, J., Yarden, Y., Mayes, E., Scrace, G., Totty, N., Stockwell, P., Ullrich, A., Schlessinger, J., and Waterfield, M. D. (1984). Close similarity of epidermal growth factor receptor and *v-erb-B* oncogene protein sequences. *Nature, 307*: 521–7

Dresch, C., Faille, A., Poirier, D. Balitrand, N. and Najean, Y. (1980). Bone marrow cell kinetics and culture in chronic and subacute myelomonocytic leukemia. Physiopathological interpretation and prognostic importance. *Leukemia Research, 4*: 129–42

Dresp, J., Schmid, E. and Bauchinger, M. (1978). The cytogenetic effect of bleomycin on human peripheral lymphocytes in vitro and in vivo. *Mutation Research, 56*: 341–53

Drummond, M. H., Gordon, M. P., Nestor, E. W. and Chilton, M. D. (1977). Foreign DNA of bacterial plasmid origin is transcribed in crown gall tumours. *Nature, 269*: 535–6

Dubochet, J. and Noll, M. (1978). Nucleosome arcs and helices. *Science, 202*: 280–6

Duckett, D. P. and Roberts, S. H. (1980). A new pericentric inversion of chromosome 6 in an abnormal infant. *Annals of Genetics, 23*: 117–18

Dufrain, R. J., Littlefield, L. G. and Wilmer, J. L. (1980). The effect of washing lymphocytes after in vivo treatment with streptonigrin on the yield of chromosome and chromatid aberrations in blood cultures. *Mutation Research, 69*: 101–5

Dulbecco, R. (1979). Contributions of microbiology to eucaryotic cell biology: new directions for microbiology. *Microbiological Reviews, 43*: 443–52

Dunn, T. B. (1954). Normal and pathologic anatomy of the reticular tissue in laboratory mice, with a classification and discussion of neoplasms. *Journal of the National Cancer Institute, 14*: 1281–1433

Dunn, T. B. (1979). Cancer and other lesions in mice receiving estrogens. *Recent Results in Cancer Research, 66*: 175–92

Du Praw, E. J. and Bahr, G. F. (1969). The arrangement of DNA in human chromosomes as investigated by quantitative electron microscopy. *Acta Cytologica, 13*: 188–205

Durack, D. T. (1981). Opportunistic infections and Kaposi's sarcoma in homosexual men. *New England Journal of Medicine, 305*: 1465–7

Durant, W. (1935). *Our Oriental Heritage*, Simon and Shuster, New York

Dykhuizen, D. and Hartl, D. (1980). Molecular clockwork. *Nature, 287*: 90

Eadie, J. S., Conrad, M., Toorchen, D., and Topal, M. C. (1984). Mechanism of mutagenesis by *O*-methylguanine. *Nature, 308*: 201–3

Early, P., Huang, M., Davis, M., Calame, K. and Hood, L. (1980). An immunoglobulin heavy chain variable region gene is generated from three segments of DNA: V, D, and J. *Cell, 19*: 981–92

Eastcott, D. F. (1963). Epidemiology of skin cancer in New Zealand. In: F. Urbach (ed.), *The Biology of Cutaneous Cancer*, National Cancer Institute Monograph Number 10, US Government Printing Office, Washington, DC, pp. 141–5

Easty, G. C. and Easty, D. M. (1976). Tissue culture methods in cancer research. In: T. Symington and R. L. Carter (eds.), *Scientific Foundations of Oncology*, Heinemann, London, pp. 15-25

Ebbel, B. (1937). *The Papyrus Ebers: The Greatest Egyptian Medical Document*, Levin and Munksgaard, Copenhagen

Eccles, S. A. and Alexander, P. (1974). Macrophage content of tumours in relation to metastatic spread and host immune reaction. *Nature, 250*: 667–9

Edgreen, J., De La Chapelle, A. and Kääriainen, R. (1966). Cytogenetic study of seventy-three patients with Down's syndrome. *Journal of Mental Deficiency Research, 10*: 47–62

Egami, N. and Ijiri, K. (1979). Effects of irradiation on germ cells and embryonic development in teleosts. *International Review of Cytology, 59*: 195–248

El Etr, M., Slatkine, S. S. and Baulieu, E. E. (1980). Initiation of meiotic maturation in *Xenopus laevis* oocytes by insulin. In: S. Iacobelli, R. J. B. King, H. R. Lindner and M. E. Lippman (eds.), *Hormones and Cancer*, Raven Press, New York, pp. 209–15

Ellerman, V. and Bang, O. (1909). Experimentelle leukämie bei Hühnern. *Centralblatt für Bakteriologie, 46*: 595–609

Ellman, L., Hammond, D. and Atkins, L. (1979). Eosinophilia, chloromas and a chromosome abnormality in a patient with a myeloproliferative syndrome. *Cancer, 43*: 2410–3

El-Shirbiny, A. F., Parkhurst, S., Bettigole, R. E. and Tourbaf, K. D. (1980). Haemoglobin E trait and probable α-thalassaemia in a black American family: a family study. *Journal of Medical Genetics, 17*: 285–7

Emanuel, B. S. (1978). Compound lateral asymmetry in human chromosome 6: BrdU-dye studies of 6q12→6q14. *American Journal of Human Genetics, 30*: 153–9

Emmett, E. A. (1974). Ultraviolet radiation as a cause of skin tumors. *CRC Critical Reviews in Toxicology, 2*: 211–55

Emperaire, J. C. and Greenblatt, R. B. (1969). L'implantation de pellets d'oestradiol dans la contraception. *Gynécologie Pratique, 5*: 327

Enesco, M. and Leblond, C. P. (1962). Increase in cell number as a factor in the growth of the organs and tissues of the young male rat. *Journal of Embryology and Experimental Morphology, 10*: 530–62

Engel, E., McGee, B. J., Flexner, J. M., Russell, M. T. and Myers, B. J. (1974). Philadelphia chromosome (Ph) translocation in an apparently Ph negative, minus G22, case of chronic myeloid leukemia. *New England Journal of Medicine, 291*: 154

Enstrom, J. E. (1979). Rising lung cancer mortality among nonsmokers. *Journal of the National Cancer Institute, 62*: 755–60

Enstrom, J. E. and Godley, F. H. (1980). Cancer mortality among a representative sample of non-smokers in the United States during 1966–68. *Journal of the National Cancer Institute, 65*: 1175–83

Epstein, M. A., Achong, B. G. and Barr, Y. M. (1964). Virus particles in cultured lymphoblasts from Burkitt's lymphoma. *Lancet, 1*: 702–3

Epstein, S. (1978). *The Politics of Cancer*, Sierra, San Francisco

Epstein, S. and Schwartz, J. B. (1981). Fallacies of lifestyle cancer theories. *Nature, 289*: 127–30

Evans, A. E., D'Angio, G. J. and Randolph, J. (1971). A proposed staging for children with neuroblastoma. *Cancer, 27*: 374–8

Evans, D. A. P., Mahgoub, A., Sloan, T. P., Idle, J. R. and Smith, R. L. (1980). A family and population study of the genetic polymorphism of debrisoquine oxidation in a white British population. *Journal of Medical Genetics, 17*: 102–5

Evans, H. J. (1974). Effects of ionizing radiation on mammalian chromosomes. In: J. German (ed.), *Chromosomes and Cancer*, Wiley and Sons, New York, pp. 191–237

Evans, H. M. and Swezy, O. (1929). The chromosomes in man: sex and somatic. *Memoirs of the University of California, 9*: 1–64

Everson, R. B., Lippman, M. E., Thompson, E. B., McGuire, W. L., Wittliff, J. L., De Sombre, E. R., Jensen, E. V., Singhakowinta, A., Brooks, S. C. and Neifeld, J. P. (1980). Clinical correlations of steroid receptors and male breast cancer. *Cancer Research, 40*: 991

Everson, T. C. and Cole, W. H. (1966). *Spontaneous Regression of Cancer*, W. B. Saunders, Philadelphia

Ewing, J. (1940). *Neoplastic Diseases: A Treatise on Tumors*, 4th edn., Saunders, Philadelphia, ch. 12

Fadly, A. M., Purchase, H. G. and Gilmour, D. G. (1981). Tumor latency in avian lymphoid leukosis. *Journal of the National Cancer Institute, 66*: 549–52

Fairlamb, D. G. (1981). Spontaneous regression of metastases of renal cancer. *Cancer, 47*: 2102–6

Falk, H., Telles, N. C., Ishak, K. G., Thomas, L. B. and Popper, H. (1979). Epidemiology of thorotrast-induced hepatic angiosarcoma in the United States. *Environmental Research, 18*: 65–73

Farber, E., Cameron, R. G., Laishes, B., Lin, J. C., Medline, A., Ogawa, K. and Solt, D. B. (1979). Physiological and molecular markers during carcinogenesis. In: A. C. Griffin and C. R. Shaw (eds.), *Carcinogens: Identification and Mechanisms of Action*, Raven Press, New York, pp. 319–35

Farber, S., Dramond, L. K., Mercer, R. D., Sylvester, R. F. and Wolff, J. A. (1948). Temporary remissions in acute leukemia in children produced by folic acid antagonist, 4-aminopteroylglutamic acid (aminopterin). *New England Journal of Medicine, 238*: 787–93

Feingold, J. (1978). Génétique et cancers humains: méthodologie d'étude. *Bulletin du Cancer* (Paris), *65*: 73–7

Fialkow, P. J., Jacobson, R. J., Singer, J. W., Sacher, R. A., McGuffin, R. W. and Neefe, J. R. (1980). Philadelphia chromosome (Ph)-negative chronic myelogenous leukemia (CML): a clonal disease with origin in a multipotent stem cell. *Blood, 56*: 70–3

Fibach, E., Landau, T. and Sachs, L. (1972). Normal differentiation of myeloid leukemic cells induced by a differentiation-inducing protein. *Nature New Biology, 237*: 276–8

Fidler, I. J., Gersten, D. M. and Hart, I. R. (1978). The biology of cancer invasion and metastasis. *Advances in Cancer Research, 28*: 149–250

Fidler, I. J. and Kripke, M. L. (1977). Metastasis results from preexisting variant cells within a malignant tumor. *Science, 197*: 893–5

Fieser, L. F. (1938). Carcinogenic activity, structure, and chemical reactivity of polynuclear aromatic hydrocarbons. *American Journal of Cancer, 34*: 37–124

Filippi, G. and McKusick, V. A. (1970). The Beckwith-Wiedemann syndrome. *Medicine, 49*: 279–98

Finan, J., Daniele, R., Rowlands, D. and Nowell, P. (1978). Cytogenetics of chronic T cell leukemia including two patients with a 14qt translocation. *Virchow's Archives B Cell Pathology, 29*: 121–7

Fisher, B. and Gebhardt, M. C. (1978). The evolution of breast cancer surgery: past, present and future. *Seminars in Oncology, 5*: 385–94

Fisher, P. B., Weinstein, B., Eisenberg, D. and Ginsberg, H. S. (1978). Interactions between adenovirus, a tumour promoter, and chemical carcinogens in transformation of rat embryo cell cultures. *Proceedings of the National Academy of Sciences (USA)*, 75: 2311–4

Fisher, R. I., Neifeld, J. P. and Lippman, M. E. (1976). Oestrogen receptors in human malignant melanoma. *Lancet*, 2: 337–8

Fishman, J. and Tulchinsky, D. (1980). Suppression of prolactin secretion in normal young women by 2-hydroxyestrone. *Science*, 210: 73–4

Flavell, R. A. (1981). Tissue-specific expression of α-amylase. *Nature*, 290: 541–2

Flemming, W. (1882). Beitrage zur Kenntniss der Zelle und ihre Lebenserscheinungen. *Archiv für Mikrobiologische Anatomie*, 20: 1–86

Floridi, A., Paggi, M. G., Marcante, M. L., Silvestrini, B., Caputo, A. and De Martino, C. (1981). Lonidamine, a selective inhibitor of aerobic glycolysis of murine tumor cells. *Journal of the National Cancer Institute*, 66: 497–9

Foa, R., Catovsky, D., Cherchi, M., Benavides I., Ganeshaguru, K. and Hoffbrand, A. V. (1980). Cell surface and enzyme markers of cord blood lymphocytes. *British Journal of Haematology*, 44: 583–92

Folca, P. J., Glascock, R. F. and Irvine, W. T. (1961). Studies with tritium-labelled hexoestrol in advanced breast cancer. *Lancet*, 2: 796–8

Foon, K. A., Herzog, P., Billing, R. J., Terasaki, P. I. and Feig, S. A. (1981). Immunologic classification of childhood acute lymphocytic leukemia. *Cancer*, 47: 280–4

Ford, C. E. and Hamerton, J. L. (1956). The chromosomes of man. *Nature*, 2: 1020–3

Ford, C. E., Jones, K. W., Polani, P. E., De Almeida, J. C. and Briggs, J. H. (1959). A sex-chromosome anomaly in a case of gonadal dysgenesis (Turner's syndrome). *Lancet*, 1: 711–13

Forrester, R. M. (1973). Wiedemann-Beckwith syndrome. *Lancet*, 2: 47

Forster, A., Hobart, M., Hengartner, H. and Rabbits, T. H. (1980). An immunoglobulin heavy-chain gene is altered in two T-cell clones. *Nature*, 286: 897–9

Foulds, L. (1969). *Neoplastic Development. Volume 1*, Academic Press, New York

Foulds, L. (1975). *Neoplastic Development. Volume 2*, Academic Press, New York

Fournier, D. V., Weber, E., Hoeffken, W., Bauer, M., Kubli, F. and Barth, V. (1980). Growth rate of 147 mammary carcinomas. *Cancer*, 45: 2198–2207

Fox, M. (1984a). Gene amplification and drug resistance. *Nature*, 307: 212–13

Fox, T. D. (1984b). Multiple forms of mitochondrial DNA in higher plants. *Nature*, 307: 415

Fraley, E. E., Lange, P. H. and Kennedy, B. J. (1979). Germ-cell testicular cancer in adults. *New England Journal of Medicine*, 301: 1370–7 and 1420–6

Francke, U. (1976). Retinoblastoma and chromosome 13. *Cytogenetics Cell Genetics*, 16: 131–4

Frantz, C. N., Stiles, C. D. and Scher, C. D. (1979). The tumor promoter 12-0-tetradecanoyl-phorbol-13-acetate enhances the proliferative response of Balb/c-3T3 cells to hormonal growth factors. *Journal of Cell Physiology*, 100: 413–24

Freeman, N. R. (1981). Quoted as a personal communication in Urbach (1983)

Fridovich, I. (1978). The biology of oxygen radicals. *Science*, 201: 875–80

Frydman, M., Shabtai, F., Barak, Y., Halbrecht, I. and Elian, E. (1979). Triple mosaicism 45.XY,−18/46,XY/47.XY,+18. *Journal of Medical Genetics*, 16: 232–3

Fuks, A., Banjo, C., Shuster, J., Freedman, S. O. and Gold, P. (1974). Carcinoembryonic antigen (CEA): molecular biology and clinical significance. *Biochimica et Biophysica Acta*, 417: 123–52

Fukuhara, S., Rowley, J. D. and Variakojis, D. (1978). Banding studies of chromosomes in a patient with mycosis fungoides. *Cancer*, 42: 2262–8

Furbetta, M., Galanello, R., Ximenes, A., Angius, A., Melis, M. A., Serra, P. and

Cao, A. (1979). Interaction of alpha and beta thalassemia genes in two Sardinian families. *British Journal of Haematology, 41*: 203–10

Fussel, C. P. (1975). The position of interphase chromosomes and late replicating DNA in centromere and telomere regions of *Allium cepa* L. *Chromosoma, 50*: 201–10

Futuyma, D. J. (1979). *Evolutionary Biology,* Sinavar Associates, Sunderland, Massachusetts

Gahrton, G., Friberg, K., Zech, L. and Lindsten, J. (1978). Duplication of part of chromosome no. 1 in myeloproliferative disease. *Lancet, 1*: 96–7

Gaille, T. (1567). *The Institucion of Chyrurgerie,* Henry Denham, London, p. 367

Galanaud, P., Chaput, J. C., Buffet, C. and Rain, B. (1976). Hépatome après oestrogénothérapie prolongée. *Nouvelle Presse Médicale, 5*: 209

Galjaard, H. (1978). Early diagnosis and prevention of genetic disease: molecules and the obstetrician. In: J. B. Scrimgeour (ed.), *Towards the Prevention of Fetal Malformation,* Edinburgh University Press, Edinburgh, pp. 3–18

Galli, M. C., De Giovanni, C., Nicoletti, G., Grilli, S., Nanni, P., Prodi, G., Gola, G., Rochetta, R. and Orlandi, C. (1981). The occurrence of multiple steroid hormone receptors in disease-free and neoplastic human ovary, *Cancer, 47*: 1297–1302

Gallo, E., Massaro, P., Miniero, R., David, D. and Tarella, C. (1979). The importance of the genetic picture and globin synthesis in determining the clinical and haematological features of thalassemia intermedia. *British Journal of Haematology, 41*: 211–21

Gallo, R. C. and Gelman, E. P. (1981). In search of a Hodgkin's disease virus. *New England Journal of Medicine, 304*: 169–70

Galloway, S. M. (1977). Ataxia telangiectasia: the effects of chemical mutagens and x-rays on sister chromatid exchanges in blood lymphocytes. *Mutation Research, 45*: 343–9

Galloway, S. M. and Buckton, K. E. (1978). Aneuploidy and ageing: chromosome studies on a random sample of the population using G-banding. *Cytogenetics Cell Genetics, 20*: 78–95

Galloway, S. M. and Evans, H. J. (1975). Sister chromatid exchange in human chromosomes from normal individuals and patients with ataxia telangiectasia. *Cytogenetics Cell Genetics, 15*: 17–29

Gardner, L. I. (1973). Pseudo-Beckwith-Wiedemann syndrome: interaction with maternal diabetes. *Lancet, 2*: 911–12

Gardner, R. L. (1983). Teratomas in perspective. *Cancer Surveys, 2*: 1

Gardner, W. U. (1947). Studies on steroid hormones in experimental carcinogenesis. *Recent Progress in Hormone Research, 1*: 217–59

Gardner, W. U. (1948). Hormonal imbalances in tumorigenesis. *Cancer Research, 8*: 397–411

Gardner, W. U. and Allen, E. (1939). Malignant and non-malignant uterine and vaginal lesions in mice receiving estrogens and estrogens and androgens simultaneously. *Yale Journal of Biology and Medicine, 12*: 213–34

Garfunkel, L. (1981). Time trends in lung cancer mortality among non-smokers and a note on passive smoking. *Journal of the National Cancer Institute, 66*: 1061

Garrison, F. H. (1929). *An Introduction to the History of Medicine,* 4th edn, W. B. Saunders, Philadelphia

Garson, O. M. (1980). Acute non-lymphocytic leukemia. *Clinics in Haematology, 9*: 39–54

Gateff, E. (1982). Cancer, genes, and development: the *Drosophila* case. *Advances in Cancer Research, 37*: 33–74

Geard, C. R., Colvett, R. D. and Rohrig, N. (1980). On the mechanisms of chromosomal aberrations. A study with single and multiple spatially-associated protons. *Mutation Research, 69*: 87–99

Gendron, C. D. (1701). *Enquiries into the Nature, Knowledge and Cure of Cancers*, J. Taylor, London

Geraedts, J. P. M., Person, P. L., Van Der Ploeg, M. and Vossepoel, A. M. (1975). Polymorphisms for human chromosomes 1 and Y. Fuelgen and UV DNA measurements. *Experimental Cell Research*, *95*: 9–14

Gerli, M., Migliorini, G., Bocchini, V., Venti, G., Ferrarese, R., Donti, E. and Rosi, G. (1979). A case of complete testicular feminisation and 47,XXY karyotype. *Journal of Medical Genetics*, *16*: 480–3

German, J. (1972). Genes which increase chromosomal instability in somatic cells and predispose to cancer. *Progress in Medical Genetics*, *8*: 61–101

German, J. (1973). Genetic disorders associated with chromosomal instability and cancer. *Journal of Investigative Dermatology*, *60*: 427–34

German, J. (1974a). Bloom's syndrome. II. The prototype of human genetic disorders predisposing to chromosome instability and cancer. In: J. German (ed.), *Chromosomes and Cancer*, John Wiley and Sons, New York, pp. 601–17

German, J. (ed.) (1974b). *Chromosomes and Cancer*, John Wiley and Sons, New York

German, J., Schonberg, S., Louie, E. and Chaganti, R. S. K. (1977). Bloom's syndrome. IV. Sister-chromatid exchanges in lymphocytes. *American Journal of Human Genetics*, *29*: 248–55

Gialnick, H. R., Galton, D. A. G., Catovsky, D., Sultan, C. and Bennett, J. (1977). Classification of acute leukemia. *Annals of Internal Medicine*, *87*: 740–53

Gilbert, W. (1978). Why genes in pieces? *Nature*, *271*: 501

Glascock, R. F. and Hoekstra, W. G. (1959). Selective accumulation of tritium-labelled hexoestrol by the reproductive organs of immature female goats and sheep. *Biochemical Journal*, *72*: 673–82

Goetsch, E. (1938). Hygroma colli cysticum and hygroma axillare; pathologic and clinical study and report of 12 cases. *Archives of Surgery*, *36*: 394–479

Golbus, M. S. (1978). Prenatal diagnosis of genetic defects — where it is and where it is going. In: J. W. Littlefield, J. de Grouchy and F. J. G. Ebling (eds.), *Birth Defects*, Excerpta Medica, Holland, pp. 330–7

Gold, P. and Freedman, S. O. (1965). Specific carcinoembryonic antigens of the human digestive system. *Journal of Experimental Medicine*, *122*: 467–81

Gold, P. and Freedman, S. O. (1975). Tests for carcinoembryonic antigen. Role in diagnosis and management of cancer. *Journal of the American Medical Association*, *234*: 190–2

Golde, D. W., Hocking, W. G., Quan, S. G., Sparkes, R. S. and Gale, R. P. (1980). Origin of human bone marrow fibroblasts. *British Journal of Haematology*, *44*: 183–7

Golden, C. J., Graber, B., Blose, I., Berg, R., Coffman, J. and Bloch, S. (1981). Difference in brain densities between chronic alcoholic and normal control patients. *Science*, *211*: 508–10

Goldenberg, V. E., Wiegenstein, L. and Mottet, N. K. (1968). Florid breast fibroadenomas in patients taking hormonal contraceptives. *American Journal of Clinical Pathology*, *49*: 52–9

Goldstein, M. N. and Plurad, S. (1980). Drug-induced differentiation of human neuroblastoma: transformation into ganglion cells with mitomycin-C. *Research Problems in Cell Differentiation*, *11*: 259–64

Goodman, R. M. and Motulsky, A. G. (eds.) (1979). *Genetic Diseases Among Askenazi Jews*, Raven Press, New York

Goodwin, D. W. (1976). *Is Alcoholism Hereditary?* Oxford University Press, New York

Goodwin, D. W. (1979). Alcoholism and heredity. *Archives of General Psychiatry*, *36*: 57–61

Gordon, D. S., Hutton, J. J., Smalley, R. V., Meyer, L. M. and Vogler, W. R.

(1978). Terminal deoxynucleotidyl transferase (TdT), cytochemistry, and membrane receptors in adult acute leukemia. *Blood, 52*: 1079–88

Gorer, P. A. (1938). Antigenic basis of tumour transplantation. *Journal of Pathology and Bacteriology, 47*: 231–52

Gorrod, J. W. (ed.) (1978). *Biological Oxidation of Nitrogen*, Elsevier/North Holland, Amsterdam

Gracey, D. R., Fish, J. E. and Divertie, M. B. (1979). Experimental squamous cell lung tumors in Sprague-Dawley and murine pneumonitis free rats. *Cancer, 44*: 598–603

Graf, W. and Diehl, W. (1966). Über den naturbedingten Normalpegel kanzerogener polyzyklischer Aromaten und seine Ursache. *Archiv für Hygiene und Bakteriologie, 150*: 49

Graham, C. F. and Wareing, P. F. (eds.) (1976). *The Developmental Biology of Plants and Animals*, Blackwell Scientific Publications, Oxford

Graham, S. (1980). Diet and cancer. *American Journal of Epidemiology, 112*: 247–52

Gralnick, H. R., Galton, D. A. G., Catovsky, D., Sultan, C. and Bennett, J. M. (1977). Classification of acute leukemia. *Annals of Internal Medicine, 87*: 740–53

Greaves, M., Brown, G., Rapson, N. T. and Lister, T. A. (1975). Antisera to acute lymphoblastic leukemia cells. *Clinical Immunology and Immunopathology, 4*: 67–8

Greaves, M., Delia, D., Janossy, G., Rapson, N., Chessells, J., Woods, M. and Prentice, G. (1980a). Acute lymphoblastic leukaemia associated antigen. IV. Expression on non-leukaemic 'lymphoid' cells. *Leukemia Research, 4*: 15–32

Greaves, M. and Janossy, G. (1978). Patterns of gene expression and the cellular origins of human leukaemias. *Biochimica et Biophysica Acta, 316*: 193–230

Greaves, M., Paxton, A., Janossy, G., Pain, C., Johnson, S. and Lister, T. A. (1980b). Acute lymphoblastic leukaemia associated antigen. III. Alterations in expression during treatment and in relapse. *Leukemia Research, 4*: 1–14

Gregmigni, V., Miceli, C. and Puccinelli, I. (1980a). On the role of germ cells in planarian regeneration. 1 Akaryological investigation. *Journal of Embryology and Experimental Morphology, 55*: 53–63

Gregmigni, V., Miceli, C. and Picano, E. (1980b). On the role of germ cells in planarian regeneration. II. Cytophotometric analysis of the nuclear fuelgen-DNA content in cells. *Journal of Embryology and Experimental Morphology, 55*: 65–76

Griffin, A. C. (1979). Role of selenium in the chemoprevention of cancer. *Advances in Cancer Research, 29*: 419–42

Grilli, G., Carbonell, F. and Fliedner, T. M. (1980). Variations in erythroid and myeloid progenitor cell numbers in normal human peripheral blood. *British Journal of Haematology, 44*: 679–81

Grodin, J. M., Siiteri, P. K. and MacDonald, P. C. (1973). Source of estrogen production in postmenopausal women. *Journal of Clinical Endocrinology and Metabolism, 36*: 207–14

Gross, L. (1970). *Oncogenic Viruses*, 2nd edn, Pergamon Press, New York

Grosse, K. P. and Schwanitz, G. (1977). Double autosomal trisomy: case report (48,XX,+18,+21) and review of the literature. *Journal of Mental Deficiency Research, 21*: 299–308

Grufferman, S., Cole, P., Smith, P. G. and Lukes, R. J. (1977). Hodgkin's disease in siblings. *New England Journal of Medicine, 296*: 248–50

Gubbins, E. J., Maurer, R. A., Lagrimini, M., Erwin, C. R. and Donelson, J. E. (1980). Structure of the rat prolactin gene. *Journal of Biological Chemistry, 255*: 8655–62

Guernsey, D. L., Ong, A. and Borek, C. (1980). Thyroid hormone modulation of x-ray induced in vitro neoplastic transformation. *Nature, 288*: 591–2

Gurdon, J. B. (1974). *The Control of Gene Expression in Animal Development*, Harvard University Press, Cambridge, Massachusetts

Gutmann, H. R. and Bell, P. (1977). *N*-Hydroxylation of arylamides by the rat and guinea pig. Evidence for substrate specificity and participation of cytochrome P-450. *Biochimica et Biophysica Acta, 498*: 229–43

Haagensen, C. D., Bodian, C. and Haagensen, D. E. (1981). *Breast Carcinoma, Risk and Detection*, Saunders, Philadelphia, p. 30

Haddow, A. (1967). Proceedings of the Ninth International Cancer Congress, Tokyo, 1966. *UICC Monograph Series, 8*: 111–16

Haddow, A. (1974). Addendum to 'molecular repair, wound healing, and carcinogenesis: tumor production a possible overhealing'? *Advances in Cancer Research, 20*: 343–66

Haddow, A., Watkinson, J. M., Patterson, E. and Koller, P. C. (1944). Influence of synthetic oestrogens upon advanced malignant disease. *British Medical Journal, 2*: 393–8

Hagberg, H., Gronowitz, S., Killander, A., Kallander, C., Simonsson, B., Sundstrom, C. and Oberg, G. (1984). Serum thymidine kinase in acute leukemia. *British Journal of Cancer, 49*: 537–40

Hagemeijer, A. and Smit, E. M. E. (1977). Partial trisomy 21. Further evidence that trisomy of band 21q22 is essential for Down's phenotype. *Human Genetics, 38*: 15–23

Hagemeijer, A., Smit, E. M. E., Lowenberg, B. and Abel, J. (1979). Chronic myeloid leukemia with permanent disappearance of the Ph chromosome and development of new clonal subpopulations. *Blood, 53*: 1–14

Hagenbüchle, O., Tosi, M., Schibler, U., Bovey, R., Wellauer, P. K. and Young, R. A. (1981). Mouse liver and salivary gland α-amylase mRNAs differ only in 5' non-translated sequences. *Nature, 289*: 643–6

Haines, A. P., Levin, A. G. and Fritsche, H. A. (1979). Ethnic-group differences in serum levels of carcinoembryonic antigen. *Lancet, 2*: 969

Hakama, M. (1983). Cancer of the uterine cervix. In: G. J. Bourke (ed.), *The Epidemiology of Cancer*, Croom Helm, London, pp. 162–75

Hakanson, R., Ekman, R., Sundler, F. and Nilsson, R. (1979). A novel fragment of the corticotropin-B-lipotropin precursor. *Nature, 283*: 789–92

Hall, T. C. (1974). Onco-cognitive autoimmunity and other paraneoplastic syndromes yet to be described. *Annals of the New York Academy of Sciences, 230*: 565–70

Haller, O., Arnheiter, H., Lindenmann, J., and Gresser, I. (1980). Host gene influences sensitivity to interferon action selectivity for influenza virus. *Nature, 283*: 660–1

Hällgren, R., Nou, E. and Lundqvist, G. (1980). Serum β_2-microglobulin in patients with bronchial carcinoma and controls. *Cancer, 45*: 780–5

Halsted, W. S. (1894). The results of operations for the cure of cancer of the breast performed at the Johns Hopkins Hospital from June 1889 to January 1894. *Annals of Surgery, 20*: 497–555

Hamada, Y., Schlaff, S., Kobayashi, Y., Santulli, R., Wright, K. H. and Wallach, E. E. (1980). Inhibitory effect of prolactin on ovulation in the in vitro perfused rabbit ovary. *Nature 285*: 161–3

Hamerton, J. L. (1971). Chromosomes and neoplastic disease. *Clinical Genetics, 2*: 407–41

Hamilton, J. M. (1974). Comparative aspects of mammary tumors. *Advances in Cancer Research, 19*: 1–37

Hammond, E. C. (1975). The epidemiological approach to the etiology of cancer. *Cancer, 35* 652–4

Hammond, S. M., Lambert, P. A. and Rycroft, A. (1984). *The Bacterial Cell Surface*, Croom Helm, London

Harington, A. and Thornley, A. (1980). Endosymbiosis, gene transfer and the mitochondrial genetic code. *South African Journal of Science*, 76: 162–5

Harnden, D., Morten, J. and Featherstone, T. (1984). Dominant susceptibility to cancer in man. *Advances in Cancer Research*, 41: 185–255

Harris, C. C., Hsu, I. C. and Stoner, G. D. (1978). Human pulmonary alveolar macrophages metabolise benzo(a)pyrene to proximate and ultimate mutagens. *Nature*, 272: 633–4

Harris, C. C., Mulvihill, J. J., Thorgeirsson, S. S. and Minna, J. D. (1980). Individual differences in cancer susceptibility. *Annals of Internal Medicine*, 92: 809–25

Harrison, R. G. (1907). Observations on the living developing nerve fiber. *Anatomical Record*, 2: 116–18

Hartl, D. and Dykhuizen, D. (1979). A selectively driven molecular clock. *Nature*, 281: 230–1

Haseltine, F. P., and Ohno, S. (1981). Mechanisms of gonadal differentiation. *Science*, 211: 1272–8

Hashem, N., Bootsma, D., Keijzer, W., Greene, A., Coriell, L., Thomas, G. and Cleaver, J. E. (1980). Clinical characteristics, DNA repair, and complementation groups in xeroderma pigmentosum patients from Egypt. *Cancer Research*, 40: 13–18

Hassold, T., Jacobs, P., Kline, J., Stein, Z. and Warburton, D. (1980). Effect of maternal age on autosomal trisomies. *Annals of Human Genetics*, 44: 29–36

Hauksdottir, H., Halldorsson, S., Jensson, O., Mikkelsen, M. and McDermott, A. (1972). Pericentric inversion of chromosome no. 13 in a large family leading to duplication deficiency causing congenital malformations in three individuals. *Journal of Medical Genetics*, 9: 413–21

Hauschka, T. S. (1952). Relationship between chromosome ploidy and histocompatibility in mouse ascites tumors. *Cancer Research*, 12: 269

Hauschka, T. S. (1953). Cell population studies on mouse ascites tumours. *Transactions of the New York Academy of Sciences*, 16: 64–73

Hauser, G. A. (1979). Das drama des ovarialkarzinomas. *Therapeutische Umschau*, 36: 532–7

Haworth, J. C., Ellestad-Sayed, J. J., King, J. and Dilling, L. A. (1980). Fetal growth retardation in smoking mothers is not due to decreased maternal food intake. *American Journal of Obstetrics and Gynecology*, 137: 719–23

Hayata, I., Sakurai, M., Kakati, S. and Sandberg, A. A. (1975). Chromosomes and causation of human cancer and leukemia. XVI. Banding studies of chronic myelocytic leukemia including five unusual Ph translocations. *Cancer*, 36: 1177–91

Hayday, A. C., Gillies, S. D., Saito, H., Wood, C., Wiman, K., Hayward, W. S. and Tonegawa, S. (1984). Activation of a translocated *c-myc* gene by an enhancer in the immunoglobulin heavy-chain locus. *Nature*, 307: 334–40

Hayes, D. M., Ellison, R. R., Glidewell, O., Holland, J. F. and Silver, R. T. (1974). Chemotherapy for the terminal phase of chronic myelocytic leukemia. *Cancer Chemotherapy Reports*, 58: 233

Hecht, F. and Case, M. (1969). Emergence of a clone of lymphocytes in ataxiatelangiectasia. Annual Meeting of the American Society on Human Genetics, San Francisco. Quoted in Sandberg (1980)

Hecht, F., Kaiser-McCaw, B. and Sandberg, A. A. (1981). Chromosome translocations in cancer. *New England Journal of Medicine*, 304: 1493

Hecht, F. and McCaw, B. K. (1977). Chromosome instability syndromes. In: J. J. Mulvihill, R. W. Miller and J. F. Fraumeni (eds.) *Progress in Cancer Research and Therapy, Genetics of Human Cancer*, Raven Press, New York, vol. 3, pp. 105–23

Heckman, J. E., Sarnoff, J., Alzner-DeWeerd, B., Yin, S. and Ray Bhandary, U.

L. (1980). Novel features in the genetic code and codon reading patterns in *Neurospora crassa* mitochondria based on sequences of six mitochondrial tRNAs. *Proceedings of the National Academy of Sciences (USA)*, 77: 3159–63

Heiberg, K. H. and Kemp, T. (1929). Über die Zahl der chromosomen in carcinomzellen beim menschen. *Virchow's Archiv für Pathologische Anatomie und Physiologie und für Klinische Medizin*, 273: 693–700

Heidelberger, C. (1973). Chemical oncogenesis in culture. *Advances in Cancer Research*, 18: 317–66

Hellstrom, K. E. and Hellstrom, I. (1974). Lymphocyte-mediated cytotoxicity and blocking serum activity to tumor antigens. *Advances in Immunology*, 18: 209–77

Hemboldt, C. F. and Fredrickson, T. N. (1978). Tumors of unknown etiology. In: M. S. Hofstad, B. W. Calnek, C. F. Hemboldt *et al.* (eds.), *Diseases of Poultry*, Iowa State University Press, Ames, pp. 468–80

Hemming, L. and Burns, C. (1979). Heterochromatic polymorphism in spontaneous abortions. *Journal of Medical Genetics*, 16: 358–62

Henderson, B. E. and Louie, E. (1978). Discussion of risk factors for nasopharyngeal carcinoma. In: G. de-Thé and Y. Ito (eds.), *Nasopharyngeal Carcinoma: Etiology and Control*, International Agency for Research on Cancer, Lyon, p. 251

Hendricks, J. D., Sinnhuber, R. O., Wales, J. H., Stack, M. E. and Hsieh, D. P. H. (1980). Hepatocarcinogenicity of sterigmatocystin and versicolorin A to rainbow trout (*Salmo gairdneri*) embryos. *Journal of the National Cancer Institute*, 64: 1503–9

Hennekens, C. H., Speizer, F. E., Lipnick, R. J., Rosner, B., Bain, C., Belanger, C., Stampfer, M. J., Willet, W. and Peto, R. (1984). A case-control study of oral contraceptive use and breast cancer. *Journal of the National Cancer Institute*, 72: 39–42

Henschen, F. (1968). Yamagiwa's tar cancer and its historical significance. *Gann*, 59: 447–51

Heppner, G. H. and Miller, B. E. (1983). *Cancer Metastasis Reviews*, 2: 5

Herbst, A. L. and Cole, P. (1978). Epidemiologic and clinical aspects of clear cell adenocarcinoma in young women. In: A. L. Herbst (ed.), *Intrauterine Exposure to Diethylstilbestrol in the Human*, American College of Obstetricians and Gynecologists, Chicago, pp. 2–7

Herbst, A. L. and Scully, R. E. (1970). Adenocarcinoma of the vagina in adolescence. A report of 7 cases including 6 clear-cell carcinomas (so-called mesonephromas). *Cancer*, 25: 745–57

Herbst, A. L., Ulfelder, H. and Poskanzer, D. C. (1971). Adenocarcinoma of the vagina. Association of maternal stilbestrol therapy with tumor appearance in young women. *New England Journal of Medicine*, 284: 878–81

Herbst, E. W., Pluznik, D. H., Gropp, A. and Uthgenannt, H. (1981). Trisomic hemopoietic stem cells of fetal origin restore hemopoiesis in lethally irradiated mice. *Science*, 211: 1175–7

Herity, B. (1983). Cancer of the breast. In: G. J. Bourke (ed.), *The Epidemiology of Cancer*, Croom Helm, London, pp. 191–213

Hertwig, O. (1911). Die radiumkrankheit tierischer keimzellen, ein beitrag zur experimentellen zeugungsund vererbungslehre. *Archiv für Mikroskopische Anatomie*, 77: 97–164

Hertz, R. (1969). The problem of possible effects of oral contraceptives on cancer of the breast. *Cancer*, 24: 1140–5

Hertz, R., Lewis, J. and Lipsett, M. B. (1961). Five years' experience with the chemotherapy of metastatic choriocarcinoma and related trophoblastic tumors in women. *American Journal of Obstetrics and Gynecology*, 82: 631–40

Heston, W. E. (1976). The genetic aspects of human cancer. *Advances in Cancer Research*, 23: 1–22

Heston, W. E. and Vlahakis, G. (1966). Factors in the causation of spontaneous hepatomas in mice. *Journal of the National Cancer Institute, 37*: 839–43

Hiasa, Y., Kitahori, Y., Enoki, N., Konishi, N. and Shimoyama, T. (1984). 4,4′-Diaminodiphenylmethane: promoting effect on the development of thyroid tumours in rats treated with N-bis (2-hydroxypropyl)nitrosamine. *Journal of the National Cancer Institute, 72*: 471

Hibbs, J. B., Granger, D. L., Cook, J. L. and Lewis, A. M. (1982). Activated macrophage mediated cytoxicity for transformed target cells. *Advances in Experimental Medicine and Biology, 146*: 315–35

Hicks, R. M., Wakefield, J. and Chowaniec, J. (1975). Evaluation of a new model to detect bladder carcinogens or co–carcinogens; results obtained with saccharin, cyclamate and cyclophosphamide. *Chemico-Biological Interactions, 11*: 225–33

Higginson, J. (1968). Present trends in cancer epidemiology. *Canadian Cancer Conference, 3*: 40–75

Higginson, J. and Muir, C. S. (1973). Epidemiology of cancer. In: J. F. Holland and E. Frei (eds.), *Cancer Medicine*, Lea and Febiger, Philadelphia, pp. 241–306

Higginson, J. and Muir, C. S. (1979). Environmental carcinogenesis: misconceptions and limitations to cancer control. *Journal of the National Cancer Institute, 63*: 1291

Higgs, D. R., Pressley, L., Old, J. M., Hunt, D. M., Clegg, J. B., Weatherall, D. J., Sergeant G. R., (1979). Negro-thalassaemia is caused by deletion of a single α-globin gene. *Lancet, 2*: 272–6

Hill, J. (1761). *Cautions Against the Immoderate Use of Snuff*, R. Baldwin, London

Hill, P. and Wynder, F. (1976). Diet and prolactin release. *Lancet, 2*: 806–7

Hirayama, T. (1978). Epidemiology of breast cancer with special reference to the role of diet. *Preventive Medicine, 7*: 173–95

Hirayama, T. (1981). Non-smoking wives of heavy smokers have a higher risk of lung cancer: a study from Japan. *British Medical Journal, 282*: 183

Hirayama, T. and Ito, Y. (1981). A new view of the etiology of nasopharyngeal carcinoma. *Preventive Medicine, 10*: 614–22

Hirono, I., Kuhara, K., Shigetoshi, H., Tomizawa, S. and Golberg, L. (1981). Induction of intestinal tumors in rats by dextran sulfate sodium. *Journal of the National Cancer Institute, 66*: 579–83

Hirshfield, M. F., Feldmeth, C. R. and Soltz, D. C. (1980). Genetic differences in physiological tolerances of Amargosa pupfish (*Cyprinodon nevadensis*) populations. *Science, 207*: 999–1001

Hitchcock, C. R. and Bell, E. T. (1952). Studies on the nematode parasite, *Gongylonema neoplasticum (Spiroptera neoplasticum)* and avitaminosis A in the forestomach of rats: comparison with Fibiger's results. *Journal of the National Cancer Institute, 12*: 1345–87

Ho, J. H.-C. (1972). Nasopharyngeal carcinoma. *Advances in Cancer Research, 15*: 57–92

Hobson, B. and Danecamp, J. (1984). Endothelial proliferation in tumours and normal tissues: continuous labelling studies. *British Journal of Cancer, 49*: 405–13

Hoch-Ligeti, C. (1978). Angiosarcoma of the liver associated with diethylstilbestrol. *Journal of the American Medical Association, 240*: 1510–11

Hod, I. and Milchan, R. (1979). Lung carcinoma of sheep (jaagsiekte): tissue-bound precipitating antibodies. *Journal of the National Cancer Institute, 62*: 371–4

Hodes, M. E., Cole, J., Palmer, C. G., and Reed, T. (1978). Clinical experience with trisomies 18 and 13. *Journal of Medical Genetics, 15*: 48–60

Hoeijmakers, J. H. J., Frasch, A. C. C., Bernards, A., Borst, P. and Cross, G. A. M. (1980). Novel expression-linked copies of the genes for variant surface antigens in trypanosomes. *Nature, 284*: 78–80

Hoekman, K., Huinink, W. W. T. B., Egbers-Bogaards, M. A., McVie, J. F., and Somers, R. (1984). Acute leukemia following therapy for teratoma. *European Journal of Cancer and Clinical Oncology, 20*: 501-2

Hoekstra, W. G. (1975). Biochemical function of selenium and its relation to vitamin E. *Federation Proceedings, 34*: 2083-9

Hoffman, L. M. and Ross, J. (1980). The role of heme in the maturation of erythroblasts: the effects of inhibition of pyridoxine metabolism. *Blood, 55*: 762-71

Hofstad, M. S., Calnek, B. W., Hemboldt, C. F. *et al.* (eds.) (1978). *Diseases of Poultry,* Iowa State University Press, Ames

Holden, C. (1980). Love Canal residents under stress. *Science, 208*: 1242-4

Holliday, R. (1965). Induced mitotic crossing-over in relation to genetic replication in synchronously dividing cells of *Ustilago maydis. Genetical Research, 6*: 104-20

Hollis, G. F., Mitchell, K. F., Battey, J., Potter, H., Taub, R., Lenoir, G. M. and Leder, P. (1984). A variant translocation places the immunoglobulin genes 3' to the *c-myc* oncogene in Burkitt's lymphoma. *Nature, 307*: 752-5

Holman, C. D'A. J. and Armstrong, B. K. (1984). Pigmentary traits, ethnic origin, benign nevi, and family history as risk factors for cutaneous malignant melanoma. *Journal of the National Cancer Institute, 72*: 257-66

Holmberg, M. (1974). No interaction between ultraviolet and X irradiation on chromosome aberrations in cells with trisomy 21. *Nature, 249*: 448-9

Holmes-Siedle, M., Kerr, S., Lindenbaum, R. H. and Bobrow, M. (1980). Dermatoglyphs and chromosome mosaicism in parents of children with trisomy 18. *Journal of Medical Genetics, 17*: 142-3

Holt, J. A., Caputo, T. A., Kelly, K. M., Greenwald, P., and Chorost, S. (1979). Estrogen and progestin binding in cytosols of ovarian adenocarcinomas. *Obstetrics and Gynecology, 53*: 50-8

Honeycombe, G. (1980). *The London Observer,* 3 August, p. 25

Hoover, R. and Cole, P. (1973). Temporal aspects of occupational bladder carcinogenesis. *New England Journal of Medicine, 288*: 1040-3

Hoover, R., Gray, L. A. and Fraumeni, J. F. (1977). Stilboestrol (diethylstilbestrol) and the risk of ovarian cancer. *Lancet, 2*: 533-4

Horuk, R., Blundell, T. L., Lazarus, N. R., Neville, R. W. J., Stone, D. and Wollmer, A. (1980). A monomeric insulin from the porcupine (*Hystrix cristata*), an old world hystricomorph. *Nature, 286*: 822-4

Hossfeld, D. K. and Köhler, S. (1979). New translocations in chronic granulocytic leukaemia: t(X;22)(p22;q11) and t(15;22)(q26;q11). *British Journal of Haematology, 41*: 185-91

Hossfeld, D. K., Han, T., Holdsworth, R. N. and Sandberg, A. A. (1971). Chromosomes and causation of human cancer and leukemia: VII. The significance of the Ph' in conditions other than CML. *Cancer, 27*: 186-92

Hozumi, M. (1983). Fundamentals of chemotherapy of myeloid leukemia by induction of leukemia cell differentiation. *Advances in Cancer Research, 38*: 121-70

Hsieh, C., Crosson, A. W., Walker, A. M., Trapido, E. J. and McMahon, B. (1984). Oral contraceptive use and fibrocystic breast disease of different histologic classifications. *Journal of the National Cancer Institute, 72*: 285-90

Hsu, L. Y. F., Pinchiaroli, D., Gibert, H. S., Wittman, R. and Hirschhorn, K. (1977). Partial trisomy of the long arm of chromosome 1 in myelofibrosis and polycythemia vera. *American Journal of Hematology, 2*: 375-83

Huebner, R. J. and Todaro, G. J. (1969). Oncogenes of RNA tumor viruses as determinants of cancer. *Proceedings of the National Academy of Sciences (USA), 64*: 1087-94

Huggins, C. and Bergenstal, D. M. (1952). Inhibition of human mammary and prostatic cancers by adrenalectomy. *Cancer Research, 12*: 134-41

Huggins, C. and Hodges, C. V. (1941). Studies on prostatic cancer. The effects of castration, of estrogen and of androgen injection on serum phosphatases in metastatic carcinoma of the prostate. *Cancer Research, 1*: 293–7

Huseby, R.A. (1980). Demonstration of a direct carcinogenic effect of estradiol on Leydig cells of the mouse. *Cancer Research, 40*: 1006–13

Hutchinson, J. (1888). On some examples of arsenic-keratosis of the skin and of arsenic-cancer. *Transactions of the Pathological Society, 39*: 352–63

Hynes, N.E., Groner, B. and Michalides, R. (1984). Mouse mammary tumor virus: transcriptional control and involvement in tumorigenesis. *Advances in Cancer Research, 41*: 155

Iacobelli, S., King, R.J.B., Lindner, H.R. and Lippman, M.E. (eds.) (1980). *Hormones and Cancer*, Raven Press, New York

IARC (1974). Sex hormones (I). *IARC Monographs on the Evaluation of Carcinogenic Risk of Chemicals to Humans*, WHO/IARC, Lyon, vol. 6

IARC (1979). Sex hormones (II). *IARC Monographs on the Evaluation of Carcinogenic Risk of Chemicals to Humans*, WHO/IARC, Lyon, vol. 21

IARC (1980). Some non-nutritive sweetening agents. *IARC Monographs on the Evaluation of Carcinogenic Risk of Chemicals to Humans*, WHO/IARC, Lyon, vol. 22

IARC Working Group (1980). An evaluation of chemicals and industrial processes associated with cancer in humans based on human and animal data: IARC monographs vols. 1 to 20. *Cancer Research, 40*: 1–12

IARC Working Group (1982). Chemicals, industrial processes and industries associated with cancer in humans, IARC Monographs vols. 1–29, Suppl. 4

Idle, J.R. Mahgoub, A., Lancaster, R., and Smith, R.L. (1978). Hypotensive response to debrisoquine and hydroxylation phenotype. *Life Sciences, 22*: 979–83

Ijiri, K. and Egami, N. (1980). Hertwig effect caused by UV-irradiation of sperm of *Oryzia latipes* (teleost) and its photoreactivation. *Mutation Research, 69*: 241–8

Ilmensee, K. and Mintz, B. (1976). Totipotency and normal differentiation of single teratocarcinoma cells cloned by injection into blastocysts. *Proceedings of the National Academy of Sciences (USA), 73*: 549–53

Imura, H. (1980). Ectopic hormone production viewed as an abnormality in regulation of gene expression. *Advances in Cancer Research, 33*: 39–75

Ingle, J.N., Ahmann, D.L., Green, S.J., Edmonson, J.H., Bisel, H.F., Kvols, L.K., Nicholas, W.C., Creagan, E.T., Hagn, R.G., Rubin, J. and Frytak, S. (1981). Randomized clinical trial of diethylstilbestrol versus tamoxifen in postmenopausal women with advanced breast cancer. *New England Journal of Medicine, 304*: 16–20

Inman, W.H.W. and Vessey, M.P. (1968). Investigation of deaths from pulmonary, coronary and cerebral thrombosis and embolism in women of child-bearing age. *British Medical Journal, 2*: 193–9

Inoue, T., Yamaguchi, K., Suzuki, H., Abe, K. and Chihara, T. (1984). Production of immunoreactive-polypeptide hormones in cervical carcinoma. *Cancer, 53*: 1509

Ip, C. and Sinha, D.K. (1981). Enhancement of mammary tumorigenesis by dietary selenium deficiency in rats with a high polyunsaturated fat intake. *Cancer Research, 41*: 31–4

Ip, C., Yip, P. and Bernardis, L.L. (1980). Role of prolactin in the promotion of dimethylbenz(a)anthracene-induced mammary tumors by dietary fat. *Cancer Research, 40*: 374–8

Irving, C.C. (1979). Species and tissue variations in the metabolic activation of aromatic amines. In: A.C. Griffin and C.R. Shaw (eds.), *Carcinogenesis: Identification and Mechanisms of Action*, Raven Press, New York, pp. 211–27

Jackson, R.S. (1979). Immunization. In: G.L. Mandell, R.G. Douglas and J.E. Bennett (eds.), *Principles and Practice of Infectious Diseases*, Wiley and Sons, New York, vol. 2, pp. 2291–305

Jacobs, P.A., Brunton, M. and Court-Brown, W.M. (1964). Cytogenetic studies in leucocytes on the general population: subjects of ages 65 years and more. *Annals of Human Genetics, 27*: 353–62

Jacobs, P.A. and Strong, J.A. (1959). A case of human intersexuality having a possibly XXY sex-determining mechanism. *Nature, 1*: 302–3

Janossy, G., Hoffbrand, A.V., Greaves, M.F., Ganeshaguru, K., Pain, C., Bradstock, K.F., Prentice, H.G., Kay, H.E.M. and Lister, T.A. (1980). Terminal transferase enzyme assay and immunological membrane markers in the diagnosis of leukemia: a multiparameter analysis of 300 cases. *British Journal of Haematology, 44*: 221–34

Janossy, G., Roberts, M. and Greaves, M.F. (1976). Target cell in chronic myeloid leukemia and its relationship to acute lymphoid leukemia. *Lancet, 2*: 1058–6

Janossy, G., Woodruff, R.K., Pippard, M.J., Prentice, G., Hoffbrand, A.V., Paxton, A., Lister, T.A., Bunch, C. and Greaves, M.F., (1979). Relation of 'lymphoid' phenotype and response to chemotherapy incorporating vincristine-prednisolone in the acute phase of Ph1-positive leukemia. *Cancer, 43*: 426–34

Jansen, H.W., Lunz, R., Bister, K., Bonner, T.I., Mark, G.E. and Rapp, U.R. (1984). Homologous cell-derived oncogenes in avian carcinoma virus MH2 and murine sarcoma virus 3611. *Nature, 307*: 281–4

Jean, P., Richer, C.L., Murer-Orlando, M., Luu, D.H. and Joncas, J.H. (1979). Translocation 8;14 in an ataxia telangiectasia-derived cell line. *Nature, 277*: 56–7

Jensen, C.O. (1903). Experimentelle untersuchungen über krebs bei mäusen. *Zentralblatt für Bakteriologie, Parasitenkunde, Infektionkrankheiten und Hygiene, 84*: 28–34

Jensen, E.V. and Jacobson, H.I. (1960). Fate of steroid estrogens in target tissues. In: G. Pincus and E.P. Vollmer (eds.), *Biological Activities of Steroids in Relation to Cancer*, Academic Press, New York, pp. 161–78

Jenssens, P.A. (1970). *Palaeopathology. Diseases and Injuries of Prehistoric Man*, John Baker, London

Johns, E.W. (ed.) (1982). *The HMG Chromosomal Proteins*, Academic Press, London, pp. 69–87

Johnson, C.D., Costa, D. and Castro, J.E. (1979). Acid phosphatase after examination of the prostate. *British Journal of Surgery, 66*: 361–3

Johnson, R.T. and Rao, P.N. (1970). Mammalian cell fusion: induction of premature chromosome condensation in interphase nuclei. *Nature, 226*: 717–22

Johnston, R.B. Godzik, L.A. and Cohn, Z.A. (1978). Increased superoxide anion production by immunologically activated and chemically elicited macrophages. *Journal of Experimental Medicine, 148*: 115–27

Jonasson, J., Povey, S. and Harris, H. (1977). The analysis of malignancy by cell fusion. VII. Cytogenetic analysis of hybrids between malignant and diploid cells and of tumours derived from them. *Journal of Cell Science, 24*: 217–54

Jonat, W., Maas, S.H., Stolzenbach, G. and Trams, G. (1980). Estrogen receptor status and response to polychemotherapy in advanced breast cancer. *Cancer, 46*: 2809–13

Jones, M.B. (1979). Years of life lost through Down's syndrome. *Journal of Medical Genetics, 16*: 379–83

Jordan, D.K., Taysi, K., and Blackwell, N.L. (1980). Familial pericentric inversion 19. *Journal of Medical Genetics, 17*: 222–5

Junien, C., DeGrouchy, J., Turleau, C. and Serville, F. (1980). Confirmation of the regional assignment of peptidase A (PEPA) to 18q23 by gene dosage studies. *Annals of Genetics, 23*: 89–90

Jussawalla, D.J., Deshpande, V.A., Haenzel, W. and Natekar, M.V. (1970). Differences observed in the site incidence of cancer between the Parsi community and the total population of greater Bombay: a critical appraisal. *British Journal of Cancer, 24*: 56–66

Kaina, B., Waller, H., Waller, M. and Rieger, R. (1977). The action of N-methyl-N-nitrosourea on non-established human cell lines *in vitro*. 1. Cell cycle inhibition and aberration induction in diploid and Down's fibroblasts. *Mutation Research, 43*: 387–400

Kakati, S, Abe, S. and Sandberg, A.A. (1978). Sister chromatid exchange in Philadelphia chromosome (Ph')-positive leukemia. *Cancer Research, 38*: 2918–21

Kakati, S., Hayata, I., Oshimura, M. and Sandberg, A.A. (1975). Chromosomes and causation of human cancer and leukemia. X. Banding patterns in cancerous effusions. *Cancer, 36*: 1729–38

Kakati, S., Hayata, I. and Sandberg, A.A. (1976). Chromosomes and causation of human cancer and leukemia. XIV. Origin of a large number of markers in a cancer. *Cancer, 37*: 776–82

Kakati, S., Song, S.Y. and Sandberg, A.A. (1977). Chromosomes and causation of human cancer and leukemia. XXII. Karyotypic changes in malignant melanoma. *Cancer, 40*: 1173–81

Kamada, N. and Uchino, H. (1978). Chronologic sequence in appearance of clinical and laboratory findings characteristic of chronic myelocytic leukemia. *Blood, 51*: 843–50

Kamp, D., Kahmann, R., Zipser, D., Broker, T.R. and Chow, L.T. (1978). Inversion of the G-DNA segment of phage Mu controls of phage infectivity. *Nature, 271*: 577–80

Kasukabe, T., Honma, Y. and Hozumi, M. (1979). Inhibition of functional and morphological differentiation of cultured mouse myeloid leukemia cells by tumor promoters. *Gann, 70*: 119–23

Kato, H. (1977a). Spontaneous and induced sister chromatid exchanges as revealed by the BudR-labeling method. *International Reviews of Cytology, 49*: 55–97

Kato, H. (1977b). Mechanisms for sister chromatid exchanges and their relation to the production of chromosomal aberrations. *Chromosoma, 59*: 179–91

Katsuki, T., Hinuma, Y., Saito, T., Yamamoto, J., Hirashima, Y., Sudoh, H., Deguchi, M. and Motokawa, M. (1979). Simultaneous presence of EBNA-positive and colony-forming cells in peripheral blood of patients with infectious mononucleosis. *International Journal of Cancer, 23*: 746–50

Kaufman, E.R. and Davidson, R.L. (1978). Bromodeoxyuridine mutagenesis in mammalian cells: mutagenesis is independent of the amount of bromouracil in DNA. *Proceedings of the National Academy of Sciences (USA), 75*: 4982–6

Kefalides, N.A. (1973). Structure and biosynthesis of basement membranes. *International Reviews of Connective Tissue Research, 6*: 63–104

Keiser, H.R., Beaven, M.A., Doppman, J., Wells, S. and Buja, L.M. (1973). Sipple's syndrome: medullary thyroid carcinoma, pheochromocytoma and parathyroid disease. *Annals of Internal Medicine, 78*: 561–79

Keleiti, J., Révész, T. and Schuler, D. (1978). Morphological diagnosis in childhood leukaemia. *British Journal of Haematology, 40*: 501–6

Kellermann, G., Cantrell, E. and Shaw, C.R. (1973a). Variations in extent of aryl hydrocarbon hydroxylase induction in cultured human lymphocytes. *Cancer Research, 33*: 1654–6

Kellermann, G., Luyten-Kellermann, M. and Shaw, C.R. (1973b). Genetic variation of aryl hydrocarbon hydroxylase in human lymphocytes. *American Journal of Human Genetics, 25*: 327–31

Kellermann, G., Luyten-Kellermann, M. and Shaw, C.R. (1973c). Genetic variation of aryl hydrocarbon hydroxylase in human lymphocytes. *Human Genetik, 20*: 257

Kellermann, G., Shaw, C.R. and Luyten-Kellerman, M. (1973d). Aryl hydrocarbon hydroxylase inducibility and bronchogenic carcinoma. *New England Journal of Medicine, 289*: 934–7

Kelsey, J.L. (1979). A review of the epidemiology of human breast cancer. *Epidemiologial Reviews, 1*: 74–109

Kemp, T. (1929). Ueber des verhälten der Chromosomen in den somatischen Zellen des Menschen. *Zeitschrift für Mikroskopish-Anatomische Forschung, 16*: 1–20

Kemp, T. (1930). Ueber die somatischen mitosen bei Menschen und warmblütigen Tieren unter normalen und pathologischen verhältnisse. *Zeitschrift für Zellforschung und Mikroscopische Anatomie, 11*: 429–44

Kendrick, K. M. and Drewett, R. F. (1980). Testosterone-sensitive neurones respond to oestradiol but not to dihydrotestosterone. *Nature, 286*: 67–8

Kessous, A. and Colombies, P. (1975). Hypodiploidy and cellular survival. *Biomedicine, 23*: 108–10

Kessous, A., Colombies, P., Pris, J. and Clement, D. (1980). Near haploid cell line in lymphoid blast crisis of Ph-positive chronic myeloid leukemia. *Cancer Research, 40*: 1354–9

Kessous, A., Corberand, J., Grozdea, J. and Colombies, P. (1975). Clone cellulaire A27 chromosomes dans une leucémie aigue humaine. *Nouvelle Revue Française d' Hématologie, 15*: 73–82

Kets de Vries, M. F. (1980). Ecological stress: a deadly reminder. *Psychoanalytical Reviews, 67*: 389–408

Khandekar, J. D., Victor, T. A. and Mukhopadhyaya, P. (1978). Endometrial carcinoma following estrogen therapy for breast cancer. Report of three cases. *Journal of the American Medical Association, 138*: 539–41

Khanolkar, V. R. (1958). Cancer in India in relation to habits and customs. In: R. W. Raven (ed.), *Cancer*, Butterworths, London, vol. 3, pp. 272–85

Kidson, C. (1980). Diseases of DNA repair. *Clinical Haematology, 9*: 141–57

Kihlman, B. A. (1971). Molecular mechanisms of chromosome breakage and rejoining. *Advances in Cell Molecular Biology, 1*: 59–107

Kikuchi, Y., Oishi, H., Tonomura, A. (1969). Translocation Down's syndrome in Japan: its frequency, mutation rate of translocation and parental age. *Japanese Journal of Human Genetics, 14*: 93–106

Kilburn, K. H. (1984). Author's reply: clarification of data on the etiological role of cigarette smoking in pulmonary fibrosis. *American Journal of Industrial Medicine, 5*: 421–2

Killmann, S. A. (1968). Acute leukemia: development, remission/relapse pattern, relation between normal and leukemic hemopoiesis, and the 'sleeper-to-feeder' stem cell hypothesis. *Seminars in Haematology, 1*: 103–28

Kimchi, A. Schulman, L., Schmidt, A., Chernajovsky, Y., Fradin, A. and Revel, M. (1979). Kinetics of the induction of three translation-regulatory enzymes by interferon. *Proceedings of the National Academy of Sciences (USA), 43*: 3208–12

King, J. J. and DiBerardino, M. A. (1965). Transplantation of nuclei from the frog renal adenocarcinoma. 1. Development of tumor nuclear transplant embryos. *Annals of the New York Academy of Sciences, 126*: 115–26

King, M. C. and Petrakis, N. L. (1977). Genetic markers and cancer. In: J. J. Mulvihill, R. W. Miller and J. F. Fraumeni (eds.), *Genetics of Human Cancer*, Raven Press, New York, p. 281

King, M. C., Go, R. C. P., Elston, R. C., Lynch, H. T. and Petrakis, N. L. (1980). Allele increasing susceptibility to human breast cancer may be linked to the glutamate-pyruvate transaminase locus. *Science, 208*: 406–8

King, R. J., Cowan, D. M. and Inman, D. R. (1965). The uptake of (6,7-3-H) oestradiol by dimethylbenzanthracene-induced rat mammary tumours. *Journal of Endocrinology, 32*: 83–90

Kirov, S. M., Kwant, W. O., Fernandez, L. A., MacSween, J. M. and Langley, G. R. (1980). Characterization of null cells in chronic lymphocytic leukaemia with B-cell allo- and hetero-antisera. *British Journal of Haematology, 44*: 235–42

Klein, G., Bregula, U., Wiener, R. and Harris, H. (1971). The analysis of malignancy by cell fusion. I. Hybrids between tumor cells and L cells derivatives. *Journal of Cell Science, 8*: 659–72

Klein, G. and Klein, E. (1956). Conversion of solid neoplasms into ascites tumors. *Annals of the New York Academy of Sciences, 63*: 640–61

Klein, G., Svedmyr, E., Jondal, M. and Persson, P. O. (1976). EBV-determined nuclear antigen (EBNA)-positive cells in the peripheral blood of infectious mononucleosis patients. *International Journal of Cancer, 17*: 21–6

Klein, J. (1975). *Biology of the Mouse Histocompatibility-2 Complex; Principles of Immunogenetics Applied to a Single System*, Springer-Verlag, New York

Knab, D. R. (1977). Estrogen and endometrial carcinoma. *Obstetrical and Gynecological Survey, 32*: 267–81

Knudson, A. G. (1977). Genetics and etiology of human cancer. *Advances in Human Genetics, 8*: 1–66

Knudson, A. G. (1979). Persons at high risk of cancer. *New England Journal of Medicine, 301*: 606–7

Knudson, A. G. (1980). Genetics and cancer. *American Journal of Medicine, 69*: 1–3

Knudson, A. G. (1981). Human cancer genes. In: F. E. Arrighi, P. N. Rao and E. Stubblefield (eds.), *Genes, Chromosomes and Neoplasia*, Raven Press, New York, p. 453

Knudson, A. G. and Strong, L. C. (1972). Mutation and cancer: neuroblastoma and pheochromocytoma. *American Journal of Human Genetics, 24*: 514–32

Knuutila, S., Helminen, E., Vuopio, P. and Delachapelle, A. (1978). Sister chromatid exchanges in human bone marrow cells. 1. Control subjects and patients with leukaemia. *Hereditas, 88*: 189–96

Kodama, M. and Kodama, T. (1981). Adolescence, a critical stage for the genesis of female cancers (review). *Anticancer Research, 1*: 93–9

Kodama, M. and Kodama, T. (1983). Relationship between steroid metabolism of the host and genesis of cancers of the breast, uterine cervix, and endometrium. *Advances in Cancer Research, 38*: 77–120

Kodani, M. (1958). Three chromosome numbers in whites and Japanese. *Science, 127*: 1339–40

Koeffler, H. P. and Golde, D. W. (1978). Acute myelogenous leukemia: a human cell line responsive to colony-stimulating activity. *Science, 200*: 1153–4

Kolata, G. B. (1980). Genes and cancer: the story of Wilms tumor. *Science, 207*: 970–1

Koller, E. J. and Fisher, C. (1980). Tooth induction in chick epithelium: expression of quiescent genes for enamel synthesis. *Science, 207*: 993–5

Koller, P. C. (1947). Abnormal mitosis in tumours. *British Journal of Cancer, 1*: 38–47

Koller, P. C. (1960). Chromosome behaviour in tumors: readjustments to Boveri's hypothesis. In: R. M. Cumley, M. Abbott and J. McCay (eds.), *Cell Physiology of Neoplasia*, University of Texas Press, Austin, pp. 9–43

Koller, P. C. (1972). *The Role of Chromosomes in Cancer Biology*, Springer-Verlag, Berlin

Kondo, I., Hamaguchi, H., Matsuura, A., Nakajima, H., Koyama, A. and Takita, H. (1979). A case of Turner's syndrome with familial balanced translocation t(1;2)(q32;q21)mat. *Journal of Medical Genetics, 16*: 321–3

Konstantinova, B. (1978). 45,X/46,XY/47,XY,+21. In: D. Borgaonkar (ed.), *Repository of Chromosomal Variants and Anomalies in Man, 5th Listing*, North Texas State University, Denton, p. 316

Korenman, S. G. (1981). The endocrine epidemiology of breast cancer. The estrogen window hypothesis. *National Cancer Institute Breast Cancer Task Force Intercommunications, 10*: 6

Koss, L. G. (1982). Precancerous lesions of the breast — theoretical and practical considerations. In: *Proceedings of the Second Symposium on Mammary Pathology*. Plenum Publishing Corporation: New York

Koss, L. G. and Greenebaum, E. (1983). Precancerous lesions. In: G. J. Bourke (ed.), *The Epidemiology of Cancer*, Croom Helm, London, pp. 31–59

Kosseff, A. L. Herrmann, J. and Opitz, J. M. (1972). The Wiedemann-Beckwith syndrome: genetic considerations and a diagnostic sign. *Lancet, 1*: 844

Kouri, R. E. (ed.) (1980). *Genetic Differences in Chemical Carcinogenesis*, CRC Press, Boca Raton, Louisiana pp. 93–128

Kriek, E. and Westra, J. G. (1979). Metabolic activation of aromatic amines and amides and interactions with nucleic acids. In: P. L. Grover (ed.), *Chemical Carcinogens and DNA*, CRC Press, Boca Raton, vol. 2, pp. 1–28

Kripko, M. L. (1979). Speculations on the role of ultraviolet radiation in the development of malignant melanoma. *Journal of the National Cancer Institute, 63*: 541–5

Kuhlmann, W., Fromme, H. G., Heege, E. H. and Ostertag, N. (1968). The mutagenic action of caffeine in higher organisms. *Cancer Research, 28*: 2375–89

Kung, I. T. M., So, K. F. and Lam, T. H. (1984). Lung cancer in Hong Kong Chinese: mortality and histological types, 1973–82. *British Journal of Cancer, 50*: 381–8

Kung, P. C., Long, J. C., McCaffrey, R. P., Ratliff, R. L., Harrison, T. A. and Baltimore, D. (1978). Terminal deoxynucleotidyl transferase in the diagnosis of leukemia and malignant lymphoma. *American Journal of Medicine, 64*: 788–94

Kuntz, R. E., Cheever, A. W. and Myers, B. J. (1972). Proliferative epithelial lesions of the urinary bladder of non-human primates infected with *Schistosoma hematobium*. *Journal of the National Cancer Institute, 48*: 223–35

Kurosawa, Y., Von Boehmer, H., Haas, W., Sakano, H., Trauneker, A. and Tonegawa, S. (1981). Identification of D segments of immunoglobulin heavy-chain genes and their rearrangement in T lymphocytes. *Nature, 290*: 565–70

Kyle, R. A. (1982). Second malignancies associated with chemotherapeutic agents. *Seminars in Oncology, 9*: 131–42

Kyritsis, A. P., Tsokas, M., Triche, T. J. and Chader, G. J. (1984). Retinoblastoma — origin from a primitive neuroectodermal cell? *Nature, 307*: 471–3

Lacassagne, A. (1932). Apparition de cancers de la mamelle chez la souris male, soumise à des injections de folliculine. *Comptes Rendus Hebdomadaires des Séances de l'Academie des Sciences* (Paris), *195*: 630–2

Lacombe, C., Casadevall, N. and Varet, B. (1980). Polycythemia vera: in vitro studies of circulating erythroid progenitors. *British Journal of Haematology, 44*: 189–99

Lacour, J., Bucalossi, P., Cacers, E., Jacobelli, G., Koszarowski, T., Le, M., Rumeau-Rouguette, C. and Veronesi, U. (1976). Radical mastectomy versus radical mastectomy plus internal mammary dissection. *Cancer, 37*: 206–14

Lajtha, L. G. (1963). On the concept of the cell cycle. *Journal of Cellular and Comparative Physiology, 62* (Suppl. 1): 143–5

Lambert, B., Hansson, K., Bui, T. H., Funes-Cravioto, F., Lindsten, J., Holmberg, M. and Strausmanis, R. (1976). DNA repair and frequency of x-ray and u.v.-light induced chromosome aberrations in leucocytes from patients with Down's syndrome. *Annals of Human Genetics, 39*: 293–303

Lambert, B., Ringborg, U. and Lindblad, A. (1979). Prolonged increase of sister-chromatid exchanges in lymphocytes of melanoma patients after CCNU treatment. *Mutation Research, 59*: 295–300

Lamm, L. U., Friedrich, U., Peterson, C. B., Jorgensen, J., Nielson, J., Therkelsen, A. J. and Kissmeyer-Nielsen, F. (1974). Assignment of the major histocompatibility complex to chromosome No. 6 in a family with a pericentric inversion. *Human Heredity, 24*: 273–84

Lampert, F. (1969). Akute lymphoblastiche leukämie bei Geschwistern mit progressiver Kleinhirnataxie (Louis-Barr-Syndrom). *Deutsche Medizinische Wochenschrift, 94*: 217–220

Langer, A. M., Rohl, A. N., Selikoff, I. J., Harlow, G. E. and Prinz, M. (1980). Asbestos as a co-factor in carcinogenesis among nickel-processing workers. *Science, 209*: 420–2

Laquer, G. L., McDaniel, E. G. and Matsumoto, H. (1967). Tumor induction in germ-free rats with methylazoxymethanol (MAM) and synthetic MAM acetate. *Journal of the National Cancer Institute, 39*: 335–71

Laquer, G. L., Mickelsen, O., Whiting, M. and Kurland, L. T. (1963). Carcinogenic properties of nuts from *Cycas circinalis L.* indigenous to Guam. *Journal of the National Cancer Institute, 31*: 919–51

Larouze, B., Blumberg, B. S., London, W. T., Lustbader, E. D., Sankale, M. and Payet, M. (1977). Forecasting the development of primary hepatocellular carcinoma by the use of risk factors: studies in West Africa. *Journal of the National Cancer Institute, 58*: 1557–61

Lathrop, A. E. C. and Loeb, L. (1916). Further investigations on the origins of tumors in mice. III. On the part played by internal secretion in the spontaneous development of tumors. *Journal of Cancer Research, 1*: 1–19

Latreille, J., Barlogie, B., Dosik, G. Johnston, D. A., Drewinko, B. and Alexanian, R. (1980). Cellular DNA content as a marker of human multiple myeloma. *Blood, 55*: 403–8

Latt, S. A. (1973). Microfluorometric detection of deoxyribonucleic acid replication in human metaphase chromosomes. *Proceedings of the National Academy of Sciences (USA), 70*: 3395–9

Latt, S. A., Stetten, G., Juergens, L. A., Buchanan, G. R. and Gerald, P. S. (1975). Induction by alkylating agents of sister chromatid exchanges and chromatid breaks in Fanconi's anemia. *Proceedings of the National Academy of Sciences (USA), 72*: 4066–70

Lattes, R. (1980). Lobular neoplasia (lobular carcinoma *in situ*) of the breast — a histological entity of controversial clinical significance. *Pathology: Research and Practice, 166*: 415

Lauritsen, J. G., Bolund, L., Friedrich, U. and Therkelsen, A. J. (1979). Origin of triploidy in spontaneous abortuses. *Annals of Human Genetics, 43*: 1–10

Lavelle, S. M. and MacIomhair M. (1984). Enhancing effect of polyamines on yield of film sarcoma. *European Journal of Cancer and Clinical Oncology, 20*: 503–6

Laver, W. G. and Webster, R. G. (1979). Ecology of influenza viruses in lower mammals and birds. *British Medical Bulletin, 35*: 29–33

Lawler, S. D. (1977). The cytogenetics of chronic granulocytic leukemia. *Clinics in Haematology, 6*: 55–75

Lawler, S. D. (1980). Cytogenetic studies in Philadelphia chromosome-negative myeloproliferative disorders, particularly polycythemia rubra vera. *Clinics in Haematology, 9*: 159–74

Lawler, S. D., Klouda, P. T., Smith, P. G., Till, M. M. and Hardisty, R. M. (1974). Survival and the HL-A system in acute lymphoblastic leukaemia. *British Medical Journal, 1*: 547–8

Lawler, S. D., O'Malley, F. and Lobbs, D. S. (1976). Chromosome banding studies in Philadelphia chromosome-positive myeloid leukaemia. *Scandinavian Journal of Haematology, 1 '*: 17–28

Lawley, P. D. (1979). Approaches to chemical dosimetry in mutagenesis and carcinogenesis: the relevance of reactions of chemical mutagens and carcinogens with DNA. In: P. L. Grover (ed.), *Chemical Carcinogens and DNA*, CRC Press, Boca Raton, Louisiana vol. 1. pp. 1–36

Layde, P. M. and Beral, V. (1981). Further analyses of mortality in oral contraceptive users. *Lancet, 1*: 541–6

Layton, M. G. and Franks, L. M. (1984). Heterogeneity in a spontaneous mouse lung carcinoma: selection and characterization of stable metastatic variants. *British Journal of Cancer, 49*: 415–502

Leavitt, W. W. (ed.) (1982). *Hormones and Cancer*, Plenum Press, New York

LeBeau, M. M. and Rowley, J. D. (1984). Heritable fragile sites in cancer. *Nature, 308*: 607–8

Le Bouffant, L., Martin, J. C., Daniel, H., Hennin, J. P. and Normand, C. (1980). Action of intensive cigarette smoke inhalations on the rat lung. Role of particulate and gaseous cofactors. *Journal of the National Cancer Institute, 64*: 273–84

Lejeune, J., Gautier, M. and Turpin, R. (1959). Etude des chromosome somatiques de neuf enfants mongoliens. *Comptes Rendus Hebdomadaires des Sciences (Paris), 248*: 1721–2

Lemanski, L. F., Paulson, D. J. and Hill, C. S. (1979). Normal anterior endoderm corrects the heart defect in cardiac mutant salamanders (*Ambystoma mexicanum*). *Science, 204*: 860–2

Lemon, P. G. and Gubareva, A. V. (1979). Tumours of the ovary. In: V. S. Turusov (ed.), *Pathology of Tumours in Laboratory Animals. Volume 2. Tumours of the Mouse.* International Agency for Research on Cancer, Lyon, pp. 385–410

Levin, D. L., Connelly, R. R. and Devesa, S. S. (1981). Demographic characteristics of cancer of the pancreas: mortality, incidence and survival. *Cancer: 47*, 1456–68

Levine, P. H., Mesa-Tejada, R., Keydar, I., Tabbane, F., Spiegelman, S. and Mourali, N. (1984). Increased incidence of mouse mammary tumor virus-related antigen in Tunisian patients with breast cancer. *International Journal of Cancer, 33*: 305

Levy, M. H. and Wheelock, E. F. (1974). The role of macrophages in defense against neoplastic disease. *Advances in Cancer Research, 20*: 131–63

Lewin, R. (1981). Tale of the orphaned genes. *Science, 212*: 530

Lezana, E. R., Bianchi, N. O., Bianchi, M. S. and Zabala-Suarez, J. E. (1977). Sister chromatid exchanges in Down's syndrome and normal human beings. *Mutation Research, 45*: 85–90

Li, C. H. and Graf, L. (1974). Human pituitary growth hormone: isolation and properties of two biologically active fragments from plasmin digests. *Proceedings of the National Academy of Sciences (USA), 11*: 1197–1201

Li, F. P., Corkery, J., Canellos, G. and Neitlich, H. W. (1981). Breast cancer after Hodgkin's disease in two sisters. *Cancer, 47*: 200–2

Li, F. P., Rapoport, M. D., Fraumeni, J. F. and Jensen, R. D. (1970). Familial ovarian carcinoma. *Journal of the American Medical Association, 214*: 1559–61

Liber, A. F. (1950). Ovarian cancer in mother and five daughters. *Archives of Pathology, 49*: 280–90

Liddle, G., Nicholson, W., Island, D., Orth, D., Abe, K. and Lowder, S. (1969). Clinical and laboratory studies of ectopic humoral syndromes. *Recent Progress in Hormone Research, 25*: 283–305

Lieber, E., Hsu, L., Spitler, L. and Fudenberg, H. H. (1972). Cytogenetic findings in a parent of a patient with Fanconi's anemia. *Clinical Genetics, 3*: 357–63

Lilleyman, J. S., Potter, A. M., Watmore, A. E., Cooke, P., Sokol, R. J. and Wood, J. K. (1978). Myeloid karyotype and the malignant phase of chronic granulocytic leukemia. *British Journal of Haematology, 39*: 317–23

Lilly, F. (1972). Mouse leukemia: a model of a multiple gene disease. *Journal of the National Cancer Institute, 49*: 927

Lin, R. S. and Kessler, I. I. (1981). A multifactorial model for pancreatic cancer in man. Epidemiologic evidence. *Journal of the American Medical Association, 245*: 147

Linch, D. C., Allen, C., Beverley, P. C. L., Bynoe, A. G., Scott, C. S. and Hogg, N. (1984). Monoclonal antibodies differentiating between monocytic and nonmonocytic variants of AML. *Blood, 63*: 566–73

Lindsay, R., MacLean, A., Kraszewski, A., Hart, D. M., Clark, A. C. and Garwood, J. (1978). Bone response to termination of oestrogen treatment. *Lancet, 1*: 1325–7

Lingeman, C. H. (1979). Hormones and hormonomimetic compounds in the etiology of cancer. *Recent Results in Cancer Research, 66*: 1–48

Liotta, L. A., Abe, S., Robey, P. G. and Martin, G. R. (1979). Preferential digestion of basement membrane collagen by an enzyme derived from a metastatic murine tumor. *Proceedings of the National Academy of Sciences (USA), 76*: 2268–72

Liotta, L. A., Tryggvason, K., Garbisa, S., Hart, I., Foltz, C. M. and Shafie, S. (1980). Metastatic potential correlates with enzymatic degradation of basement membrane collagen. *Nature, 284*: 67–8

Lipetz, P. D., Galsky, A. G. and Stephens, R. E. (1982). Relationship of DNA tertiary and quaternary structure to carcinogenic processes. *Advances in Cancer Research, 36*: 165–210

Lippman, M. E. and Allegra, J. C. (1980). Quantitative estrogen receptor analyses: the response to endocrine and cytotoxic chemotherapy in human breast cancer and the disease-free interval. *Cancer, 46*: 2829–34

Lipschitz, D. A., Udupa, K. B., Milton, K. Y. and Thompson, C. O. (1984). Effect of age on hematopoiesis in man. *Blood, 63*: 502–9

Lipsett, M. B. (1979). Interaction of drugs, hormones and nutrition in the causes of cancer. *Cancer, 43*: 1967–81

Lisker, R. and Cobo, A. (1970). Chromosome breakage in ataxia-telangiectasia. *Lancet, 1*: 618

Little, C. C. (1928). Evidence that cancer is not a simple Mendelian recessive. *Journal of Cancer Research, 12*: 30–46

Littlefield, L. G., Colyer, S. P. and DuFrain, R. J. (1980). Comparison of sister-chromatid exchanges in human lymphocytes after G_0 exposure to mitomycin in vivo vs. in vitro. *Mutation Research, 69*: 191–7

Liu, C. P., Tucker, P. W., Mushinski, J. F., and Blattner, F. R. (1980). Mapping of heavy chain genes for mouse immunoglobulins M and D. *Science, 209*: 1348–53

Lo, T. C., Salzman, F. A., Smedal, M. I. and Wright, K. A. (1980). Radiotherapy for Kaposi's sarcoma. *Cancer, 45*: 684–7

Long, E. R. (1965). *A History of Pathology*, Dover Publications, New York

Lord, B. I., Potten, C. S. and Cole, R. J. (eds.) (1978). *Stem Cells and Tissue Homeostasis*, Cambridge University Press, Cambridge

Lote, K., Andersen, K., Nordal, E. and Brennhovd, I. O. (1980). Familial occurrence of papillary thyroid carcinoma. *Cancer, 46*: 1291–7

Lotem, J. and Sachs, L. (1979). Regulation of normal differentiation in mouse and human myeloid leukemic cells by phorbol esters and the mechanism of tumor promotion. *Proceedings of the National Academy of Sciences (USA), 76*: 5758–62

Louka, M. H., Ross, R. D., Lee, J. H. and Lewis, G. C. (1978). Endometrial carcinoma in Turner's syndrome. *Gynecologic Oncology, 6*: 294–304

Lovejoy, C. O. (1981). The origin of man. *Science, 211*: 341–50

Lowenberg, B. and De Zeeuw, H. M. (1979). A method for cloning T-lymphocytic precursors in agar. *American Journal of Hematology, 6*: 35–43

Lowenberg, B., Swart, K. and Hagemeijer, A. (1980). PHA-induced colony formation in acute non-lymphocytic and chronic myeloid leukemia. *Leukemia Research, 4*: 143–9

Lower, G. M. (1978). Metabolic factors involved in bladder carcinogenesis. (Abstract) National Bladder Cancer Project Investigators' Workshop, Sarasota, Florida, p. 14

Lubinsky, M., Herrmann, J., Kosseff, A. L. and Opitz, J. M. (1974). Autosomal-dominant sex-dependent transmission of the Wiedemann-Beckwith syndrome. *Lancet, 1*: 932

Lucké, B. (1934). Carcinoma in the leopard frog. Its probable causation by a virus. *Journal of Experimental Medicine, 68*: 457–68

Luft, R. and Olivecrona, H. (1953). Experiences with hypophysectomy in man. *Journal of Neurosurgery, 10*: 301–16

Lunde, P. K., Frislid, K. and Hansteen, V. (1977). Disease and acetylation polymorphism. *Clinical Pharmacokinetics, 2*: 182–97

Lupulescu, A. (1983). *Hormones and Carcinogenesis*, Praeger Publishers, New York

Lynch, C. J. (1931). Studies on the relation between tumor susceptibility and heredity. *Journal of Experimental Medicine, 39*: 481–95

Lynch, H. T. (ed.) (1976). *Cancer Genetics*, Thomas, Springfield, Illinois

Lynch, H. T., Albano, W., Black, L., Lynch, J. F., Recabaren, J. and Pierson, R. (1981). Familial excess of cancer of the ovary and other anatomic sites. *Journal of the American Medical Association, 245*: 261–4

Lynch, H. T. and Lynch, P. M. (1979). Tumour variation in the cancer family syndrome: ovarian cancer. *American Journal of Surgery, 138*: 439–42

Lynch, H. T., Guirgis, H. A. and Harris, R. F. (1977). Familial susceptibility to lung cancer and chronic obstructive pulmonary disease. *Lancet, 2*: 815

Lynch, H. T., Mulcahy, G. M., Harris, R. E., Guirgis, H. A. and Lynch, J. F. (1978). Genetic and pathologic findings in a kindred with hereditary sarcoma, breast cancer, brain tumours, leukemia, lung, laryngeal, and adrenal cortical carcinoma. *Cancer, 41*: 2055–64

Lyon, F. A. (1975). Development of adenocarcinoma of endometrium in young women receiving long-term sequential oral contraception. *American Journal of Obstetrics and Gynecology, 123*: 299–301

Lyon, J. L., Gardner, J. W. and West, D. W. (1980). Cancer incidence in Mormons and non-Mormons in Utah during 1967–75. *Journal of the National Cancer Institute, 65*: 1055–61

Lyons, M. J. and Moore, D. H. (1962). Purification of the mouse mammary tumour virus. *Nature, 194*: 1141–2

Maas, H., Jonat, W., Stolzenbach, G. and Trams, G. (1980). The problem of non-responding estrogen-receptor-positive patients with advanced breast cancer. *Cancer, 46*: 2836–7

Mabuchi, K. (1983). Cancer of the pancreas. In: G. J. Bourke (ed.), *The Epidemiology of Cancer*, Croom Helm, London, pp. 131–44

Macdonald, J. S., Gunderson, L. L. and Cohn, I. (1982). Cancer of the pancreas. In: V. T. DeVita, S. Helman, and S. A. Rosenberg (eds.), *Cancer: Principles and Practice of Oncology*, Lippincott, Philadelphia, p. 563

McEwen, B. S. (1981). Neural gonadal steroid actions. *Science, 211*: 1303–11

McGirr, E. M., Clement, W. E., Currie, A. R. and Kennedy, J. S. (1959). Impaired dehalogenase activity as a cause of goitre with malignant changes. *Scottish Medical Journal, 4*: 232–41

McGuire, W. L., Carbone, P. P. and Vollmer, E. P. (eds.) (1975). *Estrogen Receptors in Human Breast Cancer*, Raven Press, New York

McKinnell, R. G., Deggins, B. A. and Labat, D. D. (1969). Transplantation of pluripotential nuclei from triploid frog tumors. *Science, 165*: 394–6

McKinnell, R. G., Steven, L. M. and Labat, D. D. (1976). Frog renal tumors are composed of stroma, vascular elements and epithelial cells: what type nucleus programs for tadpoles with the cloning procedure? In: N. Müller-Bérat *et al.* (eds.), *Progress in Differentiation Research*, North-Holland Publishing Company, Amsterdam, pp. 319–30

McKusick, V. A. (1975). *Mendelian Inheritance in Man: Catalogs of Autosomal*

Dominant, Autosomal Recessive and X-Linked Phenotypes, Johns Hopkins University Press, Baltimore, 4th edn.

McLaren, A. (1980). Oocytes in the testis. *Nature, 283*: 688–9

McLean, E. K. (1970). The toxic actions of pyrrolizidine (senecio) alkaloids. *Pharmacological Reviews, 22*: 429–83

MacLusky, N. J. and Naftolin, F. (1981). Sexual differentiation of the central nervous system. *Science, 211*: 1294–1303

MacMahon, B., Cole, P. and Brown J. (1973). Etiology of human breast cancer: a review. *Journal of the National Cancer Institute, 50*: 21–42

MacMahon, B., Lin, T. M., Lowe, C. R., Mirra, A. P., Ravnikar, B., Salber, E. J., Trichopoulos, D., Valaoras, V. G. and Yuasa, S. (1970). Lactation and cancer of the breast. A summary of an international study. *Bulletin of the World Health Organization, 42*: 185–94

MacMahon, B., Yen, S., Trichopoulos, D., Warren, K. and Nardi, G. (1981). Coffee and cancer of the pancreas. *New England Journal of Medicine, 304*: 630–3

McMichael, A. J. (1980). Diet and cancer: an epidemiological perspective. *Medical Journal of Australia, 2*: 10–11, 13, 16

McMichael, A. J. (1983). Cancers of the head and neck. In: G. J. Bourke (ed.), *The Epidemiology of Cancer*, Croom Helm, London, pp. 60–83

McMichael, A. J. and Potter, J. D. (1980). Endogenous and exogenous sex hormones, and colon cancer: a review and hypothesis. *Journal of the National Cancer Institute, 65*: 1201–7

McNeil, M. M., Leong, A. S. Y. and Sage, R. E. (1981). Primary mediastinal embryonal carcinoma in association with Klinefelter's syndrome. *Cancer, 47*: 343–5

McWhirter, R. (1948). Value of simple mastectomy and radiotherapy in treatment of cancer of the breast. *British Journal of Radiology, 21*: 599–610

McWhirter, W. R. and Siskind, V. (1984). Childhood cancer survival trends in Queensland 1956–80. *British Journal of Cancer, 49*: 513–19

Maciag, T., Nemore, R. E., Weinstein, R. and Gilchrest, B. A. (1981). An endocrine approach to the control of epidermal growth: serum-free cultivation of human keratinocytes. *Science, 211*: 1452–3

Mack, T. (1982). Pancreas. In: D. Schottenfeld and J. F. Fraumeni (eds.), *Cancer Epidemiology and Prevention*, Saunders, Philadelphia

Madan, K. (1976). Chromosome measurements on an XXp+ male. *Human Genetics, 32*: 141–2

Madler, L. M., Reinherz, E. L., Weinstein, H. J., D'Orsi, C. J. and Schlossman, S. F. (1980). Heterogeneity of T-cell lymphoblastic malignancies. *Blood, 55*: 806–10

Magenis, R. E., Hecht, F. and Milham, S. (1968). Trisomy 13 (D1) syndrome: studies on parental age, sex ratio and survival. *Journal of Pediatrics, 73*: 222–8

Magrath, I. T. and Ziegler, J. L. (1980). Bone marrow involvement in Burkitt's lymphoma and its relationship to acute B-cell leukemia. *Leukemia Research, 4*: 33–59

Mahgoub, A., Idle, J. R., Dring, L. G., Lancaster, R. and Smith, R. L. (1977). Polymorphic hydroxylation of debroisoquine in man. *Lancet, 2*: 584–6

Major, R. H. (1954). *A History of Medicine*, 2 vols, C. C. Thomas, Springfield, Illinois

Makino, S. (1957). The chromosome cytology of the ascites tumors of rats, with special reference to the concept of the stemline cell. *International Reviews of Cytology, 6*: 25–84

Makino, S. (1973). Historic sketches of human cytogenetics. *Heredity, 27*: 7–10

Makino, S. (1975). *Human Chromosomes*. Igaku Shoin Limited, Tokyo

Makino, S. and Sasaki, M. (1959). On the chromosome number of man. A preliminary note. *Proceedings of the Japanese Academy, 35*: 99–104

Malcolm, A. D. B. (1981). Production and processing of prolactin. *Nature, 290*: 546

Maltoni, C. and Lefemine, G. (1975). Carcinogenicity bioassays of vinyl chloride: current results. *Annals of the New York Academy of Sciences, 246*: 195–218

Manolov, G. and Manolova, Y. (1972). Marker band in one chromosome 14 from Burkitt lymphomas. *Nature, 237*: 33–4

Manson, D. (1976). Some illustrative systems of chemical carcinogenesis: (2) aromatic amines. In: T. Symington and R. L. Carter (eds.), *Scientific Foundations of Oncology*, William Heinemann Medical Books, London

Margison, G. P. and O'Connor, P. J. (1979). Nucleic acid modification by N-nitroso compounds. In: P. L. Grover (ed.), *Chemical Carcinogens and DNA*, CRC Press, Boca Raton, Louisiana. 1, pp. 111–59

Mark, J. (1973). Karyotype patterns in human meningiomas. A comparison between studies with G- and Q- banding techniques. *Hereditas, 75*: 213–19

Mark, J. (1975). Histiocytic lymphomas with the marker chromosome 14q+. *Hereditas, 81*: 289–92

Mark, J. (1977). On the specificity of medium-sized isomarker chromosomes in non-Burkitt lymphomas. *Acta Pathologica et Microbiologica Scandinavica; Section A: Pathology, 85*: 557–8

Mark, J., Ekedahl, C. and Hagman, A. (1977). Origin of the translocated segment of the 14q+ marker in non-Burkitt lymphomas. *Human Genetics, 36*: 277–82

Mark, J., Levan, G. and Mitelman, F. (1972). Identification by fluorescence of the G chromosome lost in human meningomas. *Hereditas, 71*: 163–8

Markert, C. L. (1968). Neoplasia: a disease of cell differentiation. *Cancer Research, 28*: 1908–14

Marks, S. M., Baltimore, D. and McCaffrey, R. (1978). Terminal transferase as a predictor of initial responsiveness to vincristine and prednisone in blastic chronic myelogenous leukemia. *New England Journal of Medicine, 298*: 812–14

Marmont, A. M. and Damasio, E. E. (1973). The treatment of terminal metamorphosis of chronic granulocytic leukemia with corticosteroids and vincristine. *Acta Haematologica, 50*: 1–8

Marshall, C. J. and Dave, H. (1978). Suppression of the transformed phenotype in somatic cell hybrids. *Journal of Cell Science, 33*: 171–90

Marshall, R. R., Arlett, C. F., Harcourt, S. A. and Broughton, B. A. (1980). Increased sensitivity of cell strains from Cockayne's syndrome to sister-chromatid-exchange induction and cell killing by uv light. *Mutation Research, 69*: 107–12

Martin, G. R. (1980). Teratocarcinomas and mammalian embryogenesis. *Science, 209*: 768–76

Martin, P. J., Najfeld, V., Hansen, J. A., Penfold, G. K., Jacobson, R. J. and Fialkow, P. J. (1980). Involvement of the B-lymphoid system in chronic myelogenous leukemia. *Nature, 287*: 49–50

Martland, R. E. and Humphries, R. E. (1929). Osteogenic sarcomas in dial painters using luminous paint. *Archives of Pathology, 7*: 406–17

Matsuura, N., Endo, M., Okayasu, T. and Okuno, A. (1975). Wiedemann-Beckwith syndrome. *Lancet, 2*: 508

Matthews, P. N., Millis, R. R. and Hayward, J. L. (1981). Breast cancer in women who have taken contraceptive steroids. *British Medical Journal, 282*: 774–6

Mattei, J. F., Mattei, M. G., Ayme, S. and Giraud, F. (1979). Origin of the extra chromosome in trisomy 21. *Human Genetics, 46*: 107–10

Mattocks, A. R. (1972). Toxicity and metabolism of *Senecio* alkaloids. In: J. B. Harborne (ed.), *Phytochemical Ecology*, Academic Press, London, p. 179

Maugh, T. H. (1978). Chemicals: how many are there? *Science, 199*: 162

Maurer, R. A. (1980). Dopaminergic inhibition of prolactin synthesis and prolactin messenger RNA accumulation in cultured pituitary cells. *Journal of Biological Chemistry, 255:* 8092–7

Maurer, R. A., Gubbins, E. J., Erwin, C. R. and Donelson, J. E. (1980). Comparison of potential nuclear precursors for prolactin and growth hormone messenger RNA. *Journal of Biological Chemistry, 255:* 2243

Maxson, L., Pepper, E. and Maxson, R. D. (1977). Immunological resolution of a diploid-tetraploid species complex of tree frogs. *Science, 197:* 1012–13

Mayall, B. M., Carrano, A. V., Moore, D. H. and Rowley, J. D. (1977). Quantification by DNA-based cytophotometry of the 9q+/22q− chromosomal translocation associated with chronic myelogenous leukemia. *Cancer Research, 37:* 3590–3

Meade, R. H. (1968). *An Introduction to the History of General Surgery*, W. B. Saunders, Philadelphia

Meade, T. W., Greenberg, G. and Thompson, S. G. (1980). Progestogens and cardiovascular reactions associated with oral contraceptives and a comparison of the safety of 50- and 30-mg oestrogen preparations. *British Medical Journal, 208:* 1157–61

Meisner, L. F., Gilbert, E., Ris, H. W. and Haverty, G. (1979). Genetic mechanisms in cancer predispostion. *Cancer, 43:* 679–89

Mendelson, J. H. and Mello, N. K. (1979). Biologic concomitants of alcoholism. *New England Journal of Medicine, 301:* 912–21

Menon, K. M. J. and Reel, J. R. (eds.) (1976). *Steroid Hormone Action and Cancer*, Plenum Press, New York

Mesa-Tejada, R. and Spiegelman S. (1983). Retroviruses and human breast cancer. In: L. A. Phillips (ed.), *Viruses Associated with Human Cancers*, Marcel Dekker, New York, pp. 473–500

Meselson, M. S. and Radding, C. M. (1975). A general model for genetic recombination. *Proceedings of the National Academy of Sciences (USA), 72:* 358–61

Metcalf, D., Moore, M. A. S., Sheridan, J. W. and Spitzer, G. (1974). Responsiveness of human granulocytic leukemic cells to colony-stimulating factor. *Blood, 43:* 847–59

Metcalfe, P. and Moore, M. A. S. (1971). *Haemopoietic Cells*, North Holland, Amsterdam

Mettlin, C. (1983). Cancer of the prostate and testis. In: G. J. Bourke (ed.), *The Epidemiology of Cancer*, Croom Helm, London, pp. 245–59

Miao, R. M., Fieldsteel, A. H. and Fodge, D. W. (1978). Opposing effects of tumour promoters on erythroid differentiation. *Nature, 274:* 271–2

Michael, R. O. and Williams, G. M. (1974). Chloroquin inhibition of repair of DNA damage induced in mammalian cells by methyl methane sulphonate, *Mutation Research, 25:* 391

Mikkelsen, M., Poulsen, H., Grinsted, J. and Lange, A. (1980). Non-disjunction in trisomy 21: study of chromosomal heteromorphisms in 110 families. *Annals of Human Genetics, 44:* 17–28

Miller, A. B. (1983). Cancer of the colon and rectum. In: G. J. Bourke, (ed.), *The Epidemiology of Cancer*, Croom Helm, London, pp. 145–61

Miller, D. A. and Miller, O. J. (1983). Chromosomes and cancer in the mouse: studies in tumors, established cell lines, and cell hybrids. *Advances in Cancer Research, 39:* 153–82

Miller, E. C. (1978). Some current perspectives on chemical carcinogenesis in humans and experimental animals: Presidential address. *Cancer Research, 38:* 1479–96

Miller, E. C. and Miller, J. A. (1974a). Biochemical mechanisms of chemical carcinogenesis. In: H. Busch (ed.), *Molecular Biology of Cancer*, Academic Press, New York, pp. 377–402

Miller, E. C. and Miller, J. A. (1981). Mechanisms of chemical carcinogenesis. *Cancer, 47*: 1055–64

Miller, J. A. (1970). Carcinogenesis by chemicals: an overview — G. H. A. Clowes memorial lecture. *Cancer Research, 30*: 559–76

Miller, J. A. (1979). Concluding remarks on chemicals and chemical carcinogenesis. In: A. C. Griffin and C. R. Shaw (eds.), *Carcinogenesis: Identification and Mechanisms of Action*, Raven Press, New York, pp. 455–69

Miller, J. A. and Miller, E. C. (1974b). Some current thresholds of research in chemical carcinogenesis. In: P. O. P. Ts'o and J. A. DiPaolo (eds.), *Chemical Carcinogenesis*, Marcel Dekker, New York, Part A, pp. 61–85

Miller, J. Q., Willson, K., Wyand, T. H., Jaramillo, M. A. and McConnell, T. S. (1979). Familial partial 14 trisomy. *Journal of Medical Genetics, 16*: 60–5

Miller, R. W. (1970). Neoplasia and Down's syndrome. *Annals of the New York Academy of Sciences, 171*: 636–44

Miller, R. W. (1980). Birth defects and cancer due to small chromosomal deletions. *Journal of Pediatrics, 96*: 1031

Milne, M. D. (1974). Hereditary disorders of intestinal transport. *Biomembranes, 4B*: 961–1013

Milner, G. R. and Geary, C. G. (1979). The aplasia-leukemia syndrome. In: C. G. Geary (ed.), *Aplastic Anaemia*, Baillière Tindall, London, pp. 230–43

Milunsky, A. (1980). Prenatal detection of neural tube defects. *Journal of the American Medical Association, 244*: 2731–5

Mingxin, L., Ping, L. and Baorong, L. (1980). Recent progress in research on esophageal cancer in China. *Advances in Cancer Research, 33*: 173–249

Mintz, B. and Fleischman, R. A. (1981). Teratocarcinomas and other neoplasms as developmental defects in gene expression. *Advances in Cancer Research, 34*: 211–78

Mintz, V., Vardiman, J., Golomb, H. M. and Rowley, J. D. (1979). Evolution of karyotypes in Philadelphia (Phl) chromosome-negative chronic myelogenous leukemia. *Cancer, 43*: 411–16

Miro, R., Cabalin, M. R., Marina, S. and Egozcue, J. (1978). Mosaicism in XX males. *Human Genetics, 45*: 103–6

Misset, J. L., Venuat, N. M., Nevarez, L. and Mathe, G. (1977). Crises blastiques révélatrices de leucémies myeloides chroniques et stimulant de leucémies aigues primaries, ou leucémies aigues primaires à chromosome Philadelphia? *Nouvelle Presse Médicale, 6*: 2409–13

Mitelman, F. (1974). Heterogeneity of Phl in chronic myeloid leukemia. *Hereditas, 76*: 315–16

Mitelman, F. (1980). Cytogenetics of experimental neoplasms and non-random chromosome correlations in man. *Clinical Haematology, 9*: 195–219

Mitelman, F. (1981). Marker chromosome 14q+ in human cancer and leukemia. *Advances in Cancer Research, 34*: 141–70

Mitelman, F., Klein, G., Andersson-Anuret, M., Forsby, N. and Johansson, B. (1979). 14q+ marker chromosome in an EBV-genome-negative lymph node without signs of malignancy in a patient with EBV-genome-positive nasopharyngeal carcinoma. *International Journal of Cancer, 23*: 32–6

Mitelman, F. and Levan, G. (1976). Clustering of aberrations to specific chromosomes in human neoplasms. *Hereditas, 82*: 167–74

Mitelman, F. and Levan, G. (1978). Clustering of aberrations to specific chromosomes in human neoplasms. III. Incidence and geographic distribution of chromosome aberrations in 856 cases. *Hereditas, 89*: 207–32

Mittra, I. (1980). A novel 'cleaved prolactin' in the rat pituitary: Part 1. Biosynthesis, characterization and regulatory control. *Biochemical and Biophysical Research Communications, 95*: 1750–9

Mobbs, B. G. (1966). The uptake of tritiated oestradiol by dimethylbenzanthracene-induced mammary tumours of the rat. *Journal of Endocrinology, 36*: 409–14

Mobley, P. L. and Sulser, F. (1980). Adrenal corticoids regulate sensitivity of noradrenaline receptor-coupled adenylate cyclase in brain. *Nature, 286*: 608–9

Moedjono, S. J., Crandall, B. F. and Sparkes, R. S. (1980). Tetrasomy 9p: confirmation by enzyme analysis. *Journal of Medical Genetics, 17*: 227–9

Moodie, R.L. (1923). *Paleopathology: An Introduction to the Study of Ancient Evidence of Disease*. University of Illinois Press, Urbana

Moore, D.H., Charney, J., Kramarsky, B., Lasfargues, E.Y., Sarkar, N.H., Brennan, M.J., *et al.* (1971). Search for a human breast cancer virus. *Nature, 229*; 611–14

Moore, M.A.S., Broxmeyer, H.E., Sheridan, A.P.C., Meyers, P.A., Jacobsen, N. and Winchester, R.J. (1980). Continuous human bone marrow culture: Ia antigen characterization of probable pluripotential stem cells. *Blood, 55:* 682–90

Morardet, N. and Parmentier, C. (1977). Description of a suicide technique in vitro for granulocytic stem cells (CFUc) by hydroxyurea on normal human bone marrow. *Biomedicine, 27:* 349–53

Morris, H.P. (1965). Studies on the development, biochemistry and biology of experimental hepatomas. *Advances in Cancer Research, 9:* 227–302

Morris, H. P. (1975). Biological and biochemical characteristics of transplantable hepatomas. In: E. Gründmann (ed.), *Handbuch der Allgemeinen Pathologie*, Springer-Verlag, Berlin, pp. 277–334

Morris, H. P. and Meranze, D.R. (1974). Induction and some characteristics of 'minimal deviation' and other transplantable rat hepatomas. *Recent Results in Cancer Research, 44:* 103–14

Mortimer, E. A. (1978). Immunization against infectious disease. *Science, 200:* 902–7

Mühlbock, O. and Boot, L. M. (1959). Induction of mammary cancer in mice without the mammary tumor agent by isografts of hypophyses. *Cancer Research, 19:* 402–12

Muir, C. and Parkin, D. M. (1983). The prevention of cancer. In: G. J. Bourke (ed.), *The Epidemiology of Cancer*, Croom Helm, London, pp. 343–64

Muir, E. G., Yates-Bell, A. J. and Barlow, K. A. (1966). Multiple primary adenocarcinomata of the colon, duodenum, and larynx associated with keratoacanthomata of the face. *British Journal of Surgery, 54:* 191–5

Müller, J. (1838). *Ueber den feinern Bau und die Formen der Krankhaften Geschwülste*, G. Reimer, Berlin

Müller, J. (1971). *Regulation of Aldosterone Biosynthesis*, Springer-Verlag, Berlin

Müller, R., Slamon, D. J., Tremblay, J. M., Cline, M. J. and Verma, I. M. (1982). Differential expression of cellular oncogenes during pre- and postnatal development of the mouse. *Nature, 299:* 640–4

Mulvihill, J. J. (1976). Host factors in human lung tumors: an example of ecogenetics in oncology. *Journal of the National Cancer Institute, 57:* 3–7

Mulvihill, J. J. (1980). Individual differences in cancer susceptibility. *Annals of Internal Medicine, 92:* 809–25

Murata, M. and Tanaka, N. (1983). Familial aspects of cancer. In: G. J. Bourke (ed.), *The Epidemiology of Cancer*, Croom Helm, London, pp. 17–30

Murphy, J. B. (1912). Transplantability of malignant tumors to the embryo of a foreign species. *Journal of the American Medical Association, 59:* 874–5

Murphy, M. F. (1981). Vitamin B12 deficiency due to a low cholesterol diet in a vegetarian. *Annals of Internal Medicine, 94:* 57–8

Murthy, P. B. and Rahiman, M. A. (1983). Chromosomal abnormalities in severely malnourished Indian children. *Hiroshima Journal of Medical Science, 32:* 291–4

Mustacchi, P. (1961). Ramazzini and Rigoni-Stern on parity and breast cancer. *Southern Medical and Surgical Journal, 2:* 257–93

Myers, C. E. (1980). Antitumor antibiotics I: anthracyclines. In: H. M. Pinedo (ed.), *Cancer Chemotherapy 1980*, Excerpta Medica, Amsterdam and Oxford, pp. 66–83

Nabeshima, Y., Fujii-Kuriyama, Y., Muramatsu, M. and Ogata, K. (1984). Alternative transcription and two modes of splicing result in two myosin light chains from one gene. *Nature, 308:* 333–8

Nadler, L. M., Reinherz, E. L., Weinstein, H. J., D'Orsi, C. J., and Schlossman, S. F. (1980). Heterogeneity of T-cell lymphoblastic malignancies. *Blood, 55:* 806–10

Nagasawa, H. (1979). Prolactin and human breast cancer: a review. *European Journal of Cancer, 15:* 267–79

Nagata, C., Tagashira, Y. and Kodama, M. (1974). Metabolic activation of benzo(a)pyrene: significance of the free radical. In: P. O. P. Ts'o and J. A. DiPaolo (eds.), *Chemical Carcinogenesis*, Marcel Dekker, New York, Part A, pp. 87–111

Nandi, S. and McGrath, C. M. (1973). Mammary neoplasia in mice. *Advances in Cancer Research, 17:* 353–414

Naor, D. (1979). Suppressor cells: permitters and promoters of malignancy? *Advances in Cancer Research, 29:* 45–125

Natarajan, A. T., van Zeeland, A. A., Verdegaal-Immerzeel, E. A. M. and Filon, A. R. (1980). Studies on the influence of photoreactivation on the frequencies of uv-induced chromosomal aberrations, sister-chromatid exchanges and pyrimidine dimers in chicken embryonic fibroblasts. *Mutation Research, 69:* 307-17

Nathanson, I. T. (1952). Clinical investigative experience with steroid hormones in breast cancer. *Cancer, 5:* 754-62

Nazerian, K., Lee, L. F. and Sharma, J. M. (1976). The role of herpes viruses in Marek's disease lymphoma of chickens. *Progress in Medical Virology, 22;* 123-51

Nebert, D. W., Levitt, R. C. and Pelkonen, O. (1979). Genetic variation in metabolism of chemical carcinogens associated with susceptibility to tumorigenesis. In: A. C. Griffin and C. R. Shaw (eds.), *Carcinogens: Identification and Mechanisms of Action*, Raven Press, New York, pp. 157-208

Neel, B., Jhanwar, S., Chaganti, R. and Hayward, W. S. (1982). Two human *c-onc* genes are located on the long arm of chromosome 8. *Proceedings of the National Academy of Sciences (USA), 24:* 7842-6

Nery, R. (1968). Some aspects of the metabolism of urethane and N-hydroxy-urethane in rodents. *Biochemical Journal, 106:* 1-13

Nery, R. (1976). Carcinogenic mechanisms: a critical review and a suggestion that oncogenesis may be adaptive ontogenesis. *Chemico-Biological Interactions, 12:* 145-69

Nery, R., Barsoum, A. L. Bullman, H. and Neville, A. M. (1974a). Carcinoembryonic antigen-like substances of human urethelial carcinomas: isolation of components from pathological urine and comparison with colorectal carcinoma antigens. *Biochemical Journal, 139:* 431-40

Nery, R., James, R., Barsoum, A. L. and Bullman, H. (1974b). Isolation and partial characterisation of macromolecular urinary aggregates containing carcinoembryonic antigen-like activity. *British Journal of Cancer, 29:* 413-24

Neubert, D. (1980). Teratogenicity: any relationship with carcinogenicity? *International Agency for Research on Cancer Scientific Publications, 27:* 169

Neve, A. (1900). Kangri-burn epithelioma in Kashmir. *Indian Medical Gazette, 35:* 81-3

Neve, E. F. (1923). Kangri-burn cancer. *British Medical Journal, 2:* 1255-6

Neville A.M. and O'Hare, M.J. (1982). *The Human Adrenal Cortex*, Springer-Verlag, Berlin

Nezhat, C., Karpas, A. E., Greenblatt, R. B. and Mahesh, V. B. (1980). Estradiol implants for conception control. *American Journal of Obstetrics and Gynecology, 138:* 1151-6

Nicholson, W. J. (1984). Quantitative estimates of cancer in the workplace. *American Journal of Industrial Medicine, 5,* 341

Niikawa, N., Merotto, E. and Kajii, T. (1977). Origin of acrocentric trisomies in spontaneous abortuses. *Human Genetics, 40:* 73-8

Nomura, A., Henderson, B. E. and Lee, J. (1978). Breast cancer and diet among the Japanese in Hawaii. *American Journal of Clinical Nutrition, 31:* 2020-5

Novikoff, A. B. (1957). A transplantable rat liver tumor induced by 4-dimethylaminoazobenzene. *Cancer Research, 17:* 1010-27

Nowell, P. C. and Hungerford, D. A. (1960). A minute chromosome in human chronic granulocytic leukemia. *Science, 132:* 1497

Oberling, C. (1944). *The Riddle of Cancer.* Trans. W. H. Woglom, Yale University Press, New Haven.

O'Brien, M., Catovsky, D. and Costello, C. (1980). Ultrastructural cytochemistry of leukemic cells: characterization of the early small granules of monoblasts. *British Journal of Haematology, 45:* 201-8

Odell, W. and Saito, E. (1983). Protein hormone-like materials from normal and cancer cells — 'ectopic' hormone production. *Progress in Clinical and Biological Research, 132E:* 247-58

Odell, W., Wolfsen, A., Yoshimoto, Y., Weitzman, R., Fisher, D. and Hirose, F. (1977). Ectopic peptide synthesis: a universal concomitant of neoplasia. *Transactions of the Association of American Physicians, 90:* 204-7

Oettle, A. C. (1963). Skin cancer in Africa. In: F. Urbach (ed.), *The Biology of Cutaneous Cancer,* National Cancer Institute Monograph Number 10, US Government Printing Office, Washington, DC, pp. 197-210

Ogawa, K., Solt, D. B. and Farber, E. (1980). Phenotypic diversity as an early property of putative preneoplastic hepatocyte populations in liver carcinogenesis. *Cancer Research, 40:* 725-33

O'Grady, W. P. and McDivitt, R. W. (1969). Breast cancer in a man treated with diethylstilbestrol. *Archives of Pathology, 88:* 162-5

Olsson, I. L., Sarngadharan, M. G., Breitman, T. R. and Gallo, R. C. (1984). Isolation and characterization of a T lymphocyte-derived differentiation inducing factor for the myeloid leukemic cell line HL-60. *Blood, 63:* 510-17

Omary, M. B., Trowbridge, I. S. and Minowada, J. (1980). Human cell-surface glycoprotein with unusual properties. *Nature, 286:* 888-91

Omenn, G. S. (1978). Prenatal diagnosis of genetic disorders. *Science, 200:* 925-8

Orgel, L. E. and Crick, F. H. (1980). Selfish DNA: the ultimate parasite. *Nature, 284:* 604-7

Orie, N. G. M., Sluiter, H. J. and Van Der Wal, A. M. (1977). Common familial component in lung cancer and chronic obstructive pulmonary disease. *Lancet, 2:* 1138

Osborne, C. K., Yochmowitz, M. G., Knight, W. A., and McGuire, W. L. (1980). The value of estrogen and progesterone receptors in the treatment of breast cancer. *Cancer, 46:* 2884-8

Osgood, E. E. and Brooke, J. H. (1955). Continuous tissue culture of leukocytes from human leukemic bloods by application of gradient principles. *Blood, 10:* 1010-29

Oshima, A. and Fujimoto, I. (1983). Cancer of the stomach. In: G. J. Bourke (ed.), *The Epidemiology of Cancer,* Croom Helm, London, pp. 116-30

Oshimura, M., Freeman, A. I. and Sandberg, A. A. (1977a). Chromosomes and causation of human cancer and leukemia. XXIII. Near-haploidy in acute leukemia. *Cancer, 40:* 1143-8

Oshimura, M., Freeman, A. I. and Sandberg, A. A. (1977b). Chromosomes and causation of human cancer and leukemia. XXVI. Banding studies in acute lymphoblastic leukemia (ALL). *Cancer, 40:* 1161-72

Osler, W. (1907). On multiple hereditary telangiectases with recurring haemorrages. *Quarterly Journal of Medicine, 1:* 53-8

Overzier, C. (1964). Ein XX/XY–Hermaphrodit mit einem 'intratubularen Ei' und einem Gonadoblastom Gonocytom 3. *Klinische Wochenschrift, 42:* 1052-60

Owens, D. R., Jones, M. K., Hayes, T. M., Heding, L. G., Alberti, K. G. M., Home, P. D., Burrin, J. M. and Newcombe, R. G. (1981). Human insulin: study of safety and efficacy in man. *British Medical Journal, 232:* 1264-6

Padgett, B. L., Walker, D. L., Zurhein, G. M. and Varakis, J. N. (1977). Differential neurooncogenicity of strains of JC virus, a human polyome virus, in newborn Syrian hamsters. *Cancer Research, 37:* 718-20

Paffenbarger, R. S., Fasal, E., Simmons, M. E. and Kampert, J. B. (1977). Cancer risk as related to use of oral contraceptives during fertile years. *Cancer, 39:* 1887-91

Painter, T. S. (1921). The Y-chromosome in mammals. *Science, 53:* 503-4

Pamukcu, A. M. (1963). Epidemiologic studies on urinary bladder tumors in Turkish cattle. *Annals of the New York Academy of Sciences, 108:* 938-47

Pamukcu, A. M., Erturk, E., Price, J. M. and Brown, G. (1972). Lymphatic leukemia and pulmonary tumors in female Swiss mice fed bracken fern *(Pteris aquilina)*. *Cancer Research, 32:* 1442-5

Paone, J. F., Abeloff, M. D. Ettinger, D. S., Arnold, E. A. and Baker, R. R. (1981). The correlation of estrogen and progesterone receptor levels with response to chemotherapy for advanced carcinoma of the breast. *Surgery, Gynecology and Obstetrics, 152:* 70-4

Pardon, J. F. and Wilkins, M. H. F. (1972). A super-coil model for nucleohistone. *Journal of Molecular Biology, 68:* 115-24

Parke, J. C. Grass, F. S., Pixley, R. and Deal, J. (1980). Trisomy 21 mosaicism in two successive generations in a family. *Journal of Medical Genetics, 17:* 48-9

Parmentier, C., Droz. J. P. and Tubiana, M. (1978a). Ways of expressing results of human bone marrow pregenitor cell culture. *British Journal of Haematology, 40:* 105-9

Parmentier, C., Maraninchi, D., Morardet, N. and Droz, J. P. (1978b). Observations on the distribution of granulocytic progenitor cells (CFU-C) in human bone marrow: the importance of the manner in which the results of in vitro cultures are reported. *British Journal of Haematology, 40:* 353-4

Parodi, S. and Brambilla, G. (1977). Relationship between mutation and transformation frequencies in mammalian cells treated 'in vitro' with chemical carcinogens. *Mutation Research, 47:* 53–74

Parshad, R. and Sanford, K. (1968). Effect of horse serum, bovine serum, and fetuin on neoplastic conversion and chromosomes of mouse embryo cells in vitro. *Journal of the National Cancer Institute, 41:* 767–79

Paymaster, J. C. and Gangadharan, P. (1970). Cancer in the Parsi community of Bombay. *International Journal of Cancer, 5:* 426–31

Pearson, G., Mann, J. D., Benson, J. and Bull, R. W. (1979). Inversion duplication of chromosome 6 with trisomic codominant expression of HLA antigens. *American Journal of Human Genetics, 31:* 29–34

Penman, H. G. (1970). The effect of oral contraceptives on the histology of carcinoma of the breast. *Journal of Pathology, 101:* 66–8

Penrose, L. S. (1933). Relative effects of paternal and maternal age in mongolism. *Journal of Genetics, 27:* 219–24

Pereira, M. S. (1979). Global surveillance of influenza. *British Medical Bulletin, 35:* 9–14

Peterson, L. C., Bloomfield, C. D. and Brunning, R. D. (1976). Blast crisis as an initial or terminal manifestation of chronic myelocytic leukemia. *American Journal of Medicine, 60:* 209–20

Peterson, P. A., Rask, L. and Ostberg, L. (1977). β_2-Microglobulin and the major histocompatibility complex. *Advances in Cancer Research, 24:* 115–63

Petri, S. (1933). Über familiäres Auftreten der Leukamie. *Acta Pathologica et Microbiologica Scandinavica, Section A, Pathology, 10:* 330–79

Pfeiffer, R. A., Korver, G., Sanger, R. and Race, R. R. (1964). Paternal origin of an XXYY anomaly. *Lancet, 1:* 1417–18

Philip, P., Jensen, K. M. and Pallesen, G. (1977). Marker chromosome 14q+ in non-endemic Burkitt's lymphoma. *Cancer, 39:* 1495–9

Phillips, D. H. and Sims, P. (1979). Polycyclic aromatic hydrocarbon metabolites and DNA. In: P. L. Grover (ed.), *Chemical Carcinogens and DNA*, CRC Press, Boca Raton, Louisiana vol. 2, pp. 29–57

Phillips, R. L., Garfinkel, L., Kuzma, J. W., Beeson, W. L., Lotz, T. and Brin, B. (1980). Mortality among California Seventh-Day Adventists for selected cancer sites. *Journal of the National Cancer Institute, 65:* 1097–1107

Pickthall, V. J. (1976). Detailed cytogenetic study of metastatic bronchial carcinoma. *British Journal of Cancer, 34:* 272–8

Pierce, G. B., Shrikes, R. and Fink, L. M. (1978). *Cancer: A Problem of Developmental Biology*, Prentice-Hall, Englewood Cliffs

Pierre, R. V. (1974). Preleukemic states. *Seminars in Hematology, 11:* 73–92

Pike, B. L. and Robinson, W. A. (1970). Human bone marrow colony growth in agar-gel. *Journal of Cell Physiology, 76:* 77–84

Pinedo, H. M. (ed.) (1979). *Cancer Chemotherapy*, Excerpta Medica, Amsterdam (appears annually since 1979)

Pitot, H. C., Barsness, L., Goldsworthy, T. and Kitagawa, T. (1978). Biochemical characterisation of stages of hepatocarcinogenesis after a single dose of diethylnitrosamine. *Nature, 271:* 456–8

Pitot, H. C., Shires, T. K., Moyer, G. and Garrett, C. T. (1974). Phenotypic variability as a manifestation of translational control. In: H. Busch (ed.), *The Molecular Biology of Cancer*, Academic Press, New York, pp. 523–34

Pochedly, C. (ed.) (1976). *Neuroblastoma*, Publishing Sciences Group Inc,. Acton, Massachusetts

Polani, P. E., Alberman, E., Alexander, B. J., Benson, P. F., Berry, A. C., Blunt, S., Daker, M. G., Fensoni, A. H., Garrett, D. M., McGuire, V. M., Roberts, J. A. F., Seller, M. J. and Singer, J. D., (1979). Sixteen years' experience of counselling, diagnosis, and prenatal detection in one genetic centre: progress, results, and problems. *Journal of Medical Genetics, 16:* 166–75

Ponzio, G., Demarchi, M., Gallone, G., Fonzo, D. and Carbonara, A. O., (1980). Hypomelanosis of Ito with triphalangeal thumbs: case report. *Journal of Medical Genetics, 17:* 152–4

Portier, M. M., Eddé, B., Berthelot, F., Croizat, B. and Gros, F. (1980). Effects on the cytoskeleton of a new inducer of the neuroblastoma morphological differentiation. *Biochemical and Biophysical Research Communications, 96:* 1610–18

Poste, G. and Fidler, I. J. (1980). The pathogenesis of cancer metastasis. *Nature, 283:* 139–46

Pott, P. (1775). *Chirurgical Observations Relative to the Cataract, the Polypus of the Nose, the Cancer of the Scrotum, the Different Kinds of Ruptures, and the Mortification of the Toes and Feet*, Hawkes, Clarke and Collins, London

Powell, J. R., Tabachnick, W. J. and Arnold, J. (1980). Genetics and the origin of a vector population: *Aedes aegypti*, a case study. *Science, 208:* 1385–7

Prehn, R. T. (1979). Immunological basis for differences in susceptibility to hydrocarbon oncogenesis among mice of a single genotype. *International Journal of Cancer, 24:* 789–91

Preisler, H. D. (1980). Clonogenic potential in vitro of proliferative and quiescent leukemic cells. *Leukemia Research, 4:* 245–8

Priest, J. H. Blackston, R. D., All, K. S. and Ray, S. L. (1975). Differences in human X isochromosomes. *Journal of Medical Genetics, 12:* 378–89

Priest, J. R. Robinson, L. L., McKenna, R. W., Lindquist, L. L., Warkentin, P. I., Le Bien, T. W., Woods, W. G., Kersey, J. H., Coccia, P. F. and Nesbit, M. E. (1980). Philadelphia chromosome positive childhood acute lymphoblastic leukemia. *Blood, 56:* 15–22

Priestman, T. J. (1980). Initial evaluation of human lymphoblastoid interferon in patients with advanced malignant disease. *Lancet, 2:* 113–18

Prieto, F., Badia, L., Mayans, J., Gomis, F. and Marty, M. L. (1978). Hipodiploidia de 26 cromosomas en leucémia linfoblastica aguda. *Sangre, 23:* 484–8

Prigogina, E., Fleischman, E. W., Volkova, M. A. and Frenkel, M. A. (1978). Chromosome abnormalities and clinical and morphologic manifestations of chronic myeloid leukemia. *Human Genetics, 41:* 143–56

Proctor, J. W., Yamamura, Y., Gaydos, D. and Mastromatteo, W. (1981). Further studies on endocrine factors and the growth and spread of B_{16} melanoma. *Oncology, 38:* 102–5

Pugh, T. and Goldfarb, S. (1978). Quantitative histochemical and autoradiographic studies of hepatocarcinogenesis in rats fed 2-acetylaminofluorene followed by pentobarbital. *Cancer Research, 38:* 4450–7

Pullan, P. T., Clement-Jones, V., Corder, R., Lowry, P. J., Rees, G. M., Rees, L. H., Besser, G. M., Macedo, M. M. and Galvao-Teles, A. (1980). Ectopic production of methionine enkephalin and beta-endorphin. *British Medical Journal, 280:* 758–9

Purchase, I. F. H. (1980). Inter-species comparisons of carcinogenicity. *British Journal of Cancer, 41:* 454–68

Purtilo, D. T., Paquin, L. and Gindhart, T. (1978). Genetics of neoplasia — impact of ecogenetics on oncogenesis. A review. *American Journal of Pathology, 91:* 609–88

Qasba, P. K. and Safaya, S. K. (1984). Similarity of the nucleotide sequences of rat α-lactalbumin and chicken lysozyme genes. *Nature, 308:* 377–80

Rabinowitz, Z. and Sachs, L. (1970). Control of the reversion of properties in transformed cells. *Nature, 225:* 136–9

Raghavan, D., Gibbs, J., Neville, A. M. and Peckham, M. J. (1980). Experimental germ-cell tumors. *New England Journal of Medicine, 302:* 811

Rao, P. S. S. and Inbaraj, S. G. (1979). Inbreeding effects on fertility and sterility in southern India. *Journal of Medical Genetics, 16:* 24–31

Rao, P. S. S. and Inbaraj, S. G. (1980). Inbreeding effects on fetal growth and development. *Journal of Medical Genetics, 17:* 27–33

Rather, L. J. (1978). *The Genesis of Cancer: A Study in the History of Ideas,* Johns Hopkins University Press, Baltimore

Redmond D. E. and Huang, Y. H. (1979). Current concepts. II. New evidence for a locus coeruleus-norepinephrine connection with anxiety. *Life Sciences, 25:* 2149–62

Reed, W. B., Landing, B., Sugarman, G., Cleaver, J. E. and Melnyk, J. (1969). Xeroderma pigmentosum. *Journal of the American Medical Association, 207:* 2073–9

Rees, K. R., Rowland, G. F. and Varcoe, J. S. (1965). Intranuclear changes in rat liver during the early stages of feeding the hepatocarcinogens thioacetamide and 4-dimethylaminoazobenzene. *British Journal of Cancer, 19:* 72–82

Reeves, B. R., Lobb, D. S. and Lawler, S. D. (1972). Identity of the abnormal F-group chromosome associated with polycythaemia vera. *Humangenetik, 14:* 159–61

Rehn, L. (1895). Blasengeschwülste bei Fuchsin-Arbeitern. *Archiv für Klinische Chirurgie, 50:* 588–600

Reid, D. E. and Shirley, R. L. (1974). Endometrial carcinoma associated with

Sheehan's syndrome and stilbestrol therapy. *American Journal of Obstetrics and Gynecology, 119:* 264–6

Revell, S. H. (1974). The breakage-and-reunion theory and the exchange theory for chromosomal aberrations induced by ionizing radiations: a short history. *Advances in Radiation Biology, 4:* 367–416

Revoltella, R. P. and Butler, R. H. (1980). Nerve growth factor may stimulate either division or differentiation of cloned C1300 neuroblastoma cells in serum-free cultures. *Journal of Cell Physiology, 104:* 27–33

Riccardi, V. M. (1978). Genetic etiology of retinoblastoma. *American Journal of Ophthalmology, 86:* 442

Riccardi, V. M., Svjansky, E., Smith, A. C. and Francke, U. (1978). Chromosomal imbalance in the Aniridia – Wilm's tumor association: 11p interstitial deletion. *Pediatrics, 61:* 604–10

Ridler, M. A. and McKeown, J. A. (1979). Trisomy 16q arising from a maternal 15p; 16q translocation. *Journal of Medical Genetics, 16:* 317–20

Riley, E. and Swift, M. (1979). A family with Peutz-Jehger's syndrome and bilateral breast cancer. *Cancer, 46:* 815–17

Riley, V. (guest editor) (1979). Stress and cancer. *Cancer Detection and Prevention, 2:* 159–336

Rinaldi, A., Archidiacono, N., Rocchi, M. and Filippi, G. (1975). Additional pedigree supporting the frequent origin of XXYY from consecutive meiotic non-disjunction in paternal gametogenesis. *Journal of Medical Genetics, 16:* 225–6

Rios, M. E., Kaufman, R. L., Sekon, G. S., Bucy, J. C., Bowman, J. E. and Jacobs, L. S. (1975). An XX male: cytogenetic and endocrine studies. *Clinical Genetics, 7:* 155–62

Robbins, S. L., Cotran, R. S. and Kumar, V. (1984). *Pathologic Basis of Disease*, W. B. Saunders, Philadelphia, pp. 214–53

Roberts, M., Greaves, M., Janossy, G., Sutherland, R. and Pain, C. (1978). Acute lymphoblastic leukaemia (ALL) associated antigen-1. Expression in different haematopoietic malignancies. *Leukemia Research, 2:* 105–14

Robertson, M. and Hobart, M. (1981). Antibodies, introns and biosynthetic versatility. *Nature, 290:* 543–4

Robinson, J., Smith, D. and Niederman, J. (1980). Mitotic EBNA positive lymphocytes in peripheral blood during infectious mononucleosis. *Nature, 287:* 334–5

Roemer, V. M., Neeser, E., Peters, F. D. and Wehle, H. E. (1979). Ovarialtumoren nach Hysterektomie. *Gynakologische Rundschau, 19:* (1 Suppl), 107–23

Rogentine, G. N., Trapani, R. J., Yankee, R. A. and Henderson, E. S. (1973). HL-A antigens and acute lymphocytic leukemia: the nature of the HL-A2 association. *Tissue Antigens, 3:* 470–6

Rolland, P. H., Martin, P. M., Jaquemier, J., Rolland, A. M. and Toga, M. (1980). Prostaglandin in human breast cancer: evidence suggesting that an elevated prostaglandin production is a marker of high metastatic potential for neoplastic cells. *Journal of the National Cancer Institute, 64:* 1061–70

Roos, E. and Dingemans, K. P. (1979). Mechanisms of metastasis. *Biochimica et Biophysica Acta, 560:* 135–66

Rose, G. and Shipley, M. J. (1980). Plasma lipids and mortality: a source of error. *Lancet, 1:* 523–6

Rosenthal, S., Canellos, G. P., De Vita, V. T. and Gralnick, H. R. (1977). Characteristics of blast crisis in chronic granulocytic leukemia: morphologic variants and therapeutic implications. *American Journal of Medicine, 63:* 542–7

Rosner, F. and Lee, S. L. (1972). Down's syndrome and acute leukemia: myeloblastic or lymphoblastic? Report of forty-three cases and review of the literature. *American Journal of Medicine, 53*: 203–18

Rossier, J., French, E., Rivier, C., Shibasaki, T., Guillemin, R. and Bloom, F. E. (1980). Stress-induced release of prolactin: blockade by dexamethasone and naloxone may indicate β-endorphin mediation. *Proceedings of the National Academy of Sciences (USA), 77*: 666–9

Rotkin, I. D. (1962). Relation of adolescent coitus to cervical cancer risk. *Journal of the American Medical Association, 179*: 486–91

Rous, P. (1910). A transmissible avian neoplasm. (Sarcoma of the common fowl). *Journal of Experimental Medicine, 12*: 696–705

Rous, P. (1959). Surmise and fact on the nature of cancer. *Nature, 183*: 1357–61

Rous, P. and Kidd, J. G. (1941). Conditional neoplasms and sub-threshold neoplastic states. A study of the tar tumors of rabbits. *Journal of Experimental Medicine, 73*: 365–90

Rovera, G., O'Brien, T. and Diamond, L. (1977). Tumor promoters inhibit spontaneous differentiation of friend erythroleukemia cells in culture. *Proceedings of the National Academy of Sciences (USA), 74*: 2894–8

Rovera, G., O'Brien, T. and Diamond, L. (1979). Induction of differentiation in human promyelocytic leukemia cells by tumor promoters. *Science, 204*: 868

Rovera, G., Olashaw, N. and Meo, P. (1980). Terminal differentiation in human promyelocytic leukemic cells in the absence of DNA synthesis. *Nature, 284*: 69–70

Rowley, J. D. (1975). Non-random chromosomal abnormalities in hematologic disorders of man. *Proceedings of the National Academy of Sciences (USA), 72*: 152–6

Rowley, J. D. (1976). The role of cytogenetics in hematology. *Blood, 48*: 1–7

Rowley, J. D. (1978a). The cytogenetics of acute leukemia. *Clinics in Haematology, 7*: 385–406

Rowley, J. D. (1978b). Abnormalities of chromosome no. 1 in haematological malignancies. *Lancet, 1*: 554–5

Rowley, J. D. (1980). Ph-positive leukaemia, including chronic myelogenous leukaemia. *Clinics in Haematology, 9*: 55–86

Rowley, J. D. and Testa, J. R. (1982). Chromosome abnormalities in malignant hematologic diseases. *Advances in Cancer Research, 36*: 103

Rozencweig, M., Von Hoff, D. D., Abele, R. A. and Muggia, F. M. (1980). Cisplatin. In: H. M. Pinedo (ed.), *Cancer Chemotherapy 1980*, Excerpta Medica, Amsterdam and Oxford, pp. 107–17

Rubin, H. (1980). Is somatic mutation the major mechanism of malignant transformation? *Journal of the National Cancer Institute, 64*: 995–1000

Rubin, H. (1984). Adaptive changes in spontaneously transformed *Balb/3T3* cells during tumor formation and subsequent cultivation. *Journal of the National Cancer Institute, 72*: 375–81

Rubin, R. T., Reinisch, J. M. and Haskett, R. F. (1981). Postnatal gonadal steroid effects on human behaviour. *Science, 211*: 1318–24

Ruoslahti, E. and Seppälä, M. (1979). α-Fetoprotein in cancer and fetal development. *Advances in Cancer Research, 29*: 275–346

Rupert, C. S. (1975). Enzymatic photoreactivation: overview. In: P. C. Hanawalt and R. B. Setlow (eds.), *Molecular Mechanisms for Repair of DNA*, Plenum Press, New York, Part A, pp. 73–87

Russell, M. A. H., Jarvis, M. J. and Feyerabend, C. (1980). A new age for snuff? *Lancet, 1*: 474–5

Rygaard, J. and Povlsen, C. O. (1976). The nude mouse vs. the hypothesis of immunological surveillance. *Transplantation Reviews, 28*: 43–61

Sabine, J. R., Horton, B. J. and Wicks, M. B. (1973). Spontaneous tumours in *C3H-A vy* and *C3H-A vyfB* mice: high incidence in the United States and low incidence in Australia. *Journal of the National Cancer Institute, 50*: 1237–42

Sachs, L. (1978). Control of normal cell differentiation and the phenotypic reversion of malignancy in myeloid leukaemia. *Nature, 274*: 535–9

Sadoff, L., Winkley, J. and Tyson, S. (1973). Is malignant melanoma an endocrine-dependent tumor? The possible adverse effect of estrogen. *Oncology, 27*: 244–57

Safai, B., Mike, V., Giraldo, G., Beth, E. and Good, R. A. (1980). Association of Kaposi sarcoma with second primary malignancies. Possible etiopathogenic implications. *Cancer, 45*: 1472–9

Sakano, H., Huppi, K., Heinrich, G. and Tonegawa, S. (1979). Sequences at the somatic recombination sites of immunoglobulin light-chain genes. *Nature, 280*: 288–94

Sakurai, J., Hayata, I. and Sandberg, A. A. (1976). Prognostic value of chromosomal findings in Ph-positive chronic myelocytic leukemia. *Cancer Research, 36*: 313–18

Sallan, S. E., Ritz, J., Pesando, J., Gelber, R., O'Brien, C., Hitchcock, S., Coral, F. and Schlossman, S. F. (1980). Cell surface antigens: prognostic implications in childhood acute lymphoblastic leukemia. *Blood, 55*: 395–402

Salmon, S. E. and Seligmann, M. (1974). B-cell neoplasia in man. *Lancet, 2*: 1230–3

Sandberg, A. A. (1980). *The Chromosomes in Human Cancer and Leukemia*, Elsevier, New York.

Sandberg, A. A. (1983). Chromosomes in human neoplasia. *Current Problems in Cancer, 8*: 1–52

Sandberg, A. A. and Abe, S. (1980). Cytogenetic techniques in haematology. *Clinics in Haematology, 9*: 19–38

Sandberg, A. A., Cohen, M. M., Rimm, A. A. and Levin, M. L. (1967). Aneuploidy and age in a population survey. *American Journal of Human Genetics, 19*: 633–43

Sandberg, A. A., Cortner, J., Takagi, N., Moghadam, M. A. and Crosswhite, L. H. (1966). Differences in chromosome constitution of twins with acute leukemia. *New England Journal of Medicine, 275*: 809–12

Sandberg, A. A. and Hossfeld, D. K. (1970). Chromosomal abnormalities in human neoplasia. *Annual Reviews of Medicine, 21*: 379–408

Sanders-Haigh, L., Anderson, W. F., and Franke, U. (1980). The β-globin gene is on the short arm of human chromosome 11. *Nature, 283*: 683–6

Sandra, A., Paltzer, W. B. and Thomas, M. J. (1981). Morphological differentiation of murine neuroblastoma induced by liposomes. *Experimental Cell Research, 32*: 473–7

Sanes, J. R. (1984). More nerve growth factors? *Nature, 307*: 500

Sanger, R., Tippett, P., Gavin, J., Teesdale, P. and Daniels, G. L. (1977). Xg groups and sex chromosome abnormalities in people of northern European ancestry: an addendum. *Journal of Medical Genetics, 14*: 210–11

Sankaranarayanan, K. and Volkers, W. S. (1980). Exposure fractionation effects for x-ray-induced dominant lethals in immature (stage 7) oocytes of *Drosophila melanogaster*: a re-analysis. *Mutation Research, 69*: 249–62

Sasaki, M. and Hara, Y. (1973). Paternal origin of the extra chromosome in Down's syndrome. *Lancet, 2*: 1257

Sasaki, M., Ikeuchi, T. and Makino, S. (1968). A feather pulp culture technique for avian chromosomes, with notes on the chromosomes of the peafowl and the ostrich. *Experientia, 24*: 1292–3

Sasaki, M. S. (1978). Fanconi's anaemia. A condition possibly associated with a defective DNA repair. In: P. C. Hanawalt, E. C. Friedberg and C. F. Fox (eds.), *DNA Repair Mechanism*, Academic Press, New York, pp. 675–84

Sass, B., Rabstein, L. S., Madison, R., Nims, R. M., Peters, R. L. and Kelloff, G. J. (1975). Incidence of spontaneous neoplasms in F344 rats throughout the natural life-span. *Journal of the National Cancer Institute, 54*: 1449–53

Schaefer, O. (1969). Cancer of the breast and lactation. *Canadian Medical Association Journal, 100*: 625–6

Schally, A. V., Comaru-Schally, A. M., and Redding, T. W. (1984). Antitumor effects of analogs of hypothalamic hormones in endocrine-dependent cancers. *Proceedings of the Society of Experimental Biology and Medicine, 175*: 259–81

Scheid, W. and Traut, H. (1971). Visualization by scanning electronmicroscopy of achromatic lesions ('gaps') induced by X-rays in chromosomes of *Vicia faba*. *Mutation Research, 11*: 253–5

Schibler, U., Tosi, M., Pittet, A. C., Fabiani, L. and Wellauer, P. K. (1980). Tissue-specific expression of mouse α-amylase genes. *Journal of Molecular Biology, 142*: 93–116

Schild, G. C. (ed.) (1979). Influenza: introduction. *British Medical Bulletin, 35*: 1–2

Schilling, J., Clevinger, B., Davie, J. M. and Hood, L. (1980). Amino acid sequence of homogeneous antibodies to dextran and DNA rearrangements in heavy chain V-region gene segments. *Nature, 283*: 35–40

Schimke, R. N. (1978). *Genetics and Cancer in Man*, Churchill Livingstone, New York

Schlesinger, M., Levin, S., Handzel, Z., Hahn, T., Altman, Y., Cherabilski, B., and Bos, J. (1976). Clinical immunological and histopathological evidence for thymic deficiency in Down's syndrome (mongolism). *Advances in Experimental Medicine and Biology, 66*: 665–71

Schmid, W., Tenconi, R., Baccichetti, C., Caufin, D. and Schinzel, A. (1983). Ring chromosome 21 in phenotypically apparently normal persons: report of two families from Switzerland and Italy. *American Journal of Medical Genetics, 16*: 323–9

Schwab, M., Varmus, M. E., Bishop, J. H., Grzeschik, K. H., Naylor, S. L., Sakaguchi, A. Y., Brodeur, G. and Trent, J. (1984). Chromosome localization in normal human cells and neuroblastomas of a gene related to *c-myc*. *Nature, 308*: 288–91

Schwartz, J. H., Canellos, G. P., Young, R. C. and De Vita, V. T. (1975). Meningeal leukemia in the blastic phase of chronic granulocytic leukemia. *American Journal of Medicine, 59*: 819–28

Scott, G. M., Secher, D. S., Flowers, D., Bate, J., Cantell, K. and Tyrrell, D. A. J. (1981). Toxicity of interferon. *British Medical Journal, 282*: 1345–8

Scotto, J. and Bailar, J. C. (1969). Rigoni-Stern and medical statistics. A nineteenth-century approach to cancer research. *Journal of the History of Medicine and Allied Sciences, 24*: 65–75

Scriver, C. R., Laberge, C., Clow, C. L. and Fraser, F. C. (1978). Genetics and medicine: an evolving relationship. *Science, 200*: 946–52

Sears, M. E. and Olson, K. B. (1980). Extramural review of clinical response of breast cancer to cytotoxic chemotherapy. *Cancer, 46*: 2928–9

Segaloff, A., Hankey, B. F., Carter, A. C., Bundy, B. and Masnyk, I. J. (1980). Identification of breast cancer patients with high risk of early recurrence after radical mastectomy. *Cancer, 46*: 1087–92

Seger, R., Buchinger, G. and Stroder, J. (1977). On the influence of age on immunity in Down's syndrome. *European Journal of Pediatrics, 124*: 77–87

Seidman, J. G. and Leder, P. (1980). A mutant immunoglobulin light chain is formed by aberrant DNA- and RNA-splicing events. *Nature, 286*: 779–83

Selikoff, I. J., Hammond, E. C. and Chung, J. (1968). Asbestos exposure, smoking and neoplasia. *Journal of the American Medical Association, 204*: 106–12

Sell, S. (ed.) (1980). *Cancer Markers*, The Humana Press, Clifton, New Jersey

Sellakumar, A. R., Montesano, R., Saffiotti, U. and Kaufman, D. G. (1973). Hamster respiratory carcinogenesis induced by benzo(a)pyrene and different dose levels of ferric oxide. *Journal of the National Cancer Institute, 50*: 507–10

Seo, I. S., Warren, J., Mirkin, L. D., Weisman, S. J., and Grosfeld, J. L. (1984).

Mucoepidermoid carcinoma of the bronchus in a 4-year-old child. *Cancer, 53*: 1600–4

Serjeant, G. R., Mason, K. P. and Serjeant, B. E. (1980). Negro alpha-thalassemia: genetic studies in homozygous sickle cell disease. *Journal of Medical Genetics, 17*: 281–4

Seuanez, H. N. (1979). *The Phylogeny of Human Chromosomes*, Springer, Berlin

Seuanez, H. N., Evans, H. G., Marlin, D. E. and Fletcher, J. (1979). An inversion of chromosome 2 that distinguishes between Bornean and Sumatran orangoutans. *Cytogenetics Cell Genetics, 23*: 137–40

Shabad, L. M. (1950). *Novinsky, Forefather of Experimental Oncology*, Academia Medica Nauk USSR, Moscow

Shalev, M., Murphy, J. C., Fox, J. G., Wallstrom, B. C. and Gottlieb, L. S. (1980). Myxoma of bone in a nonhuman primate. *Cancer, 45*: 2573–82

Sharkis, S. J., Spivak, J. L., Ahmed, A., Misiti, J., Stuart, R. K., Wiktor-Jedrzejczak, W., Sell, K. W. and Sensenbrenner, L. L. (1980). Regulation of hematopoiesis: helper and suppressor influences of the thymus. *Blood, 55*: 524–7

Sharma, G. P., Gupta, B. L. and Kumbkarni, C. G. (1961). Cytology of spermatogenesis in the honey-bee, *Apis indica* (F.). *Journal of the Royal Microscopic Society, 79*: 337

Sheppard, J. R., Koestler, T. P., Corwin, S. P., Buscarino, C., Doll, J., Lester, B., Grieg, R. G. and Poste, G. (1984). Experimental metastasis correlates with cyclic AMP accumulation in B16 melanoma clones. *Nature, 308*: 544–7

Shibata, S. (1961). Hemoglobinopathy, with special reference to the abnormal hemoglobins found in Japan. *Acta Haematologica Japan, 24*: 141–55

Shimkin, M. B. (1977). *Contrary to Nature*, National Institute of Health, Bethesda, Maryland

Shirai, T., Oshima, M., Masuda, A., Tamano, S. and Ito, N. (1984). Promotion of 2-(ethylnitrosamino)ethanol-induced renal carcinogenesis in rats by nephrotoxic compounds: positive responses with folic acid, basic lead acetate and N-(3,5-dichlorophenyl)succinimide but not with 2,3-dibromo-1-propanol phosphate. *Journal of the National Cancer Institute, 2*: 477–80

Shope, R. E. (1933). Infectious papillomatosis of rabbits. *Journal of Experimental Medicine, 58*: 607–24

Shoubridge, E. A. and Hochachka, P. W. (1980). Ethanol: novel end-product of vertebrate anaerobic metabolism. *Science, 209*: 308–9

Shows, T. B. and McAlpine, P. J. (1978). The catalog of human genes and chromosome assignments. A report on human genetic nomenclature and genes that have been mapped in man. *Cytogenetics Cell Genetics, 22*: 132–45

Silverberg, S. G. and Makowski, E. L. (1975). Endometrial carcinoma in young women taking oral contraceptive agents. *Obstetrics and Gynecology, 46*: 503–6

Simmons, H. E. (1979). *The Psychogenic Biochemical Aspects of Cancer*, Psychogenic Disease Publishing Company, Sacramento

Sims, P. and Grover, P. L. (1974). Epoxides in polycyclic aromatic hydrocarbon metabolism and carcinogenesis. *Advances in Cancer Research, 20*: 166–274

Singer, C. and Underwood, E. A. (1962). *A Short History of Medicine*, 2nd edn, Oxford University Press, New York

Sivak, A. (1977). Induction of cell division in *BALB/c-3T3* cells by phorbol myristate acetate or bovine serum: effects of inhibitors of cyclic AMP phosphodiesterase and Na^+-K^+-ATPase. *In vitro, 13*: 337–43

Skinner, L. G., Barnes, D. M. and Ribeiro, G. G. (1980). The clinical value of multiple steroid receptor assays in breast cancer management. *Cancer, 46*: 2939–45

Sklar, L. S. and Anisman, H. (1980). Special stress influences tumor growth. *Psychosomatic Medicine, 42*: 347–65

Sledge, G. W. and McGuire, W. L. (1983). Steroid hormone receptors in human breast cancer. *Advances in Cancer Research, 38*: 61–76

Sloan, T. P., Mahgoub, A., Lancaster, R., Idle, J. R. and Smith, R. L. (1978). Polymorphism of carbon oxidation of drugs and clinical implications. *British Medical Journal, 2*: 655–7

Slye, M. (1928). The relation of heredity to cancer, with regard to the communication of President C. C. Little of the University of Michigan. *Journal of Cancer Research, 12*: 83–133

Smith, A. and Troop, P. A. (1983). Cancer of the lung. In: G. J. Bourke (ed.), *The Epidemiology of Cancer*, Croom Helm, London, pp. 84–101

Smith, E. F. and Townsend, C. O. (1907). A plant-tumour of bacterial origin. *Science, 25*: 671–3

Smith, K. A., Crabtree, G. R., Gillis, S. and Munck, A. (1980). Glucocorticoid control of T-cell proliferation. In: S. Iacobelli, R. J. B. King, H. R. Lindner and M. E. Lippman (eds.), *Hormones and Cancer*, Raven Press, New York, pp. 125–34

Smith, K. L. and Johnson, W. (1974). Classification of chronic myelocytic leukemia in children. *Cancer, 34*: 670–9

Sommer, A., Cutler, E. A., Cohen, B. L., Harper, D. and Backes, C. (1977). Familial occurrence of the Wiedemann-Beckwith syndrome and persistent fontanel. *American Journal of Medical Genetics, 1*: 59–q

Sonnenschein, C. and Soto, A. M. (1980). But . . . are estrogens per se growth promoting hormones? *Journal of the National Cancer Institute, 64*: 211–15

Sonta, S., Oshimura, M., Sakurai, M., Freeman, A. I. and Sandberg, A. A. (1976). Chromosome and causation of human cancer and leukemia. XXI. Cytogenetically unusual cases of leukemia. *Blood, 48*: 697–705

Sonta, S. and Sandberg, A. A. (1977). Chromosomes and causation of human cancer and leukemia. XXIV. Unusual and complex Ph translocations and their clinical significance. *Blood, 50*: 691–7

Sonta, S. and Sandberg, A. A. (1978). Chromosome and causation of human cancer and leukemia. XXIX. Further studies on karyotypic progression in CML. *Cancer, 41*: 153–63

Soudek, D. and Laraya, P. (1976). C and Q bands in long arm of Y chromosomes; are they identical? *Human Genetics, 32*: 339–41

Sparagana, M., Wong, P. W., Dorsch, T. R., Casten, C., Rauer, M. and Szego, K. (1980). 45,X/46,XY/47,XY,+21 Mosaicism in a hypogonadal phenotypic male. *Journal of Medical Genetics, 17*: 319–21

Sparkes, R. S., Muller, H., Klisak, I. and Abram, J. A. (1979). Retinoblastoma with 13q− chromosomal deletion associated with maternal paracentric inversion of 13q. *Science, 203*: 1027–9

Spencer, J. D., Millis, R. R. and Hayward, J. L. (1978). Contraceptive steroids and breast cancer. *British Medical Journal, 1*: 1024–6

Spitzer, G., Verma, D. S., Fisher, R., Zander, A., Vellekoop, L., Litam J., McCredie, K. B. and Dicke, K. A. (1980). The myeloid progenitor cell — its value in predicting hematopoietic recovery after autologous bone marrow transplantation. *Blood, 55*: 317–23

Sporn, M. B. (1983). Retinoids and cancer. *Cancer Surveys, 2*: 221

Spratt, J. S., Kaltenbach, M. L. and Spratt, J. A. (1977). Cytokinetic definition of acute and chronic breast cancer. *Cancer, 37*: 226–30

Squartini, F. (1979). Tumours of the mammary gland. In: V. S. Turusov (ed.), *Pathology of Tumours in Laboratory Animals. Vol. 2. Tumours of the Mouse*, World Health Organization/International Agency for Research on Cancer, Lyon, p. 43

Srivastava, B. I. S., Khan, S. A., and Henderson, E. S., (1976). High terminal deoxynucleotidyl transferase activity in acute myelogenous leukemia. *Cancer Research, 36*: 3847–50

Stanton, M. F. (1979). Tumours of the bone. In: V. S. Turusov (ed.), *Pathology of*

Tumours in Laboratory Animals. Vol. 2. Tumours of the Mouse, World Health Organization, International Agency for Research on Cancer, Lyon, p. 577

Stanton, M. F., Layard, M., Tegeris, A., Miller, E., May, M. and Kent, E. (1977). Carcinogenicity of fibrous glass: pleural response to fiber dimension. *Journal of the National Cancer Institute, 58*: 587–603

Starr, D. S., Lawrie, G. M. and Morris, G. C. (1981). Unusual presentation of bronchogenic carcinoma. *Cancer, 47*: 398–401

Steinheitz, M. and Zachau, H. G. (1980). Two rearranged immunoglobulin kappa light chain genes in one mouse myeloma. *Nucleic Acids Research, 18*: 1693–1707

Stellman, S. D. and Garfinkel, L. (1984). Cancer mortality among woodworkers. *American Journal of Industrial Medicine, 5*: 343

Stenbäck, F., Sellakumar, A. and Shubik (1975). Magnesium oxide as carrier dust in benzo(a)pyrene-induced lung carcinogenesis in Syrian hamsters. *Journal of the National Cancer Institute, 54*: 861–5

Stewart, A. (1971). Low dose radiation cancers in man. *Advances in Cancer Research, 14*: 359–90

Stewart, F. W. (1971). Retirement in New York: prognosis and reminiscences of a non-optimist. *Bulletin of the New York Academy of Medicine, 47*: 1342–9

Stewart, H. L. (1966). Pulmonary cancer and adenomatosis in captive wild animals and birds from the Philadelphia zoo. *Journal of the National Cancer Institute, 36*: 117–38

Stewart, H. L. (1976). Comparative aspects of certain cancers. In: F. F. Becker (ed.), *Cancer*, Plenum Publishing Corporation, New York

Stewart, H. L., Dunn, T. B., Snell, K. C. and Deringer, M. K. (1979). Tumours of the respiratory tract. In: V. S. Turusov (ed.), *Pathology of Tumours of Laboratory Animals. Vol. 2 Tumours of the Mouse*, World Health Organization/International Agency for Research on Cancer, Lyon, pp. 251–88

Stewart, S. E., Eddy, B. E. and Borgese, N. G. (1958). Neoplasms in mice inoculated with a tumor agent carried in tissue culture. *Journal of the National Cancer Institute, 200*: 1223–43

Strathern, J. N., Newlon, C. S., Herskowitz, I. and Hicks, J. B. (1979). Isolation of a circular derivative of yeast chromosome III. Implications for the mechanism of mating type interconversion. *Cell, 18*: 309–19

Strathern, J. N., Spatola, E., McGill, C. and Hicks, J. B. (1980). Structure and organization of transposable mating type cassettes in Saccharomyces yeasts. *Proceedings of the National Academy of Science (USA), 77*: 2839–43

Straus, D. S., Jonasson, J. and Harris, H. (1977). Growth in vitro of tumor cell x fibroblast hybrids in which malignancy is suppressed. *Journal of Cell Science, 25*: 73–86

Streissguth, A. P., Landesman-Dwyer, S., Martin, J. C. and Smith, D. W. (1980). Teratogenic effects of alcohol in humans and laboratory animals. *Science, 209*: 353–61

Stroebe, H. (1892). Zur Zenntris verschiedener cellulärer Vorgänge und Erscheinungen in Geschwülsten. *Beitraege zur Pathologischen Anatomie und Allgemeinen Pathologie, 11*: 1–38

Strong, L. C. (1977). Genetic and environmental interactions. *Cancer, 40*: 1861–6

Strong, L. C. (1978). Inbred mice in science. In: H. C. Morse (ed.), *Origins of Inbred Mice*, Academic Press, New York, 3rd edn, pp. 45–67

Strong, L. C. (1981). Genetic-environment interactions in human cancer. In: F. E. Arrighi, P. N. Rao and E. Stubblefield (eds.), *Genes, Chromosomes and Neoplasia*, Raven Press, New York, p. 463

Strong, L. C. (1985). The establishment of the *C3H* inbred strain of mice for the study of spontaneous carcinoma of the mammary gland. *Genetics, 20*: 586–91

Stryckmans, P. A. (1974). Current concepts in chronic myelogenous leukemia. *Seminars in Hematology, 11*: 101–27

Stutman, O. (1975). Immunodepression and malignancy. *Advances in Cancer Research, 22*: 261–422

Sugiura, K. (1971). Reminiscence and experience in experimental chemotherapy of cancer. *Medical Clinics of North America, 55*: 667–82

Sugiyama, T., Uenaka, H., Ueda, N., Fukuhara, S. and Maeda, S. (1978). Reproducible chromosome changes of polycyclic hydrocarbon-induced rat leukemia: incidence and chromosome banding pattern. *Journal of the National Cancer Institute, 60*: 153–60

Sulewski, J. M., Dang, T. P., Ward, S. and Ladda, R. L. (1980). Gonadal dysgenesis in a 46,XY female mosaic for double autosomal trisomies 8 and 21. *Journal of Medical Genetics, 17*: 321–3

Sullivan, P. D., Calle, L. M., Shafer, K. and Nettleman, M. (1978). Effect of antioxidants on benzo(a)pyrene free radicals. In: P. W. Jones and R. I. Freudenthal (eds.), *Carcinogenesis: A Comprehensive Survey*, Raven Press, New York, pp. 1–8

Summitt, R. L. (1980). Amniotic fluid α-fetoprotein in the prenatal diagnosis of fetal neural tube defects. *Journal of the American Medical Association, 244*: 2754–5

Sutherland, G. R., Gardiner, A. J. and Carter, R. F. (1976). Familial pericentric inversion of chromosome 19, inv(19)(p13q13), with a note on genetic counseling of pericentric inversion carriers. *Clinical Genetics, 10*: 54–9

Svennevig, J. L., Lovik, M. and Svaar, H. (1979). Isolation and characterization of lymphocytes and macrophages from solid, malignant human tumours. *International Journal of Cancer, 23*: 626–31

Svennevig, J. L. and Svaar, H. (1979). Content and distribution of macrophages and lymphocytes in solid malignant human tumours. *International Journal of Cancer, 24*: 754–8

Swan, S. H. and Brown, W.L. (1981). Oral contraceptive use, sexual activity, and cervical carcinoma. *American Journal of Obstetrics and Gynecology, 139*: 52–7

Tabor, E., Gerety, R. J., Needy, C. F., Elisberg, B. L., Colon, A. R., and Jones, R. (1981). Carcinoembryonic antigen levels in asymptomatic adolescents. *European Journal of Cancer, 17*: 257–8

Tache, Y., Vale, W. and Brown, M. (1980). Thyrotropin-releasing hormone-CNS action to stimulate gastric acid secretion. *Nature, 287*: 149–5

Taha, A. and Ball, K. (1980). Smoking and Africa: the coming epidemic. *British Medical Journal, 280*: 991–3

Takasuki, K., Uchiyama, T., Ueshima, Y. and Hattori, T. (1979). Adult T-cell leukemia: further clinical observations and cytogenetic and functional studies of leukemic cells. *Japanese Journal of Clinical Oncology, 9 (Suppl.)*: 317–24

Talmadge, J. E. (1983). The selective nature of metastasis. *Cancer Metastasis Reviews, 2*: 25–40

Tanzer, J., Najean, Y., Frocrain, C. and Bernheim, A. (1977). Chronic myelocytic leukemia with a masked Ph chromosome. *New England Journal of Medicine, 296*: 571–2

Tatemoto, K. and Mut, V. (1980). Isolation of two novel candidate hormones using a chemical method for finding naturally occurring polypeptides. *Nature, 285*: 417–18

Taylor, J. H., Woods, P. S. and Hughes, W. L. (1957). The organization and duplication of chromosomes as revealed by autoradiographic studies using tritium-labelled thymidine. *Proceedings of the National Academy of Sciences (USA), 43*: 122–7

Taysi, K., Bobrow, M., Balsi, S., Madan, K., Atasu, M. and Say, B. (1973). Duplication-deficiency product of a pericentric inversion in man: a cause of D1 trisomy syndrome. *Journal of Pediatrics, 82*: 263–8

Temin, H. M. and Mizutani, S. (1970). RNA-dependent DNA polymerase in virions of Rous sarcoma virus. *Nature, 226*: 1211–13

Terao, K. (1978). Mesotheliomas induced by sterigmatocystin in Wistar rats. *Gann, 69*: 237–47

Terracini, B. and Campobasso, O. (1979). Tumours of the kidney, renal pelvis and ureter. In: V. S. Turusov (ed.), *Pathology of Tumours in Laboratory Animals. Vol. 2. Tumours of the Mouse*, World Health Organization/International Agency for Research on Cancer, Lyon, pp. 289–300

Terrell, T. G., Gribble, D. H. and Osburn, B. I. (1980). Malignant lymphoma in macaques: a clinicopathologic study of 45 cases. *Journal of the National Cancer Institute, 64*: 561–8

Thompson, D. M. P., Tataryn, D. N., Weatherhead, J. C., Friedlander, P., Rauch, J., Schwartz, R., Gold, P. and Shuster, J. (1980). A human colon tumour antigen associated with β_2-microglobulin and isolated from solid tumour, serum and urine is unrelated to carcinoembryonic antigen. *European Journal of Cancer, 16*: 539–51

Thorwald (1962). *Science and Secrets of Early Medicine: Egypt, Mesopotamia, India, China, Mexico, Peru*, Thames and Hudson, London

Till, J. E. and McCulloch, E. A. (1961). A direct measurement of the radiation sensitivity of normal mouse bone marrow cells. *Radiation Research, 14*: 213–22

Timson, J. (1977). Caffeine. *Mutation Research, 47*: 1–52

Tjio, J. H. and Levan, A. (1956). The chromosome number of man. *Hereditas, 42*: 1–6

Tokuhata, G. K. and Lilienfeld, A. M. (1963). Familial aggregation of lung cancer in humans. *Journal of the National Cancer Institute, 30*: 289–312

Tomatis, L., Agthe, C., Bartsch, H., Huff, J., Montesano, R., Saracci, R., Walker, E. and Wilbourn, J. (1978). Evaluation of the carcinogenicity of chemicals: a review of the Monograph program of the International Agency for Research on Cancer (1971 to 1977). *Cancer Research, 38*: 877–85

Tomura, T. and Van Lancker, J. L. (1980). DNA repair of u.v. damage in heterochromatin and euchromatin of rat liver. *International Journal of Radiation Biology, 38*: 231–5

Tonegawa, S. (1983). Somatic generation of antibody diversity. *Nature, 302*: 575–81

Topham, J. C. (1980). The detection of carcinogen-induced sperm head abnormalities in mice. *Mutation Research, 69*: 149–55

Torre, D. (1968). Multiple sebaceous tumours. *Archives of Dermatology, 98*: 549–51

Tough, I. M., Court-Brown, W. M., Baikie, A. G., Buckton, K. E., Harnden, D. G., Jacobs, P. A., King, M. J. and McBride, J. A. (1961). Cytogenetic studies in chronic myeloid leukemia and acute leukemia associated with mongolism. *Lancet, 1*: 411–17

Trent, J. M. and Davis, J. R. (1979). D-Group chromosome abnormalities in endometrial cancer and hyperplasia. *Lancet, 2*: 361

Ts'o, P. O. P., Caspary, W. J., Cohen, B. I., Leavitt, J. C., Lesko, S. A., Lorentzen, R. J. and Schechtman, L. M. (1974). Basic mechanisms in polycyclic hydrocarbon carcinogenesis. In: P. O. P. Ts'o and J. A. DiPaolo (eds.), *Chemical Carcinogenesis*, Marcel Dekker, New York, Part A, pp. 113–44

Tsuchida, T., Yokomori, K., Saito, S., Kaku, H. and Bessho, F. (1984). Stage IV-S neuroblastoma involving the liver and ectopic liver. *Cancer, 53*: 1609–11

Tsukimoto, I., Wong, K. Y. and Lampkin, B. C. (1976). Surface markers and prognostic factors in acute lymphoblastic leukemia. *New England Journal of Medicine, 294*: 245–8

Tubiana, N., Derre, M., Carcossone, Y. and Martin, P. M. (1984). Sex steroid binding to human lymphocytes plasma membrane. *British Journal of Cancer, 49*: 531–6

Turner, M. (1980). How trypanosomes change coats. *Nature, 284*: 13–14

Turner, M. J. and Cordingley, J. S. (1980). Esoteric DNA? *Nature, 286*: 756–7

Tursz, T., Hors, J., Lipinski, M. and Amiel, J. L. (1978). HLA phenotypes in long-term survivors treated with BCG immunotherapy for childhood ALL. *British Medical Journal, 1*: 1250–4

Turusov, V. S., Breslow, N. E. and Tomatis, L. (1974). Frequency and organ distribution of lung tumor metastases in CF-1 mice. *Journal of the National Cancer Institute, 52*: 225–32

Turusov, V. S. and Takayama, S. (1979). Tumours of the liver. In: V. S. Turusov (ed.), *Pathology of Tumours in Laboratory Animals. Vol. 2. Tumours of the Mouse*, World Health Organization/International Agency for Research on Cancer, Lyon, p. 193

Tuyns, A. J. (1979). Epidemiology of alcohol and cancer. *Cancer Research, 39*: 2840–3

Uchida, I. A. (1973). Paternal origin of the extra chromosome in Down's syndrome. *Lancet, 2*: 1258

Uchida, S., Watanabe, S., Aizawa, T., Furuno, A. and Muto, T. (1979). Polyoncogenicity and insulinoma-inducing ability of BK virus, a human papova-virus, in Syrian golden hamsters. *Journal of the National Cancer Institute, 63*: 119–26

Uenaka, H., Ueda, N., Maeda, S. and Sugiyama, T. (1978). Involvement of chromosome No. 2 in chromosome changes in primary leukemia induced in rats by *N*-nitroso-*N*-butylurea. *Journal of the National Cancer Institute, 60*: 1399–1404

Underwood, J. C. E. (1974). Lymphoreticular infiltration in human tumours: prognostic and biological implications: a review. *British Journal of Cancer, 30*: 538–48

Urbach, F. (1983). Cancer of the skin. In: G. J. Bourke (ed.), *The Epidemiology of Cancer*, Croom Helm, London, pp. 102–15

Urban, J. A. and Marjani, M. A. (1971). Significance of internal mammary lymph node metastases in breast cancer. *American Journal of Roentgenology, Radium Therapy and Nuclear Medicine, 3*: 130–6

Uriel, J. (1979). Retrodifferentiation and the fetal patterns of gene expression in cancer. *Advances in Cancer Research, 29*: 127–74

Urtega, O. and Pack, G. T. (1966). On the antiquity of melanoma. *Cancer, 19*: 607–10

Usdin, E., Borchardt, R. T. and Creveling, C. R. (eds.) (1979). *Transmethylation*, Elsevier/North Holland, New York

Van Den Berghe, H., Louwagie, A., Broeckaert-Van Orshoven, A., Verwilghen, R., Michaux, J. L. and Sokal, G. (1979). Philadelphia chromosome in human multiple myeloma. *Journal of the National Cancer Institute, 63*: 11–16

Van Rensburg, S. J. (1981). Epidemiological and dietary evidence for a specific nutritional predisposition to esophageal cancer. *Journal of the National Cancer Institute, 67*: 243

Van Valen, L. M. (1980). Molecular clockwork. *Nature, 287*: 89–90

Van Wering, E. R. and Vissers-Praalder, E. C. (1979). Distribution of childhood leukemia according to the fab-classification. *British Journal of Haematology, 45*: 482

Veale, A. M. O. (1965). *Intestinal Polyposis Series 40. Eugenics Laboratory Memoirs*, Cambridge University Press, London

Vecchi, V., Rosito, P., Vivarelli, F., Mancini, A. F., Pession, A. and Paolucci, G. (1980). Prognostic significance of lymphoblast morphology in acute lymphoblastic leukemia (ALL) in childhood. *British Journal of Haematology, 45*: 178–81

Velpeau, A. (1854). *Traité des Maladies du Sein et de la Région Mammaire*, V. Masson, Paris

Verhest, A. and Lustman, F. (1980). Y-chromosome structural rearrangement in

Philadelphia chromosome-negative chronic myelogenous leukemia. *New England Journal of Medicine, 303*: 53–4

Verhoeyen, M., Fang, R., Joll, W. M., Devos, R., Huylebroeck, J., Saman, E. and Fiers, W. (1980). Antigenic drift between the haemagglutinin of the Hong Kong influenza strains A/Aichi/2/68 and A/Victoria/3/75. *Nature, 286*: 771–6

Verma, R. S. and Dosik, H. (1980). Heteromorphism of the Philadelphia (Ph') chromosome in patients with chronic myelogenous leukemia (CML). *British Journal of Haematology, 45*: 215–22

Veronesi, U. and Valagussa, P. (1981). Inefficacy of internal mammary nodes dissection in breast cancer surgery. *Cancer, 47*: 170–5

Vessey, M. P., Doll, R., Jones, K., McPherson, K. and Yeates, D. (1979). An epidemiological study of oral contraceptives and breast cancer. *British Medical Journal, 1*: 1757–60

Vessey, M. P., Doll, R. and Sutton, P. M. (1971). Investigation of the possible relationship between oral contraceptives and benign and malignant breast disease. *Cancer, 28*: 1395–9

Vessey, M. P., McPherson, K. and Yeates, D. (1981). Mortality in oral contraceptive users. *Lancet, 1*: 549–50

Vianna, N. J. and Strauss, D. (1983). Lymphoreticular malignancies. In: G. J. Bourke (ed.), *The Epidemiology of Cancer*, Croom Helm, London, pp. 214–44

Vogel, F. (1979). Genetics of retinoblastoma. *Human Genetics, 52*: 1–54

Von Hansemann, D. (1890). Ueber asymmetrische Zeltheilung in Epithelkrebsen und deren biologische Bedewtung. *Virchow's Archives, 119*: 299–326

Von Hoff, D. D., Kuhn, J. and Harris, G. J. (1980a). New anticancer drugs. In: H. M. Pinedo (ed.), *Cancer Chemotherapy 1980*, Excerpta Medica, Amsterdam and Oxford, pp. 118–33

Von Hoff, D. D., Kuhn, J. and Harris, G. J. (1980b). Miscellaneous anticancer agents. In: H. M. Pinedo (ed.), *Cancer Chemotherapy 1980*, Excerpta Medica, Amsterdam and Oxford, pp. 134–8

Von Siebold, A. E. (1824). *Ueber den Gebärmutterkrebs, dessen Entstenhung und Verhütung*, F. Dummler, Berlin

Vuitch, M. F. and Mendelsohn, F. (1981). Relationship of ectopic ACTH production to tumour differentiation: a morphologic and immunohistochemical study of prostatic carcinoma. *Cancer, 47*: 296–9

Wachtel, S. S. and Ohno, S. (1979). The immunogenetics of sexual development. *Progress in Medical Genetics, 3*: 109–42

Wagner, J. C., Griffiths, D. M. and Hill, R. J. (1984). The effect of fibre size on the in vivo activity of UICC crocidolite. *British Journal of Cancer, 49*: 453–8

Wagner, J. C., Sleggs, C. A. and Marchand, P. (1960). Diffuse pleural mesothelioma and asbestos exposure in the northwestern Cape Province. *British Journal of Industrial Medicine, 17*: 260

Wagoner, J. K., Archer, V. E., Carroll, B. E., Holaday, D. A. and Lawrence, P. A. (1964). Cancer mortality patterns among U. S. uranium miners and millers, 1950 through 1962. *Journal of the National Cancer Institute, 32*: 787–801

Wahl, G. M., de Saint Vincent, B. R. and De Rose, M. L. (1984). Effect of chromosomal position on amplification of transfected genes in animal cells. *Nature, 307*: 516–20

Wakabayashi, K., Inagaki, T., Fujimoto, Y. and Fukuda, Y. (1978). Induction by degraded carrageenan of colorectal tumours in rats. *Cancer Letters, 4*: 171–6

Waldenstrom, J. G. (1978). *Paraneoplasia. Biological Signals in the Diagnosis of Cancer*, John Wiley and Sons, New York

Waldeyer, W. (1872). Die Entwicklung der Carcinoma. *Virchow's Archives, 55*: 67–159

Wallach, D. and Revel, M. (1980). An interferon-induced cellular enzyme is incorporated into virions. *Nature, 287*: 68–70

Wang, N. and Schoffner, R. N. (1980). Induction of heteroploidy in *Gallus domesticus*. *Mutation Research, 69*: 263–73

Wang, N., Trend, B., Bronson, D. L. and Fraley, E. E. (1980). Nonrandom abnormalities in chromosome 1 in human testicular cancers. *Cancer Research, 40*: 796–802

Ward, C. W. and Dopheide, T. A. (1979). Primary structure of the Hong Kong (H3) haemagglutinin. *British Medical Bulletin, 35*: 51–6

Ward, H. W. C. (1973). Anti-oestrogen therapy for breast cancer: a trial of tamoxifen at two dose levels. *British Medical Journal, 1*: 13–14

Ward, J. M., Goodman, D. G., Squire, R. A., Chu, K. C. and Linhart, M. S. (1979). Neoplastic and nonneoplastic lesions in aging (C57BL/6NxC3H/HeN) F₁(B6C3F1) mice. *Journal of the National Cancer Institute, 63*: 849–54

Warner, R. H. and Rosett, H. L. (1975). The effects of drinking on offspring. An historical survey of the American and British literature. *Journal of Studies on Alcohol, 36*: 1395–1420

Warthin, A. S. (1913). Heredity with reference to carcinoma. *Archives of Internal Medicine, 12*: 546–55

Warthin, A. S. (1925). The further study of a cancer family. *Journal of Cancer Research, 9*: 279–86

Waterhouse, J., Muir, C., Correa, P. and Powell, J. (1976). *Cancer Incidence in Five Continents*, Vol. 3, International Agency for Research on Cancer, Lyon

Watson, D. M. A., Kelly, R. W., Hawkins, R. A. and Miller, W. R. (1984). Prostaglandins in human mammary cancer. *British Journal of Cancer, 49*: 459–64

Watt, J. L., Hamilton, P. J. and Page, B. M. (1977). Variation in the Philadelphia chromosome. *Human Genetics, 37*: 141–8

Wattenberg, L. W. (1980). Inhibition of chemical carcinogenesis by antioxidants. In: T. J. Slaga (ed.), *Carcinogenesis: A Comprehensive Survey*, Raven Press, New York, vol. 5, p. 85

Weber, T. H., Wegelius, R., Borgstrom, G. H., Gahmberg, C. G. and Andersson, L. C. (1979). A case of pure monocytic leukemia in a child — characterization of cellular morphology, membrane markers, surface glycoproteins and karyotype. *Scandinavian Journal of Haematology, 22*: 47–52

Wehner, A. P., Olson, R. J. and Busch, R. H. (1976). Increased lifespan and decreased weight in hamsters exposed to cigarette smoke. *Archives of Environmental Health, 31*: 146–53

Weichselbaum, R. R., Nove, J. and Little, J. B. (1980). X-ray sensitivity of fifty-three human diploid fibroblast cell strains from patients with characterized genetic disorders. *Cancer Research, 40*: 920–5

Weinberg, R. A. (1982). Oncogenes of spontaneous and chemically induced tumors. *Advances in Cancer Research, 36*: 149–64

Weinberg, R. A. (1983). Oncogenes and the molecular biology of cancer. *Journal of Cell Biology, 97*: 1661–2

Weinstein, I. B., Yamasaki, H., Wigler, M., Lee, L. S., Fisher, P. B., Jeffrey, A. and Grunberger, D. (1979). Molecular and cellular events associated with the action of initiating carcinogens and tumor promoters. In: A. C. Griffin and C. R. Shaw (eds.), *Carcinogens: Identification and Mechanisms of Action*, Raven Press, New York, pp. 399–418

Weisburger, J. H. and Weisburger, E. K. (1973). Biochemical formation and pharmacological, toxicological and pathological properties of hydroxylamines and hydroxamic acids. *Pharmacological Reviews, 25*: 1–66

Weiss, W. (1984). Presentation of data on pulmonary fibrosis and cigarette smoking. *American Journal of Industrial Medicine, 5*: 417–19

Welsch, C. W. (1978). Prolactin and the development and progression of early neoplastic mammary gland lesions. *Cancer Research, 38*: 4054–8

West, S. C., Cassuto, E. and Howard-Flanders, P. (1981). Homologous pairing can occur before DNA strand separation in general genetic recombination. *Nature, 290*: 29–33

Whang-Peng, J. and Knutsen, T. (1980). Lymphocytic leukemias, acute and chronic. *Clinics in Haematology, 9*: 87–127

Wickström, B. O. (1979). *Cigarette Smoking and the Third World*. University of Gothenberg, Sweden

Wieacker, P., Mueller, C. R., Mayerova, A., Grzeschik, K. H. and Ropers, H. H. (1980). Assignment of the gene coding for human catalase to the short arm of chromosome 11. *Annals of Genetics, 23*: 73–7

Wiedemann, H. R. (1964). Complex malformatif familial avec hernie embilicale et macrogrossiea — un syndrome nouveau? *Journal Génétique Humaine, 13*: 223–32

Wiedemann, H. R. (1973). E. M. G. syndrome. *Lancet, 2*: 626–7

Wieland, H. and Dane, E. (1933). Untersuchungen über die Konstitution der Gallensäuren. LII. Mitt. Über die Haftostelle der Seitenkette. *Zeitschrift für Physiologische Chemie, 219*: 240–4

Wiener, F., Ohno, S., Spira, J., Haran-Ghera, N. and Klein, G. (1978a). Chromosome changes (trisomies 15 and 17) associated with tumour progression in leukemias induced by radiation leukemia virus. *Journal of the National Cancer Institute, 61*: 227–37

Wiener, F., Spira, J., Ohno, S., Haran-Ghera, N. and Klein, G. (1978b). Chromosome changes (trisomy 15) in murine T-cell leukemia induced by 7,12-dimethylbenz(a)anthracene. *International Journal of Cancer, 22*: 447–53

Wilkinson, E. J., Friedrich, E. G., Mattingly, R. F., Regali, J. A. and Garancis, J. C. (1973). Turner's syndrome with endometrial adenocarcinoma and stilbestrol therapy. *Obstetrics and Gynecology, 42*: 193–200

Williams, N., Jackson, H., Sheridan, A. P. C., Murphy, M. J., Elste, A. and Moore, M. A. S. (1978). Regulation of megakaryopoiesis in long-term murine bone marrow cultures. *Blood, 51*: 245–55

Williams, R. O., Young, J. R. and Majiwa, P. A. O. (1979). Genomic rearrangement correlated with antigenic variation in *Trypanosoma brucei*. *Nature, 282*: 847–51

Williams, R. R., Sorlie, P. O., Feinlab, M., McNamara, P. M., Kannel, W. B., and Dawber, T. R. (1981). Cancer incidence by levels of cholesterol. *Journal of the American Medical Association, 245*: 247–52

Williams, R. T. (1959). *Detoxification Mechanisms*, 2nd edn, Chapman and Hall, London

Williamson, E. M., Miller, J. F. and Seabright, M. (1980). Pericentric inversion (13) with two different recombinants in the same family. *Journal of Medical Genetics, 17*: 309–12

Willis, R. A. (1952). *The Spread of Tumours in the Human Body*, Butterworths, London

Willis, R. A. (1967). *Pathology of Tumours*, Butterworths, London

Wilson, A. C., Carlson, S. S. and White, T. J. (1977). Biochemical evolution. *Annual Reviews of Biochemistry, 46*: 573–639

Wilson, J. D., George, F. W. and Griffin, J. E. (1981). The hormonal control of sexual development. *Science, 211*: 1278–84

Wilson, M. G., Fujimoto, A. and Alfi, O. S. (1974). Double autosomal trisomy and mosaicism for chromosomes no. 8 and no. 21. *Journal of Medical Genetics, 11*: 96–101

Woglom, W. H. (1913). *The Study of Experimental Cancer*, Columbia University Press, New York

Wolff, S., Rodin, B. and Cleaver, J. E. (1977). Sister chromatid exchanges induced by mutagenic carcinogens in normal and xeroderma pigmentosum cells. *Nature, 265*: 347–9

Wolman, S. R., Horland, A. A. and Becker, F. F. (1973). Altered karyotypes of transplantable 'diploid' tumours. *Journal of the National Cancer Institute, 51*: 1909–14

Wolpert, L. (1978). Cell position and cell lineage in pattern formation and regulation. In: B. I. Lord, C. S. Potten and R. J. Cole (eds.), *Stem Cells and Tissue Homeostasis*, Cambridge University Press, Cambridge, pp. 29–47

Wood, G. W. and Gollahon, K. A. (1977). Detection and quantitation of macrophage infiltration into primary human tumours with the use of cell surface markers. *Journal of the National Cancer Institute, 59*: 1081–7

Wood, M. and Bonser, G. M. (1979). Tumours of the urinary bladder. In: V. S. Turusov (ed.), *Pathology of Tumours in Laboratory Animals. Vol. 2. Tumours of the Mouse*, World Health Organization/International Agency for Research on Cancer, Lyon, p. 301

Woodruff, R. K., Malpas, J. S., Wrigley, P. F. M., Lister, T. A., Paxton, A. M. and Janossy, G. (1977). Meningeal leukemia in lymphoid blast crisis of chronic myeloid leukemia. *British Medical Journal, 2*: 1375–6

World Health Organization (1964). Report of a WHO expert committee on the prevention of cancer. *WHO Technical Report Series, 276*

World Health Organization (1978). Information Bulletin on the Survey of Chemicals Being Tested for Carcinogenicity, Number 7. IARC, Lyon

World Health Organization (1978). Steroid contraception and the risk of neoplasia. *WHO Technical Report Series, 619*

World Health Organization (1979). Tobacco smoking in the third world. *WHO Chronicle, 33*: 94–7

Wurster-Hill, D. H., Cornwell, G. G. and McIntyre, O. R. (1979). Chromosome aberrations of myeloid and lymphoid cells in cancer patients and family members without evidence of cancer. *Cancer Detection and Prevention, 2*: 125

Wynder, E. L. and Gori, G. B. (1977) Contribution of the environment to cancer incidence. An epidemiologic exercise. *Journal of the National Cancer Institute, 58*: 825–32

Wynder, E. L. and Graham, E. A. (1950). Tobacco smoking as a possible etiologic factor in bronchiogenic carcinoma. A study of six hundred and eighty-four proved cases. *Journal of the American Medical Association, 143*: 329–36

Wynder, E. L. and Hoffmann, D. (1967). *Tobacco and Tobacco Smoke*, Academic Press, New York

Wynder, E. L. and Hoffmann, D. (1976). Tobacco and tobacco smoke. *Seminars in Oncology, 3*: 5–15

Wynder, E. L., MacCornack, F. A. and Stellman, S. D. (1978). The epidemiology of breast cancer in 785 United States Caucasian women. *Cancer, 41*: 2341–54

Yalow, R. S. (1979). Big ACTH and bronchogenic carcinoma. *Annual Reviews of Medicine, 30*: 241–8

Yamagiwa, K. and Ichikawa, K. (1915). Experimentelle Studie über die Pathogenese der Epithelial geschwülste. *Mitteilungen Med. Facultat Kaiserl. University of Tokyo, 15*: 295–344

Yaoita, Y. and Honjo, T. (1980). Deletion of immunoglobulin heavy chain genes from expressed allelic chromosome. *Nature, 286*: 850–3

Yoder, J., Watson, M. and Bender, W. W. (1973). Lymphocyte chromosome analysis of agricultural workers during extensive occupational exposure to pesticides. *Mutation Research, 21*: 335–40

Yogeeswaran, G. (1983). Cell surface glycolipids and glycoproteins in malignant transformation. *Advances in Cancer Research, 38*: 289

Yoshida, T. H. (1952). Cytological studies on cancer v. heteroplastic transplantation of the Yoshida sarcoma, with special regard to the behaviour of tumour cells. *Gann, 43*: 35–42

Young, D. A., Nicholson, M. L., Voris, B. P. and Lyons, R. T. (1980). Mechanisms involved in the generation of the metabolic and lethal actions of glucocorticoid hormones in lymphoid cells. In: S. Iacobelli, R. J. B. King, H. R. Lindner and M. E. Lippman (eds.), *Hormones and Cancer*, Raven Press, New York, pp. 135–56

Young, R. A., Hagenbüchle, O. and Schibler, U. (1981). A single mouse alpha-amylase gene specifies two different tissue-specific mRNAs. *Cell, 23*: 451–8

Yu, M. C., Ho, J. H. C., Ross, R. K. and Henderson, B. E. (1981). Nasopharyngeal carcinoma in Chinese — salted fish or inhaled smoke? *Preventive Medicine, 10*: 15–24

Yunis, J. J., Bloomfield, C. D. and Ensrud, K. (1981). All patients with acute nonlymphocytic leukemia may have a chromosomal defect. *New England Journal of Medicine, 305*: 135–9

Yunis, J. J. and Chandler, M. E. (1977). The chromosomes of man — clinical and biologic significance. A review. *American Journal of Pathology, 88*: 466–95

Yunis, J. J. and Ramsey, N. (1978). Retinoblastoma and subband deletion of chromosome 13. *American Journal of Diseases of Childhood, 132*: 161–3

Yunis, J. J., Sawyer, J. R. and Ball, D. W. (1978). Characterization of banding patterns of metaphase-prophase G-banded chromosomes and their use in gene mapping. *Cytogenetics Cell Genetics, 22*: 679–83

Zambryski, P., Holsters, M., Kruger, K., Depicker, A., Schell, J., Van Montagu, M. and Goodman H. M. (1980). Tumor DNA structure in plant cells transformed by *A. tumefaciens. Science, 209*: 1385

Zech, L., Haglund, U., Nilsson, K. and Klein, G. (1976). Characteristic chromosomal abnormalities in biopsies and lymphoid-cell lines from patients with Burkitt and non-Burkitt lymphomas. *International Journal of Cancer, 17*: 47–56

Zembrzycka, H. (1979). Nowotwory jajników ze szczególnym uwzglednieniem psów. *Patologica Polska (Warsaw), 30*: 245–51

Ziff, E. B. (1980). Transcription and RNA processing by the DNA tumour viruses. *Nature, 287*: 491–9

Zur Hausen, H. (1980). The role of viruses in human tumours. *Advances in Cancer Research, 33*: 77–107

Zur Hausen, H., Bornkamm, G. W., Schmidt, R. and Hecker, E. (1979). Tumor initiators and promoters in the induction of Epstein-Barr virus. *Proceedings of the National Academy of Sciences (USA), 76*: 782–5

INDEX

Acetlylaminofluorene 133, 339, 342
Adrenalectomy 161
Adrenocorticotropic hormone
    (ACTH) 139, 150, 327
Aetius of Amida 49
Aflatoxins 133–4, 330
Ageing 28–30, 322–4
Agricola 92
Agrobacterium tumefaciens 84, 362
Ali-al-Tabari 49
ALL-type therapy 311
Alternation of generations 268
Amiloride 364
Amine-precursor-uptake-and-
    decarboxylation (APUD) 327
Androgens 139
Animal recipients: Novinsky 125–6
Antigenic drift 243
Antigenic shift 243
Antimetabolites 121
Antiquity and ubiquity of neoplasia 36,
    83–6, 321–2
Arecaidine 330
Arecoline 330
Aristotle 37–48 *passim*
Arylhydrocarbon hydroxylase 201–4,
    227
Asbestos 98–9
Ascorbic acid 341
Asprin 330
Asymmetrical karyokinesis 237, 351
Ataxia telangiectasia 272, 274–5
Autonomy 14, 16
Avicenna 50

Bacillus Calmette Guèrin 118
Bard 70
Baron Carro de Vaux 50
Barr bodies 271
Beatson 155
Bence-Jones proteins 58
Beniveni 54
Benzo(a)pyrene 13, 158
Biological environment and
    cancer 102–11
    complexity of host-virus response in
        viral oncogenesis 107–8
    non-viral parasites 102–4
    oncogenic viruses 105–11

two chemical classes of
    oncoviruses 106–7
viruses and human cancer 110–11,
    324, 329
viruses in cancer etiology 105–6
see also Environment as almost
    exclusive cause of cancer
B-K mole 224
Bladder cancer 194, 331
Blood group A and stomach cancer 214
Bloom's syndrome 271–8 *passim*
Bombay Parsi women and breast
    cancer 230–1
Boveri 236–8, 318, 350
Bracken fern 134
Breast cancer
    among Italian nuns 92
    ancient claim of cure 113
    'bulging tumours' (in ancient
        Egypt) 36
    comparative aspects 187–8, 196–9
    complexity of risk factors 228, 336–7
    discriminant functions 162
    hormones and 148–8
    hormone receptors 162–3
    therapeutic ovariectomy 160–1
    variable inborn susceptibility 228–31
Buddha 136, 369
Bulinus 103
Butylated hydroxyanisole 341

Cachexia 144, 327
Caffeine 350
Cancer enigma: outline 1–31
    comparative studies: a special human
        predilection for neoplasia 20–3
    definitions and the question of
        benign and malignant
        neoplasms 11–12
    growth and its control: the question
        of autonomy 14–17
    heterogeneity of neoplasms 12–14,
        350–1
    incidence, mortality and
        civilisation 17–20
    latency and preneoplasia 10–11
    physiologic mimicries 6–10, 325–8
    problems of definition and
        diagnosis 1–3, 6–17

problems of etiology 27–30
problems of prevention and
   treatment 23–7
scope 1–6
Cancer-predisposing mendelian
   disorders in man 207–8, 213–22
Carageenans 346
Carbamates 344
Carcinogenic mechanisms: clues from
   experimental carcinogenesis 339–
   47
CAUTION 136–7
Charaka Samhita 36
Chemical carcinogenesis 128–9
Chemical environment and cancer 92–
   9, 329–34
   alcohol 96–8
   arsenic and arsenicals 93
   asbestos 98–9
   chimney soot 92
   dyestuffs 93
   mining dust 92
   tobacco 93–6; 'origins' of
      tobacco 93–4; 'chutta' and
      'supari' 96; snuff 95; pipe, cigar
      and cigarette 95
   vinyl chloride 99
   see also Environment as almost
      exclusive cause of cancer
Chemotherapy 118–21
Chronic obstructive pulmonary disease
   (COPD) 227
Chromosomes and cancer 235–318
   anomalies and mosaicism 263–6
   anomalies and viability 263–6
   anomalies involving entire
      chromosomes: role of non-
      disjunction 257–9
   anomalies involving parts of
      chromosomes 259–61
   anomalies involving sex
      chromosomes and autosomes: a
      comparison 261–3
   anomalous chromosomes in human
      cancer 279–318; non-random
      anomalies 288–90; random
      anomalies 290–7
   banding and its problems 253–5
   Boveri's hypothesis 236–8
   chromosomal instability 238–42
   chromosomal morphology 250
   enumeration of human
      chromosomes 248–9
   extrinsic agents 247–8
   heritability 268–71

metaphase paucity: the direct and
   indirect methods, and the use of
   mitogens 250–1
   methodology 248–56
   problems intrinsic to the indirect
      method 251–3
   recombinations and related
      features 245–7
   spontaneous changes and
      anomalies 256–68
   structural subunits 238–45
   variants and anomalies in physiologic
      states 266–8
   see also Philadelphia
      chromosome 302–10
Chromosome anomalies in spontaneous
   abortions 180
Circumcision 147
Citrovorum factor 121
Clemmeson's hook 229
Clomiphene citrate 141, 157
Clonorchis sinensis 329
Coagulating lymph 59
Coal-tar and polycyclic
   arylhydrocarbons 129–30
Colon cancer 224–6
   ethnic features 225
   Muir's syndrome 226
   mucus-associated antigens 225
   polyposis syndromes 215, 224–6
Colony forming units (CFUs) 314
Complexity of developmental gene
   control 353
Conditional neoplasms 132, 360–1
Conheim 72–3, 320
Conservatism in evolution and
   development 358–9
Critical cellular target in
   oncogenesis 343–6
Cycasin 134
Cyclamate 346
Cysticercus sarcoma 103
Cytochrome P450-dependent
   monooxygenases 342
Cytoxan 120

Dedifferentiation 367
Democedes and Atossa 113
Denman's thirteen questions 80–2
Denver classification (of
   chromosomes) 254
Deviant genetic code 357
Diet and cancer 335
Diethylstilbestrol (DES) 150–2, 158,
   173, 174

Dichlorodiphenyltrichloroethane (DDT) 156, 158
Dimethylsulfoxide (DMSO) 364
Dioxin 157
Discriminant functions 162
Divergent differentiation 176
DNA constancy rule 75–7, 359
Doll (Sir Richard) 93, 95, 178, 325, 332, 335, 336
Double threshold theory 168
Doubling time 282
Down's syndrome 269–74 *passim*
Drosophila melanogaster 329
Dyestuffs and arylamines 131–3

Ebers papyrus 36
Edwin Smith papyrus 36
Ecdysone 164
Ectopic tumour products 6–10, 173–6, 327–8, 359, 367
Ehrlich 118–19, 326
Electrophiles 340, 343
Embryofetal expressions 6–7
Embryonal carcinoma 362
Environment as almost exclusive cause of cancer 177–8, 332–3
Endosymbiosis theory (mitochondrial evolution) 357
Epidemiology and cancer etiology 333–8
Epidemiology and cancer-risk factors 332–3
Estrogen replacement therapy 162
Estrophilin 162
Ethnicity and cancer 18–19
and other diseases 181–5
Ethoxyquin 341
Evolutionary adaptation 28
Experimental oncology: historical aspects 123–34
Expressivity 208
Extrapolative difficulties 329–31

Fanconi's anemia 275
Farmers' neoplasms 337
Fetal alcohol syndrome 97
Feudalism 51
Fibiger 104
Folliculin 148
Foreign body tumorigenesis 98–9, 343, 345
Foulds 11, 16, 74–5, 320
Friend erythroleukemia 346

Ganglioneuroma 12, 363

Gene amplification 355–6
Genetic colonisation 85
Genetic epidemiology 338
Genetic paradigm 177
Genetic susceptibility and cancer 328–9
Glutamate pyruvate transaminase (GPT-1) 222
Glycoconjugates 344
Greece 37–48, 86–8
anatomy and physiology 45–6
classification and treatment of tumours 44–5, 86–8
Galen and Galenism 46–8
Greek synthesis 37–43
humoralism and the origin of tumours 44
Growth factors 281
Growth fraction 281

Hemoglobinopathies 183
Hepatomas 15
Hepatoscopy 36
Heredity and cancer 177–234
Hertwig effect 260
Heterochromatin 354
Heterogeneity of single neoplasms 350–1
High mobility group (HMG) proteins 170–1
Hill 95, 136
Hippocrates' aphorism no.38 113
Histones 170–1, 354
Historical sources 33
History of cancer 32–137
HLA haplotypes and cancer 233
Hormonal influences upon dietary and other cancer-risk factors 145–8
Hormonal manipulations 148–54
Hormones 138–76
in tumour development 144–60
in tumour regression 160–3
in gene regulation 163–72
Hormones and chemical carcinogens: some structural and other analogies 158–9
Hormones and legislation 154–5
Human gene mapping 239
Humanism 53
Hunter 59
Hutchinson 93

Immunity and cancer 363–4
Incurability 36–7, 113–16, 322
Induced neoplasia 193–5, 200–1
Infectious mononucleosis 110–11

Initiation 339–40
Intercellular matrix 344
Interferon 244
Interhuman transference 124–5
Interspecific comparisons 185–95
Interspecific comparisons 195–204
Islam 48–51
    contributions to western culture
        50–1
    culture 48
    oncology and medicine 49–50
    science 48–9

John of Arderne 115

Kaposi sarcoma 18, 36
Khanolkar 96
Klinefelter's syndrome 229, 262
Koelliker 77
Kwashiorkor 179

Lactation 147
Landmarks in the history of hormones
    and cancer 142–3
Leukeran 120
Lissauer of Bendorff 118
Liver angiosarcoma 195
Lobular carcinoma *in situ* 230
Long road ahead 368–70
Lung cancer
    among non-smokers 226
    among smokers 3, 226
    comparative aspects 191
    human genetic aspects 226–8, 325
    in a 4-year-old child 325
    metastasis to brain and adrenal
        gland 191
    poor prognosis 227–8
    preventability 228

Maldifferentiation 367
McKinnell 362
Mammary neoplasia 187–8, 196–9,
    228–31
    see also breast cancer
Magna Carta 53
Marco Polo 52
Mark Twain 25
Marker chromosome 3
Mathematics 34–5
Maturation promoting factor 165
Medical paradigm 177
Meiotic recombination 325, 347
Melphalan 120
Metabolic activation 339–40

and cancer prevention 341
    limitations 341–3
Methotrexate 120
Methylation 344–5
Methylazoxymethanol 344
Mitochondrion 356–7
    deviant genetic code 357
    possible role in tumorigenesis 357
Mitomycin C 365
Mobile genes 244
Models for the study of human cancer:
    limitations of non-human
        systems 352–3
Modern West 51–77
    anatomy and surgery 54–5
    Astruc's biochemical 'disproof' of
        atrabilism and spagyricism 57–8
    blastema hypothesis 65–7
    cancer as a degenerative growth 55–6
    cancer cells and cancer 'seeds' 64–5
    cellular theory 62–4, 67–70
    contagiousness of cancer 55
    embryology and cell rests 72–3
    etiology and histogenesis 74–5
    histogenetic specificity 70
    historical background 51–4
    lymphatic theory 58–60
    molecular genetics and the DNA
        constancy rule 75–7
    spagyric theory 56–8
Molecular mechanisms in the
    developmental hypothesis 365–8
Morgagni 54
Mueller 64–5
Mulvihill 207, 338
Myelofibrosis 315–16

Naegeli 75, 76, 77, 359
2-Naphthylamine 93, 342
Nasopharyngeal carcinoma 231–3
    Epstein-Barr virus and other risk
        factors 232
    HLA haplotypes 233
    in Southern China and Malaysia 232
Natural specificities 324–5
Neoplasia 1–2
Neoplastic genome 361–2
Nerve growth factor 365
Neuroblastoma 363
Neve and Neve 101
N-Hydroxylation 339, 342
NIH3T3 cells 349
Nigerian cancer experience 334
Normal developmental capabilities of
    the neoplastic genome 361–2

Nucleosome assembly factor 171
Nucleosomes 171, 354

Oat-cell carcinoma 193
Omnis cellula a cellula 67–73 *passim*
*Omnis cellula a cellula ejusdem
    naturae* 67–73 *passim*
Oncogenes 207, 234, 328–9, 348–50,
    358
Oncologic theories
    atrabilism (black bile theory) 44
    blastema theory 65–7
    cell rest theory 73
    cellular theory 67–70
    connective tissue theory
        (Virchow's) 69–70
    degenerative membrane theory 55–6
    developmental theory 310–16, 359–65
    lymphatic theory 58–60
    rise and fall 319–21
    somatic mutation theory 236–8,
        347–52
    see also Modern West
Operons 353
Opisthorchis felineus 329
Oral contraceptives 141, 148, 152
Orphons 245
Oxidative metabolism 341–2

Panax ginseng 362
Paracelsus 56, 92, 99
Paraneoplasia 144, 174–6
Pasteur 326
Paul of Aegina 50
Penetrance 208
Phenacetin 331
Philadelphia (PH') chromosome 254,
    302–9
    clinical aspects 304–10
    rarity in childhood CML 309
    structural heterogeneity 302–4
Phorbol esters (promotors) 159, 364
Physical environment and cancer
    'Kangri' cancers 101
    mechanistic speculations 100–1
    radiation cancers 99–100, 185
    see also Environment as almost
        exclusive cause of cancer
Physiologic mimicries 6–10, 325–8, 360
Pill lesion 151
Plant neoplams 21
Plethora of experimental
    carcinogens 329–31
Pluripotent hematopoietic stem
    cell 310–16

Polycyclic arylhydrocarbons and
    structure-activity
    relationships 130–1
Pott 32, 92
Preembryonic expressions 9, 358–9
Pre-Grecian contributions to oncology
    and civilisation 33–7
    general aspects 33–5
    oncology 35
Premarin 154
Prezygotic mutations 348
Printing 34
Procarcinogens 339–40
Progression 3, 16
Progynon 148
Proliferation of synthetic
    hormones 155–8
Promotion 346–7
Propagation *in vitro* 126–8
Proximate carcinogens 339–40
Psychiatric malignancy 5
Pure gonadal dysgenesis 263
Pyrrolizidine alkaloids 330

Qualitative basis of modern medical
    successes 326

Radiotherapy 117
Ramazzini 92
Rehn 93
Retinoids 121–2, 341, 364
Rhazes 49
Rigoni-Stern 17, 332
Rous 370
Rufus of Ephesus 50

Salmonella typhimurium 347
Salvarsan 326
SBLA syndrome 227
Schistosoma haematobium 103, 177
Schistosoma mansoni 103
Schleiden and Schwann 62–4
Schultes 55
Schwartz 96
Second messenger 169
Second primaries 213–14, 322
Selenium 341
Seveso 247
Sipple's syndrome 211, 229–30
Skin cancers 222–4
Smoking and cancer *see* lung cancer,
    tobacco
Socioeconomic status 111
Soft agar colony technique 252

Somatic mutation theory 236–8, 347–52, 369–70
  bacterial mutagenicity and carcinogenicity 347
  limitations 350–2
  oncogenes and cancer 348–50
  problems of definition 347–8
  see also oncologic theories
Special creation (mitochondria) 357
Spirochaeta pallida 119
Spiroptera neoplasticum 105
Spontaneous neoplasia 127–8, 185–93, 195–200
Statistics (Tanchou and Rigoni-Stern) 112–13
Stem cells 14, 310–16, 361, 366
Sterigmatocystin 133
Stress (psychosomatic) 5, 138
Superoxide ion and dismutase 13
Surgery 116
Synthetic chemicals 18, 331

Tanchou 17, 112–13, 332
Teratocarcinoma 362
Testicular feminization syndrome 263
12-Tetradecanoylphorbol 13-acetate (TPA) 346
The Riddle of Cancer 105
Third World (smoking and cancer) 22–3
Thorotvast 195
Three Mile Island 247
Thalassemias 183–4
Thioproline in cancer therapy 122, 364
Ti plasmids 85
Tobacco and
  adrenocorticotropic hormone (ACTH) 8
  alcohol 96–8
  asbestos 98–9
  carcinoembryonic antigen (CEA) 7
  experimental cancers 324–5
  human cancers 3, 10, 20, 25–7, 93–6, 206–7, 226–8, 324–5, 337–8
  smoke components 331
  see also chemical environment and cancer

Transcription units 239
Transformation and carcinogenesis 351
Transformed phenotypes 9

Ubiquity of neoplasia 83–6
Uhrglas theory 63–4
Ultimate carcinogens 339–40
Underestimation of inherited human cancer predisposition 206–12
Unity, diversity and the genetic and medical paradigms 177–85

Van Helmont 57
Vasa lymphatica 59
Versicolorina 133
Vesalius 54
Virchow 67–70, 80–1, 319–20, 325–6
  Archives 68
  cellular pathology 67–70
  connective tissue theory 69–70
  homologous and heterologous neoplasms 68–9, 80–1
  omnis cellula a cellula 67
  tubercle 67
Viruses and cancer 105–11, 248, 329
  see also Biological environment and cancer
Vitamin A 341

Waldeyer 70, 320
Warburg effect 13
Weismann's postulates 76, 320, 359
Writing 34

Xeroderma pigmentosum 224, 273–5 *passim*
  see also Skin cancer

Yamagiwa and Ichikawa 128–9, 339
Yin and Yang 28

Zahn 74, 320
Zur Frage der Entstehung maligner Tumoren 236, 237